AF673193

Encyclopedia of Ethnomedicine

Printed and bound in India by Thomson Press Ltd., New Delhi

Encyclopedia of Ethnomedicine

Dr. S.K. Singh

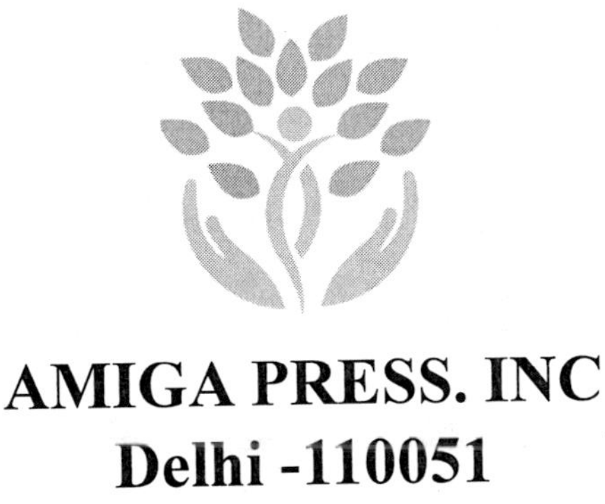

AMIGA PRESS. INC
Delhi -110051

AMIGA PRESS. INC
H.O :- 28-A, Indra Park, Chander Nagar
Delhi :- 110051 (India)
Tel :- 011-22504028, +91-98736-57000
Email :- amigapress@gmail.com
Website: www.amigapress.co.in

This edition is published by Amiga Press.Inc

ISBN : 978-93-84533-03 8

First Published 2018

Printed and bound in India by Thomson Press Ltd., New Delhi

Preface

Ethnomedicine is a sub-field of ethnobotany or medical anthropology that deals with the study of traditional medicines: not only those that have relevant written sources (e.g. Traditional Chinese Medicine, Siddha, Ayurveda), but especially those, whose knowledge and practices have been orally transmitted over the centuries. Ethnomedicine practices are becoming a rising new trend in urban areas. With the migration of individuals from diverse geographical locations, metropolitan cities are starting to see a sudden increase in the amount of traditional healing clinics.

Ethnobiology itself, as a distinctive practice, only emerged during the 20th century as part of the records then being made about other peoples, and other cultures. As a practice, it was nearly always ancillary to other pursuits when documenting others' languages, folklore, and natural resource use: At it earliest and most rudimentary, this comprised listing the names and uses of plants and animals in native non-Western or 'traditional' populations often in the context of salvage ethnography..[ie] ethno-biology as the descriptive biological knowledge of 'primitive' peoples. This 'first phase' in the development of ethnobiology as a practice has been described as still having an essentially utilitarian purpose, often focusing on identifying those 'native' plants, animals and technologies of some potential use and value within increasingly dominant western economic systems.

Ethnomedicine is a study or comparison of the traditional medicine practiced by various ethnic groups, and especially by indigenous peoples. The word ethnomedicine is sometimes used as a synonym for traditional medicine. Ethnomedical research is interdisciplinary; in its study of traditional medicines, it applies the methods of ethnobotany and medical anthropology. Often, the medicine traditions it studies are preserved only by oral tradition. Scientific ethnomedical studies constitute either anthropological research or drug discovery research. Anthropological studies examine the cultural perception and context of a traditional medicine. The purpose of drug discovery research is to identify and develop a marketable pharmaceutical product.

Ethnomedicine explores the medical institutions and the manner in which peoples cope with illness and disease as a result of their cultural perspective. A broad field of study, ethnomedical study is a cumulative product of various fields of study, including ecology, epidemiology, and medical history. The study of ethnomedicine largely involves the collection of empirical data, especially that of the patterns of illness and treatment from cultures and peoples outside of the practicing biomedicine world. An important issue ethnomedicine addresses is the overlap between disease and illness and how one person may distinguish between the two based on cultural influences.

Ayurvedic medicine is a system of traditional medicine native to the Indian subcontinent and practiced in other parts of the world as a form of alternative medicine. In Sanskrit, the word ayurveda consists of the words âyus, meaning "longevity", and veda, meaning "related to knowledge" or "science". Evolving throughout its history, ayurveda remains an influential system of medicine in South Asia. The earliest literature on Indian medical practice appeared during the Vedic period in India. The Sucœruta Sanhitâ and the Charaka Sanhitâ were influential works on traditional medicine during this era. Over the following centuries, Ayurvedic practitioners developed a number of medicinal preparations and surgical procedures for the treatment of various ailments and diseases.

This book gives an account of medicinal plants of all the countries on planet earth.

—Editor

Contents

1

Ethnomedicinal Plants

ETHNOMEDICINAL PLANTS IN ARUNACHAL PRADESH

The natural flora and fauna used by the specific ethnic group in the form of medicines in curing and preventing different aliments and diseases are known as ethnomedicine. From time immemorial, indigenous people of different parts of the world have been gathering knowledge about these forms of medicine and medication, which has been handed down for generations merely on verbal tradition. The art is not so compact today because of the allopathic form of modern medicine, which is neither cost-effective nor having easy accessibility at remote Siang villages of Arunachal Pradesh rather still governing the *Adi* way of medication to its people.

The changing aspects of socio-geographic and economic scenario claim a rigorous multidimensional study on the problem of starting the farming of ethno-botanical knowledge and plants on ground of their holistic needs of economic, environmental and ethical types. Certainly, the studied area concerned is the world's richest store house of medicinal plants and the people who determine their physique form the totality of nature, still have immense belief on the Mother Nature to a large extent.

It is not the economic botany rather more of pure economics as associated with the tribal medicine; it is at a very young stage of study as far as the studied area concerned. Economic farming of ethno-medicinal plants has been started in the developed nations since a century back and a crude amount of investment coming from both the government and large Pharmaceuticals Companies and Drug Houses is increasing at every minutes of day. Today, the realization comes to our national level planners too from the evidences revealed in the different agro-climatic regions of the world. Instead of having huge potential of farming of medicinal plants at ours own, India is presently importing nearly 90% of total demand from the countries like Nepal, Indonesia, Bulgaria and others. The 10th Five Year Plan (2002-2007) has set a goal to achieve a sum of Rupees

4200 crore targeted economy from the cultivation of medicinal plants. And accordingly, Medicinal Plants Boards at the Centre and State level have been constituted under the Ministry of Health and Family Welfare of the Union Government and State Governments respectively, in order to monitor and to provide the overall guidance for the farming of medicinal plants.

STUDY AREA AND METHODOLOGY

The area of this study is Siang region, named after the mighty Siang river, the down stream of the Tsang-po and upper tributary of the Bhrammaputra, comprising of West Siang, East Siang and Upper Siang districts of Arunachal Pradesh located within the geographical ambit of about $27^{0}32^{/}$ N to 29^{0} $20^{/}$ N latitudinal and 93^{0} $48^{/}$ E to 95^{0} $36^{/}$ E longitudinal extents bordering the historic Mc Mohon line to its north and Demaji district of Assam state to its south. The east and west are fringed by the sister districts Dibang valley and lower and upper Sabansiri, respectively. The topographical feature varies form southern plains to the snow clad mountains in the north. The area is located in the subtropical temperate zone with forest coverage of about 63% of the present territorial occupancy, inhabited by 224470 people at a rate of density of 12.12 people per km^2 to its total geographical area of 18518 km^2. The indigenous people is known as the *Adi,* a Mongoloid racial community originated with the Tibeto-Burmese linguist genealogy, leads the livelihood basically on forest resources hitherto. Apart form hunting, gathering, fishing and other related activities associated with the forest resources, the *Adis* use to practice *Adiavik,* known as the shifting cultivation or *Jhum* in the Indio logy. Shifting cultivation as a system of cropping practice represents the indigenous from of agriculture being the most commonly and customarily accepted in the region both by virtue of its physical compass and by virtue of heavy reliance of the settlers for their total livelihood. But the practice, which involves cutting and slashing and burning of invaluable forest resources that is hitherto providing a culturally rich bio-diversity of the region, may leads to a severity by courting the extinction of different species of flora and fauna not only having economic values; also it is an alarming rate of subtraction of environmental qualities.

From a general observation and a causal form of oral investigation from the elderly people of the area arising the hope and scope of farming of ethno medicinal plants by which the local farmers may improve their standard of living not only in terms of income generation in the short run, but the practice as proved in the other familiar agro-climatic zones of the world that it could evolve a healthy environment for the mother earth by minimizing the social cost as incurred for *jhumming* and bringing a larger benefit for the society as a whole.

Scope of Study

The earliest treatise on Indian Medicine, the *Charak Samhita* (1000 B C) recorded some 340 drugs of vegetable origin and developed the *Indian Materia Medica*. However, since the early 20th Century, rapid extensions of Allopathic system of medication throughout the world generated a huge commercial demand for the pharmacopocial drugs and their products. The actual history of agronomic practice of growing medicinal plants starts form this time. The *Indian Pharmacopoeia* (1966) recognizes some odd eighty-five drug plants grow abundantly and naturally with the prevailing agro-climatic condition in the selected parts of the country. However, no full phased literature on medicinal plants on the studied area is available. As far as Siang region, the land is still a virgin one to the limit of present study. The first ever task of textualization of available medicinal plants in the area was recorded by the Botanical Survey of India in its years long effort. However, the task is yet to be finished because of the difficult terrain and wilderness of the area. Very recently Mibang and Chowdhari: 2003, have recorded the proceedings of the Seminar on Ethno Medicinal Plants of Arunachal Pradesh, where some scholarly works are found. Apart form these, Singh et. al: 2003, and Dhiman: 2003 are also some helpful documentation on medicinal plants of tribal use in general and the studied area in particular. Riba: 2003, has pointed out some relevant socio-economic changes of the tribal life resulted due to a number of reasons, are very much relevant to the context of the present study. However, literature on ethno-medicine is scared as scared for ethno-medicinal plants and economic use of these plants is yet to be revealed in the said region.

Although the ideology of the present study is at the very hypothetical stage, farming of medicinal plants used by the tribal for curing his diseases and ailments is having much economic importance as far as the studied area concerned. The practical evidence of economic farming is yet to be started. The Central Institute of Medicinal and Aromatic Plants (CIMAP) have been carrying on a number of researcher works but Siang region is undiscovered. Very recently, the *Adis* have undertaken the cultivation of medicinal plants successfully in Gagin hills, Lissing hills, Riga-top of Boleng Circle of East Siang District. The District Horticulture Department, East Siang District at Pasighat has undertaken some pilot projects of farming of medicinal plants. It is also providing guidance to the aspiring farmers for introducing the cultivation of medicinal plants, on which they inherited a vast traditional knowledge. An NGO at Mirbuk village at Pasighat has introduced the cultivation of medicinal plants on experimental basis. But private entrepreneurial initiatives of large scale production of medicinal plants, which grow naturally in the study area, are to be found lethargic.

Finding out the economic value of ethno-medicinal plants is a holistic approach indeed and use of those plants as industrial inputs except cinchona and some others is undiscovered to the people. Arunachal Pradesh as a whole and Siang region in particular is literarily having no industry at all. Although the factor endowment and the existing infrastructure for some industrial setup might set another story, industrial development is still at a slumbering state so it is for any Pharmaceutical Plant and Drug House.

The existing scenario of industrial backwardness retards the tremendous growth prospects of medicinal plants at its commercial use. No doubt, the advanced world realizes the healing touch of ethno-botanical plants to a great extent because this form of medicine is proved to be more cost effective and humane friendly up to the extent of some diseases like Aids and Cancer. Plants having medicinal values used by the Aids are not cultivated. These plants grow naturally with no weeding and no effort at all. They are harvested as per household need at any particular point of time. These plants are not so scared so far. A basic hypothesis may gavels that the economic farming is also feasible for these plants in the area by these people.

Discussion

The Arunachal economy as a whole is still succumbing to the severe backwardness for a number of factors, which is not to mention within this limited jargon, but it is not very inappropriate to note that the people are backward because they are backward. For Arunachal economy, agriculture is the prime source livelihood and *jhumming* shares the lion part of the total agrarian practice. *Jhum is* not only the form of cultivation but also a way of life for the Arunachalees. Arunachal Pradesh, being a land locked state of Indian Union with her difficult topographical features does not have a vast scope of setting up large industries and with low level of technological base along with other constraints does not provide avenues for rapid expansion of service sector, may gets a boost if the prevailing agricultural resources are used in a planned way. The Government initiatives in these regard is noteworthy that after achieving the statehood status in 1987, the Government has put emphasis on various types of agricultural extension projects and program like animal husbandry, horticulture, agro-forestry and other allied schemes either as the joint venture with the Union Government or with its own limited resources. There is a number of projects has been being implemented as the substitute of jhum, a primitive form of agrarian practice, but they are not proved to be very effective ones from the ground of its physical relevance. Therefore, the jhumming is going on as it was there at the hundreds of years back. The Jhumias, on the other hand, on the way of carrying out the practice are incurring a huge amount of social cost in terms of different types of natural hazards vis-à-vis, soil erosion, flood and others alike, which can't be compensated in the near future. In the jhum land, the Jhumias were once producing merely the amount to sustain rather indulging by the modern life style and other exogenous factors alike, they reduced the spun of jhum cycle in order to produce marketable cash crops. Thus, they are courting more and more ruins for their own. It is evidenced from the present study that the cultivation of medicinal plants as an alternative to jhumming is viable for Arunachal Pradesh as a whole and the studied area, Siang region in particular, where medicinal plants grow abundantly and the ethnic group associated, the Adis, could be better off if they do under take the project, initially with the support of the government and other NGOs, which are working for the upliftment of the society. However, the benefit associated with the farming of medicinal plants in the studied area may be summarized as follows:

1. Medicinal Plants-*An august source of employment generation:* The overall employment scenario in Arunachal Pradesh is as worse as for any other Indian state. Higher growth of population, fast increase of literacy rate along with massive in-migration are the main reasons for increasing figure of unemployment scenario in the state. Since the government with its limited resources is virtually incapable to provide rooms for much employment opportunity in the organized sectors, farming of medicinal plants alike of other agricultural extension programs may open up the scope for unemployed youth to earn their bread from an august source.
2. Medicinal Plants-*An approach to commercialization and modernization of agriculture*: The tribal economy in general is succumbing to its subsistence level hitherto and so it is the Arunachal economy as well. The Jhumias are still producing for their own consumption and no marketable surplus. Although the womenfolk brings a very trivial quantity at the market for raising cash in order to meet the non-food demand, it does not consist a considerable amount of the state Gross Domestic Product (SGDP). On the contrary, if the medicinal plants, which grow naturally in the state could accumulate a fair deal of cash inflow into the economy if they were brought into commercial cultivation applying the modern technology and technological know-how. Thus, the farming of medicinal plants may be an approach to transform the subsistence Arunachal agriculture into a commercialized one. Another way, it is a stir of modernizing the primitive economy as well.
3. Medicinal Plants-*A stimulant for raising the standard of living*: Growing population pressure along with under utilization of natural resources force the mass to live below poverty line. The farming of medicinal

plants may compensate the 69% of the total population in the state, who depends on agriculture and more particularly on jhumming, very often succumbs to crop failure due to different sort of natural calamities. The cultivation of medicinal plans would give them readymade cash to purchase their livelihood. Moreover, it is unlike the household need that they get from the jhum land, the farming of medicinal plants, which will attach the people with market mechanism, would give them better understanding of the outer world.

4. Medicinal Plants-*A catalyst for Industrialization*: Perhaps the difficult terrains and low level of infrastructures hinder the process of industrialization at this north-east extremity of India. Medicinal plants on the other hand, an endowed factor along with traditional knowledge of the *Kennapanna ami* (the village medicine men) may be the economic agents to begin the history of industrialization in the land of the rising sun. The existing Citronella plant at Pasighat in East Siang District may raise the hope further.
5. Medicinal Plants-*The source of Government revenue, not bathos*: A recent study shows that medicinal plant worth of millions of US $ are imported in the country from Nepal annually. In the era of economic globalization, the phenomenon is virtually contradictory for Indian economy, when we have vast resources for the same products at our own. If the resources are explored properly, import substitution in this arena could save the worthy foreign exchange reserves of millions of dollar. Above all, setting up of industries of medicinal plants will raise huge revenue for the government as well.
6. Medicinal Plants-*Manifestation of indigenous knowledge system:* Primitive local tribal people have vast and extended knowledge about the various medicinal plants available in this region which certainly helps in conserving the biodiversity.
7. Medicinal Plants-*Protecting the patent rights of indigenous plant species*: Participation in the rat race of globalize economic yard might bring some positive results for Indian economy; rather we loose the rights on *Basmati* or *Neem*, the species of our own. Hence, it is a sort of responsibility to protect the patent rights of the invaluable medicinal plants growing exclusively on the Siang soil.
8. Medicinal Plants-*An ecological agent of immense value! Save our only earth*: The jhum practice, no doubt, feeds the Arunachalees although at subsistence level, but the method of practicing jhum is too cruel to the Mother Nature because it involves slashing and burning of the forest resources without realizing the far reaching consequences of the

environment. An alarming rate of deforestation leads to severity for the natural vegetation not only for the area concerned, but the frequent flood and other natural hazards alike mostly caused by this massive deforestation program claim lives and property of billions of rupees as a yearly fiesta. '*Modus operandi* of jhumming first leads to ecological disequilibrium by depleting forest cover, aggravating chances of soil erosion to cause removal of top soil, silting river beds and threatening the existence of life itself and all these by putting grain crop as the only levy on the earth'. However, we cannot escape from the reality that jhumming remains here not merely as a farming method but constitutes as *modus vivendi* of people who operate it. Thus, various alternative projects even did not yield any expected results for the region. Cultivation of medicinal plants, if undertaken commercially, would not only save the natural vegetation but also it is to prevent from flood and other natural disasters caused by the massive deforestation program.

ETHNOBIOLOGY

Ethnobiology is the scientific study of the way plants and animals are treated or used by different human cultures. It studies the dynamic relationshipsbetween peoples, biota, and environments, from the distant past to the immediate present.

"People-biota-environment" interactions around the world are documented and studied through time, across cultures, and across disciplines in a search forvalid, reliable answers to two 'defining' questions: "How and in what ways do human societies use nature, and how and in what ways do human societies view nature?"

History : Beginnings (15th century-19th century)

Naturalists have been interested in local biological knowledge since the time Europeans started colonising the world, from the 15th century onwards.

Europeans not only sought to understand the new regions they intruded into but also were on the look-out for resources that they might profitably exploit, engaging in practices that today we should consider tantamount to biopiracy. Many new crops.. entered into Europe during this period, such as the potato, tomato, pumpkin, maize, and tobacco.

Local biological knowledge, collected and sampled over these early centuries significantly informed the early development of modern biology:

- during the 17th century Georg Eberhard Rumphius benefited from local biological knowledge in producing his catalogue, *"Herbarium Amboinense"*, covering more than 1 200 species of the plants of Indonesia;

- during the 18th century, Carl Linnaeus relied upon Rumphius's work, and also corresponded with other people all around the world when developing the biological classification scheme that now underlies the arrangement of much of the accumulated knowledge of the biological sciences.
- during the 19th century, Charles Darwin, the 'father' of evolutionary theory, on his Voyage of the Beagle took interest in the local biological knowledge of peoples he encountered.

Phase I (1900s-1940s)

Ethnobiology itself, as a distinctive practice, only emerged during the 20th century as part of the records then being made about other peoples, and other cultures. As a practice, it was nearly always ancillary to other pursuits when documenting others' languages, folklore, and natural resource use:

At it earliest and most rudimentary, this comprised listing the names and uses of plants and animals in native non-Western or 'traditional' populations often in the context of salvage ethnography..[ie] *ethno*-biology as the descriptive biological knowledge of 'primitive' peoples.

This 'first phase' in the development of ethnobiology as a practice has been described as still having an essentially utilitarian purpose, often focusing on identifying those 'native' plants, animals and technologies of some potential use and value within increasingly dominant western economic systems.

Phase II (1950s-1970s)

Arising out of practices in Phase I (above) came a 'second phase' in the development of 'ethnobiology', with researchers now striving to better document and better understand how other peoples' themselves "conceptualise and categorise" the natural world around them.

By the mid-20th century.. utilitarian-focussed studies started to give way to more cognitively framed ones, notably studies that centred on elucidating classificatory schemes.

This 'second' phase is marked:

- in Northern America (mid 1950s) with Harold Conklin's completing his doctorate entitled *"The relation of Hanunóo culture to the plant world"*
- in Britain (mid 1960s) with the publication of Claude Lévi-Strauss' book *The Savage Mind* legitimating "folk biological classification" as a worthy cross-cultural research endeavour
- in France (mid 1970s) with André-Georges Haudricourt's linguistic studies of botanical nomenclature and R. Porteres' and others work in economic biology.

Present (1980s-2000s)

By the turn of the 20th century ethnobiological practices, research, and findings have had a significant impact and influence across a number of fields of biological inquiry including ecology, conservation biology, development studies, and political ecology.

The Society of Ethnobiology advises on its web page:

Ethnobiology is a rapidly growing field of research, gaining professional, student, and public interest.. internationally

Ethnobiology has come out from its place as an ancillary practice in the shadows of other core pursuits, to arise as a whole field of inquiry and research in its own right: taught within many tertiary institutions and educational programmes around the world; with its own methods manuals, its own readers, and its own textbooks

SUBJECTS OF INQUIRY

Usage

All societies make use of the biological world in which they are situated, but there are wide differences in use, informed by perceived need, available technology, and the culture's sense of morality and sustainability. Ethnobiologists investigate what lifeforms are used for what purposes, the particular techniques of use, the reasons for these choices, and symbolic and spiritual implications of them.

Taxonomy

Different societies divide the living world up in different ways. Ethnobiologists attempt to record the words used in particular cultures for living things, from the most specific terms (analogous to species names in Linnean biology) to more general terms (such as 'tree' and even more generally 'plant'). They also try to understand the overall structure or hierarchy of the classification system (if there is one; there is ongoing debate as to whether there must always be an implied hierarchy.

Cosmological, Moral and Spiritual Significance

Societies invest themselves and their world with meaning partly through their answers to questions like "how did the world happen?", "how and why did people come to be?", "what are proper practices, and why?", and "what realities exist beyond or behind our physical experience?" Understanding these elements of a societies' perspective is important to cultural research in general, and ethnobiologists investigate how a societies' view of the natural world informs and is informed by them.

Traditional Ecological Knowledge

In order to live effectively in a given place, a people needs to understand the particulars of their environment, and many traditional societies have complex and subtle understandings of the places in which they live. Ethnobiologists seek to share in these understandings, subject to ethical concerns regarding intellectual property and cultural appropriation.

Cross-cultural Ethnobiology

In cross cultural ethnobiology research, two or more communities participate simulatenously. This enables the researcher to compare how a bio-resource is used by different communities.

SUBDISCIPLINES

Ethnobotany

Ethnobotany investigates the relationship between human societies and plants: how humans use plants- as food, technology, medicine, and in ritual contexts; how they view and understand them; and their symbolic and spiritual role in a culture.

Ethnozoology

The subfield ethnozoology focuses on the relationship between animals and humans throughout human history. It studies human practices such as hunting, fishing and animal husbandry in space and time, and human perspectives about animals such as their place in the moral and spiritual realms.

Ethnoecology

Ethnoecology refers to an increasingly dominant 'ethnobiological' research paradigm focused, primarily, on documenting, describing, and understanding how other peoples perceive, manage, and use whole ecosystems.

Other Disciplines

Studies and writings within ethnobiology involve and draw upon the research and researchers from across such disciplines and fields of knowledge as;

- archaeology,
- geography,
- linguistics,
- systematics,
- population biology,

- ecology,
- cultural anthropology,
- ethnography,
- pharmacology,
- nutrition,
- conservation, and
- sustainable development.

Ethics

Through much of the history of ethnobiology, its practitioners were primarily from dominant cultures, and the benefit of their work often accrued to the dominant culture, with little control or benefit invested in the indigenous peoples whose practice and knowledge they recorded.

Just as many of those indigenous societies work to assert legitimate control over physical resources such as traditional lands or artistic and ritual objects, many work to assert legitimate control over their intellectual property.

In an age when the potential exists for large profits from the discovery of, for example, new food crops or medicinal plants, modern ethnobiologists must consider intellectual property rights, the need for informed consent, the potential for harm to informants, and their "debt to the societies in which they work".

Furthermore, these questions must be considered not only in light of western industrialized nations' common understanding of ethics and law, but also in light of the ethical and legal standards of the societies from which the ethnobiologist draws information.

2

The Propagation of Medicinal Plants

Information on the propagation of medicinal plants is available for less than 10% and agro-technology is available only for 1% of the total known plants globally. This trend shows that developing agro-technology should be one of the thrust areas for research. Furthermore, in order to meet the escalating demand of medicinal plants, farming of these plant species is imperative. Apart from meeting the present demand, farming may conserve the wild genetic diversity of medicinal plants. Farming permits the production of uniform material, from which standardized products can be consistently obtained. Cultivation also permits better species identification, improved quality control, and increased prospects for genetic improvements.

Selection of planting material for large-scale farming is also an important task. The planting material therefore should be of good quality, rich in active ingredients, pest- and disease-resistant and environmental tolerant. For the large scale farming, one has to find out whether monoculture is the right way to cultivate all medicinal plants or one has to promote polyculture model for better production of medicinal plants. Studies conducted on the agro-forestry of medicinal plants elsewhere suggest that since many medicinal plant species prefer to grow under forest cover, agroforestry offers a convenient strategy for their cultivation as well as conservation through: (1) integrating shade tolerant medicinal plants as lower strata species in multistrata system, (2) cultivating short cycle medicinal plants as intercrops in existing stands of tree crops, (3) growing medicinal tree as shade providers and boundary markers, and 4) inter-planting medicinal plants with food crops. Notwithstanding, it is understood that the cultivation of medicinal plants is not an easy task as the history of medicinal plants farming reflects.

Many farmers in trans-Himalayan region of northern India have replaced the medicinal plants farming with common crops [*i.e.*, peas (Pisum sativum), potatos (Solanum tuberosum) and hops (Humulus lupulus)] due to the lengthy cultivation cycle of medicinal plants like Saussurea costus. The cost of many medicinal plants in northern India is lower than many seasonal vegetables, which is a cause of scanty farming of medicinal plants.

Attempts are being made by different organizations to cultivate various medicinal plant species, including rare and endangered categories. Agro-technology for about 20 species of rare and endangered medicinal plants of the northern India has been developed by different organizations. However, the per hectare cost of cultivation, total annual production and cost benefit ratio fluctuate with different medicinal plant species. Out of 10 selected rare and endangered medicinal plant species, Rheum emodi was calculated as a most beneficial cash crop of the medicinal plant in terms of net income generation in northern India.

At present, however, the farming of most of the medicinal plant species is being operated on a small scale and is restricted to a few hectares of land in various states of northern India. There is an uncertainty of obtaining the necessary permits from government agencies for cultivation of medicinal plants. Additionally, many farmers are unaware about the agency responsible for issuing permits. If the farmers are not granted permits needed to cultivate, they are forced to sell their products on the illegal market, which exposes them to action by government agencies and the exploitation by middlemen.

Bio-prospecting and Bio-piracy

The former remote green forests have now become part of a dynamic, profit-seeking economy and demanding pluralistic politics worldwide. Reducing the pressure on various forest products, especially on the medicinal plants, is therefore a tough challenge both for policy makers and for economists. Medicinal plants are the local heritage with global importance.

The Convention on Biological Diversity at Rio had agreed on a framework that would help the biodiversity to be utilized in a prudent and controlled way. Bio-prospecting, at present, occurs in an environment of suspicions and growing tensions between the bio-piracy and rights of sharing benefits between the developing and developed countries. Most of the issues relating to the protection of the legal status for indigenous knowledge and compensation of the indigenous herbal practitioners for that knowledge are extremely complicated. There are arguments for the present state of compensation or benefit sharing under the intellectual property rights, which is being considered a new legal form of bio-piracy by one group, whereas other groups argue that the intellectual property right is a legal tool to protect the rights of knowledge holders.

Different ways and systems for awarding patents on the medicinal plants in India, United States, Europe, Canada and other countries have widened the confusion. In many countries, the plants and inventions directed to the plants and the plant products (*i.e.*, seeds, flowers, gums, and resins) are not eligible for filing a patent. In United States, however, any living organism derived by human invention, such as by breeding or by laboratory-based manipulation, can be filed for awarding patent. The Indian Protection of Plant Varieties and Farmers Rights Act of 2001 recognizes the contribution of farmers who actively participate in the breeding programmes. Furthermore, this act contains provisions for benefit sharing whereby local communities are acknowledged as a contributor of plants.

Unfortunately, there is a wide gap between developed and developing nations such as India on patenting the products. For example, out of the 3,125,603 patents filed in 91 countries, only 301,177 or 9.6% are registered in developing countries while the rest is in industrialized countries. Of these, only 0.2% of the total and 2.3% of those registered in developing countries belong to residents. In addition, 97.7% of the total patents filed thus far are in the name of non-residents, who apply solely to control export markets in developing countries.

Developing nations and many scientists who want to exploit medicinal plants demand more specific rules about the recording of nationality of samples and sharing of their benefits between the nations of origin, the inventor, and the commercial sponsors. Some developed nations are not inclined to accept such provisions. These conflicts have frustrated many scientists who believe that natural products remain the most promising source for new drugs. To mitigate such conflicts and gear up to find out new sources for drugs, the representatives of 188 nations at Kuala Lumpur Conference in 2004 agreed to try to build such a framework that would be acceptable to all signatories and thus the proposed framework will be placed for consideration at the next meeting in 2006 going to be held in Brazil.

Strengthening Legalized Market System

Besides government agencies, there are numbers of stake-holders ranging from herb gatherers, local middlemen, urban traders, wholesalers, manufacturers, exporters and herbal healers in the medicinal plants trade sector. The marketing system in medicinal plants sector is largely unregulated and inequitable. The medicinal plant collectors are generally the marginal farmers and labourers. They get cash income to meet their basic requirements for food, health and children education by selling medicinal plants.

They are often unaware about the real market prices of many medicinal plant species. Generally, in medicinal plants sector, there is a top down approach and even the many stake-holders at the bottom are not aware of the rising demand of their product and the availability of its market. In some villages of Chamoli district of Uttaranchal, the farmers had cultivated Kut (Saussurea costus) and Dolu (Rheum emodi) but they were unable to sell them due to lack of knowledge on the marketing system. Conversely, many medicinal plant species are traded through illegal channels.

The other constraints in the medicinal plants sector are: (1) slow rate of production of many medicinal plants, (2) long gestation period, (3) shortage of suitable cultivation technology, (4) production of small quantity, (5) unscientific harvesting, (6) paucity of research on the high yielding varieties, (7) inefficient processing techniques, (8) fluctuation in demand and supply, (9) poor quality control procedures, (10) scarcity of good manufacturers, (11) poor marketing infrastructure, and (12) poor coordination among different stake-holders.

On many occasions, the wild medicinal plants are preferred by manufactures compared to the cultivated ones, as there is a general feeling that wild plant species contain better chemical contents. The variation in chemical contents also depends upon the harvesting seasons of species and different stages of species growth. The medicinal plant sector is largely less documented and inadequately regulated. The economy generated by this sector is therefore, not precise because of the enormous illegal trade. The economic benefits and management cost for wild populations are poorly estimated on several occasions.

PRINCIPLES OF BIODYNAMIC CULTIVATION

The main aim of biodynamic cultivation is to improve the quality of either food, fibre or medicinal plants. Of course, it also aims at improving the yields but, most importantly, it concentrates on quality.

In this century, more and more chemical fertilisers have been developed to produce maximum yields. The main objective has been to increase the yields. The reason is simple: bigger yields bring more money. Most vegetable producers have been cheating the consumer by selling them water for the price of vegetables. For example, dried carrots which have been chemically fertilised show less weight than organic carrots.

Adding fertilisers, which are salts, to plants, means that the plants draw more water from the soil in order to balance the ratio of fibre to salt inside. Consequently, as the plant cells expand and swell with water, the ratio of proteins and even vitamins decreases, and the essential oils, which have important medicinal properties, deteriorate. It has been scientifically proven that the amount of vitamins is less in chemically fertilised products. There is an imbalance of vitamins because the fertilised plants draw only one kind of nutrient and not all the trace elements. Hence, it does not produce the entire range of vitamins, and its whole value changes.

Quality of Medicinal Plants

What we want to achieve in biodynamic farming of medicinal plants, is the cultivation of the inherent quality of the plant. That is the very subtle active principle, which the plant has in very minute quantities. Instead of substance, here we are dealing with essential oils, which are almost not substantial, sometimes present only in parts per million. What is quality, and how can we provide quality in food or in medicinal plants?

What are the indicators for quality in medicinal plants? Quality comprises certain active principles, such as taste, juice, colour, seed content in the fruits, nutritional value, the vitamin and protein content. The question is, do we know how to evaluate subtle medicinal properties?

How do we define the taste, the aroma, the smell of flowers? How do we increase the scent of a rose, and how do we make oranges more sweet? How do we increase the content of active principles in medicinal plants? Does science know how to produce the best quality of food?

Modern agricultural sciences are based on how to work with yields. We know how to produce quantity but we don't know how to produce quality.

We are facing the tragedy that roses don't have any smell any more; oranges have lost their taste; tomatoes are not sweet any more; carrots are bitter, and cultivated medicinal plants have less active principles.

Characteristics of the Himalayan Flora and Fauna

Each plant develops in a particular ecological zone. Here in the Darjeeling Hills we meet with this fantastic possibility of having land from very low elevations up to very high summits. Additionally the climate provides a lot of warmth and moisture. This combination of moisture and warmth creates very specific kinds of chemicals in the plants. In high altitude mountains the principles are mainly dry and cold, with a lot of light. In contrast, the valleys are full of moisture, heat with a lot of vegetation and rather dark forests. Those extremes produce substances that are very different from each other.

In the higher regions of the Himalayas plants grow on very dry alpine soils. These, in many cases, are sandy and not very fertile. The cold climate limits the plants' growth. On lower elevations, the plants produces a lot of leaf, and in higher altitude they prominent with the flowers.

Polarities in Biodynamics

There is a polarity between yields and quality, between substance and un-substance, between big quantity of products and very small quantities of subtle ethereal oils. Regarding the definition of quality, a polarity can be observed between something very physical, such as the weight, substance-and something very subtle, such as ethereal oils.

In biodynamic farming we are trying to rediscover what is important in agriculture.

EARTH AND SUN

The entire plant life is a product of the earth and the sun-as some people say, the Mother Earth, and the Father Sun. In many cultures, the sun is masculine and the earth is feminine.

Sun	Earth
Warmth, Heat	Coolness, minerals,
Seasonal Rhythm	Gravity, Water,
Space	Soil
Light	Darkness

The Principle of Light

The colours of the beautiful high altitude flowers are a powerful manifestation of light. Colour is the resistance of substances to light, the tension between the light and the earth. The alpine regions are full of light.

This leads to very special structures of medicinal plants: the flowers are very colourful and bright, the leaves are very delicate-and with a lot of medicinal value. With hardly any substance alpine medicinal plants tend to be small but very powerful. The light that they accumulate is all transformed into essential oils. The more light, the more essential oils are produced. These medicinal plants pass through the whole winter with very little water. They are processing all this light, and they have to concentrate everything into essential oils. The tannin in the tea leaf, for example, is nothing but concentrated sunlight. It is this sunlight which activates our senses, working on very subtle principles.

Using Polarity Principles in Biodynamic Agriculture

An example: Curcure (Equisetum arvense L.) is a plant without leaf. It consists only of stem. It grows in shady places, and is very rich in silica. The amount of silica, almost 90%, is one of the highest in the plant world. Silica is a mineral, belonging to the earth, but it lets the light go through.

Where do we find silica? In sand. Sixty or seventy per cent of the earth's crust is silica. And if you want to know how silica is connected to life, just look at a window: the glass is pure silica. There is silica in spectacles, silica in the eyes and skin, in the hair-and in leaves. Silica has an affinity to light. In fact, it draws light.

With silica as a carrier of light, we can make use of the polarity of light and darkness in agriculture. Equisetum arvense contains a lot of silica, and therefore belongs to the realm of light. On the contrary, fungus belongs to the realm of cold, moisture and darkness. We can use a product from one realm to control an imbalance in another. Equisetum arvense is an excellent fungicide.

Biodynamic Preparations

Out of his own insight, Rudolf Steiner introduced what is known as biodynamic preparations. Naturally occurring plant and animal materials are combined in specific recipes in certain seasons of the year and then placed in compost piles. These preparations bear concentrated forces within them and are used to organise the chaotic elements within the compost piles. When the process is complete, the resulting preparations are medicines for the Earth which draw new life forces from the cosmos. Effects of the preparations have been verified scientifically.

One of the preparations is made from silica powder, processed in a special way. It is applied to the plants at the time when they are producing the part that shall be harvested. In case of medicinal plants, if, for example, the root is harvested for medicinal purposes, silica is applied when the root is forming. The same applies for the flower, leaf, etc.

This silica powder preparation helps to increase the concentration of silica in the plant. With silica, the plant increases its rate of photosynthesis, draws more light, and produces more of those finer aspects. The medicinal value of plants cultivated under such conditions will be naturally higher and their pests lesser.

Silica is an excellent remedy for the foggy Darjeeling climate. The monsoon mists hold back the plant, whereas silica will activate the plant growth. Too much shade also creates a situation for fungus, which silica counteracts. In this way one can balance an unfavourable climatic situation with biodynamic preparations.

One of the biodynamic preparation is made from quartz crystals: the crystal form of silica. These crystals have geometric forms, perfect hexagonal shapes. The geometry shows another polarity of form and formlessness: in silica we have these beautiful shapes, and in fungus we have amorphous shapes, without form.

Geometric Principles and Medicinal Values

Alpine flowers are of the most perfect shapes, like stars: they have the most beautiful, artistic quality. The same applies for this quartz. These perfect shapes are based on the same geometric principle. It belongs to the heights, near the light, close to the stars. In pentagonal and hexagonal flowers we find the same geometrical principles as in crystals.

The differences between the root and the flower of such alpine medicinal plants reveal the polarity that we are talking about. The flower is very nicely shaped, though every species is different. But why do we not study the roots to differentiate those plants?

Because they are all more-or-less the same. There is no differentiation at the root level, and yet there is this high differentiation at the flower level.

How do these plants know that they have to grow like this? Why are they shaped and coloured like this? For example, this plant has five petals, five sepals, five stamens, so it is shaped by the principle of five, but where does it come from? It is these principles that form the plant, and along with it its medicinal values.

We can release this formative principle in our plants and understand how it starts shaping them and bringing forth these fine aspects of scent, aroma, taste, colour and medical properties.

In comparison, in tropical plants the principle of flower has been pushed into the leaf. Tropical climate produces fleshy plants that would never grow in the Alpine regions. These plants need moisture. It is warmth, which, combined with light, manifests in these plants in the leaves instead of in the flower.

Many plants, where this principle of warmth pushing into the leaf operates, develop a lot of poison. When this principle, that belongs to the flower, has been pushed as far as into the root, it colours even the roots. Colour at the root level means that what belongs to the flower has been pushed deep inside the plant.

COSMIC INTEGRATION

The Zodiac Principles

The ultimate fine-tuning of biodynamic principles lies in harnessing cosmic influences for cultivation. Only at particular times of the month or year are the cosmic influences are most supportive to the growth of a particular part of the plant. The cosmic factor that determines a month is the moon. The movement of the moon in relation to the Zodiac is most interesting. The Zodiac symbols are Greek in origin. The Chinese developed a different system, and the Tibetans created their own amalgamation of the Indian and Chinese systems.

All the different systems have twelve constellations, though represented by different archetype figures and animals. Within these twelve signs there are four groups of three constellations each which have the same qualities. They are related to the four elements, earth, water, fire, air. These four elements can be placed in relation to the four parts of the plant: the root, the leaf, the flower and the fruit.

- The roots are associated with the earth: there is no base and ground without earth.
- The leaves relate to the water element: the more water, the more leaf.
- The flower corresponds to air and light: there is no light without air. (There is no light on the moon because there is no atmosphere.)
- Fruits are associated with fire: there is no ripening without warmth.

Cultivating the soil on specific days means harnessing the cosmic influences for the particular plant. Recent research has shown that in one month there are three periods which are variously beneficial for the root, the leaf, the flower and the fruit. These period are governed by the moon cycle. The different parts of the plant are stimulated, one at a time, three times in a month. Researchers discovered this by planting radishes every day and then observing their growth. Radishes from one day would be of very of good quality while those from another day would be smaller and less healthier. In between would be radishes with shrivelled roots or too much leaf. Anybody can try this experiment. The researchers found that the yields can be increased 20 to 30% just by cultivating at the right time.

IMPORTANCE OF MEDICINAL PLANTS

The most common diseases during the middle ages were dysentery, epilepsy, influenza, diphtheria, scurvy, typhoid, smallpox, scabies, impetigo, leprosy, pneumonia, stroke, heart attack, scrofula (chronically swollen lymph nodes, later identified as a form of tuberculosis), St. Vitus' Dance (rheumatic chorea, a temporary disorder of the parts of the brain that control movement and coordination), and St. Anthony's Fire (ergotism, caused by ingesting toxic amounts of alkaloids produced by a fungus that infests rye - symptoms included gangrene with burning pain in the extremities, convulsions, hallucinations, and severe psychosis). Plants listed in this section are those used most frequently to treat these and other illnesses. Quoted excerpts of treatments from medical texts were translated from Middle English.

Aloe: Greek physician Dioscorides recommended aloe externally for wounds, hemorrhoids, ulcers and hair loss. Pliny prescribed it internally as a laxative.

Angelica (Wild Celery): Angelica leaf necklaces were worn as protection against illness and witchcraft. Angelica was reputed to be the only herb witches never used and its presence in a woman's garden or cupboard was successfully used as a defense against charges of witchcraft. Gilbert Anglicus' Compendium of Medicine gives the following prescription for using angelica as a cough remedy: And if the cough is of sticky thick phlegm, give him a syrup made with horehound, the root of fennel, radish, wild celery and anise.

Anise: Hippocrates recommended anise to help clear mucus from the respiratory system. It was also recommended by other renowned physicians as a breath freshener, digestive aid, a cure for "hicket" (hiccups), headache, asthma, insomnia, nausea, lice and infant colic. Anise was so popular in medieval England as a spice, medicine and perfume that in 1305 Edward I placed a special tax on it to raise money to repair London Bridge.

Apple: Hildegard of Bingen prescribed raw apples as a tonic for healthy people and cooked apples as the first treatment for any sickness.

Balm (Melissa): Lemon balm and bee balm were prescribed for nervousness and anxiety in the form of Melissa water or Eau de Melisse. Recommended for treatment of insomnia, arthritis, headache, toothache, sores, digestive problems and cramps, balm was considered to be something of a cure-all. Greek physicians recommended applying balm leaves to wounds and added the herb to wine to treat a variety of illnesses. Pliny prescribed it to stop bleeding.

Basil: The ancient physicians disagreed on the merits of basil. Dioscorides and Galen warned that taking basil internally would cause insanity and the spontaneous generation of internal worms. Pliny used it to treat stomach ailments. Hildegard of Bingen used basil in a concoction that included powder from a vulture's beak to treat tumors.

Blackberry: Blackberry was also known as "goutberry" as its most popular use was as a treatment for gout. Leaves and bark were chewed for bleeding gums, leaves were applied to the skin to sooth burns and scalds. Blackberry syrup was recommended for treatment of dysentery.

Buckthorn : Buckthorn became popular around the 13th century and was primarily used to purge the body of "foul humors". Buckthorn bark seeped in water produced a powerful laxative. It was also recommended for jaundice, hemorrhoids, gout and arthritis.

Burdock : In the 14th century burdock leaves were used to treat leprosy. Hildegard of Bingen used it to treat cancerous tumours. Burdock root was also prescribed for fever, ringworm and skin infections.

Caraway : Caraway seeds were recommended for the treatment of indigestion, gas and infant colic. Gilbertus Anglicus prescribed the following decoction for a syrup to treat ailments of the lungs: Take barley water which has been strained, raisins, violets, jujube, seed of melon and gourd, wheat starch, licorice, black plums, fennel root, parsley, wild celery, anise, caraway, and make thereof a syrup. That is to say, seep all these in water until the virtue of them be in the water. Then strain it and add sugar or honey. And then set it over the fire to steep softly. Then take the white of four eggs and beat them well and add them. And always skim it until it is clear. Then take it down and strain it clean so that no dregs remain therein. Put it in a closed vessel.

Chamomile : Used to treat headaches, kidney, liver and bladder problems and as an aid for digestive upsets.

Cinnamon : Hildegard of Bingen recommended cinnamon to treat colds, flu, cancer and "inner decay and slime."

Coltsfoot : Used for treating coughs, wheezing, shortness of breath, fever and inflammation.

Comfrey : Boiling comfrey root in water produced a thick paste in which cloth was soaked and then wrapped around broken bones. Internally, comfrey was used for treating respiratory and gastrointestinal problems.

Dandelion : Dandelion was prescribed to treat colds, boils, ulcers, dental problems, itching, jaundice and gallstones.

Dill : Digestive aid and gas remedy. Also a cure for hiccups. From Gilbertus Anglicus' Compendium of Medicine this treatment for squinacy (quinsy):

But if a postem be of phlegm, after his blood-letting and his purging, make him a gargle of sap from a hazelnut tree, dill, poppy, either the water that bark from a nut or mulberry tree has been seeped in, or the juice of bittersweet, with dried honeysuckle leaves and aloe.

Elecampane : Prescribed to treat coughs, bronchitis, asthma and indigestion.

Fennel : The ancient physicians prescribed fennel to treat infant colic, as an appetite suppressant and recommended the seeds to nursing mothers to boost milk production. Pliny believed that fennel was a cure for eye problems, including blindness. Hildegard of Bingen recommended fennel for treating colds, heart ailments and to aid in good digestion and body odour. Folk healers mixed fennel with strong laxatives such as buckthorn to counteract intestinal cramps.

Fenugreek : Fenugreek seeds mixed with water was used as a salve to soothe inflamed or irritated tissue. Internally, it was used to treat fever and digestion and respiratory ailments. Gilbertus Anglicus considered a plaster using fenugreek (femigreke) in combination with a gargle made of other ingredients to be somewhat of a cure-all: Good for every postem both within a man's body and without: Take the root of hollyhock and lily roots and seep them in water. Then crush them with fresh grease and butter and add meal of flax seed (linseed) and fenugreek and snails and crush them together. And give him a gargle of vinegar that barley has lain in and water that pomegranate or sumac or roses or oak galls or lentils have soaked in.

Garlic : Greek and Roman physicians recommended garlic for infections, wounds, cancer, leprosy, heart problems, colds, and epilepsy among many other ailments. In the middle ages the upper class shunned the use of garlic, but the peasantry viewed it as a preventative medicine and cure-all.

Horehound **:** First used in ancient Rome as an ingredient in poison antidotes lead medieval Europeans to believe horehound provided protection from wtiches' spells. Hildegard of Bingen considered it one of the best herbs for colds. Galen was the first to recommend horehound for coughs and respiratory problems.

Hyssop **:** Prescribed for use in a tea for coughs, wheezing and shortness of breath and in plasters and salves for chest decongestion. Hildegard of Bingen recommended a meal of chicken stewed in hyssop and wine as a treatment for depression.

Licorice **:** Hippocrates recommended licorice for cough, asthma and other respiratory diseases. Hildegard of Bingen prescribed it for stomach problems.

Mint **:** Spearmint was the original medicinal mint and was used to aid in digestion and the treatment of gout. In Gilbertus Anglicus' Compendium of Medicine the following treatment is recommended for "stinking of the mouth":

If there be no rotten flesh, let the mouth be washed with wine that birch or mint has been soaked in. And let the gums be well rubbed with a rough linen cloth until they bleed. And let him eat marjoram, mint and parsley till they be well chewed. And let him rub well his teeth with the herbs he chewed and also his gums.

Motherwort **:** Used to treat heart palpitations and depression; later to stimulate contractions during childbirth.

Myrrh **:** Myrrh was valued primarily as an oral treatment for bleeding gums, mouth ulcers and sore throat. It was also used as an expectorant for colds and congestion.

Oregano **:** Used as a digestive aid, arthritis treatment, expectorant for cough, colds and chest congestion.

Parsley **:** Galen prescribed parsley for epilepsy and as a diuretic to treat water retention. Hildegard of Bingen recommended parsley compresses for arthritis and parsley boiled in wine for chest and heart pain.

Pennyroyal (Fleabane) **:** Pliny first discovered that when rubbed on the skin or strewn, penyroyal repelled fleas. He also recommended it as a cough remedy and digestive aid. Taken with honey, pennyroyal was said to cleanse the lungs and clear the chest of "all gross and thick humours".

Roses **:** Hippocrates recommended rose flowers mixed with oil for diseases of the uterus. Hildegard of Bingen prescribed rose hip tea as the initial treatment for many complaints including headache, dizziness and cramps. For difficulty in swallowing, Gilbertus Anglicus recommended a syrup called "honey roset" which consisted of a pound of minced roses soaked in a pound of honey over a fire.

Rosemary **:** In 1235 Queen Elizabeth of Hungary became paralyzed. According to legend, a hermit soaked a pound of rosemary in a gallon of wine for several days then rubbed it on her limbs, curing her. Rosemary/wine combinations became known as Queen of Hungary's Water and were used externally to treat skin problems, gout, dandruff, and prevention of baldness.

Saffron : Rare in Europe until after the Crusades, by the 14th century saffron was recommended to treat jaundice, insomnia and cancer.

Sage : Sage was considered to be something of a cure-all. Pliny prescribed it for snakebite, epilepsy, intestinal worms and chest ailments. Dioscorides recommended using sage leaves as bandages for wounds. Gilbertus Anglicus recommends the following for aching eyes:

And if it (the ache of the eyes) comes of phlegm purge it as I told in the headache and in other sicknesses of the head. And if it be of melancholy, purge it. And afterward let him be stood over a stew five or seven times, that is made of wormwood, betony, fennel, sage, flowers of thyme, chamomile flowers, melilot flowers, hock, and wild celery. All these must be soaked in wine and water together, half wine and the other half water. And let him hold his eyes and his head over the stew. And afterward take a linen cloth or cotton and wet in the water. And annoint therewith his eyes.

St. John's Wort : Early physicians prescribed St. John's Wort taken internally with wine as a cure for poisonous snakebite and externally as a treatment for burns. Christians believed that St. John's wort repelled evil spirits and burned it in bonfires on St. John's Eve to purify the air, drive away evil spirits and ensure healthy crops.

Thyme : Thyme was used as a cough remedy, digestive aid and treatment for intestinal worms. Hildegard of Bingen favoured it for skin problems. Thyme was also recommended to those who suffered from depression; they were advised to sleep on thyme-stuffed pillows. Gilbertus Anglicus recommended the following involved treatment for a soft spleen:

For softness of the spleen, if it be of cold humours give him oximel (medicine made of two parts vinegar and one of honey) to defy the humours. Afterward give him iera pigra Galieni (a decoction made of valerian, cinnamon, saffron, camel hay, hazelwort, bark of cassia and balsa, violets, wormwood, roses, gourds and alloes among other spices) to purge the humours. After the third day treat with a bath of hot herbs such as oregano, mint, horehound, thyme, rosemary and such others. And the next day let him bleed under the ankle in the underside of the left foot. And make him hot plasters of rue, celandine, and nettles to consume the humours and lay to the spleen.

Valerian : Ancient physicians recommended valerian as a diuretic, antidote to poisons, for pain relief and as a decongestant. Hildegard of Bingen prescribed it as a tranquilizer and sleeping aid.

Vervain : In the middle ages healing herbs were called simples. Vervain was prescribed so often and for so many different ailments that it became known as "simpler's joy." It was recommended for fever, tumours, blood infections, toothache, and acne among many other ailments.

Yarrow : Used to treat inflammations, to stop bleeding, as a digestive aid, for pain relief and as a mild sedative.

BIOENGINEERING OF MEDICINAL PLANTS

Pharmaceutical importance/therapeutic value of medicinal plants is due to specific constituents/combination of secondary metabolites present in them. Changes in the proportion of secondary metabolites are often required for the improvement of therapeutic values of medicinal plants. For example, increase in the artemisinin content of Artemisia annua in proportion to its immediate precursors and other terpenes is required to make the production of antimalarials from this plant more economically.

The biosynthetic pathways for the biologically active chemical compounds in medicinal plants are usually complex and high branches. Genetic manipulations can help increase/decrease the contents of specific compounds in medicinal plants. Detailed understanding of these pathways will be a prerequisite for the identification, cloning and genetic engineering of the concerned structural and regulatory genes. These genetic techniques will also help develop designer medicinal plants. For example it will be possible to produce medicinal plants that will help raise the immunity towards infectious diseases in the use of such plants.

In Vitro Propagation Techniques

The biotechnological tools are important to select, multiply and conserve the critical genotypes of medicinal plants by adopting techniques such as micropropagation, creation of somacional varations and genetic transformations. Biotechnological tools can also be harnessed for production of secondary metabolites using plants as bioreactors.

In vitro propagation involves cell culture systems of a range of ex-plant tissues and mostly micropropagation is achieved from organised tissues by multiplication of meristems and auxillary buds. In many cases it provides an opportunity to maintain type-to type plant species and the propagation system can produce a large number of plants from a single clone. Plant regeneration from shoot and stem meristems has yielded encouraging results in medicinal plants like Catharanthus roseus, Cinchona ledgeriana and Digitalis spp.

The production of tropane alkaloids by hairy root culture has been resorted in several medicinal plants like Atropa, Datura and Hyoscyamus. Plant cell suspension culture is the selection of variant cell lines for the genetic improvement of plants. High secondary product yields in plant cell cultures of medicinal plants like Catharanthus roseus, Coleus blumei, Coptis japonica and Panax ginseng have been reported.

Cryopreservation has been used successfully to store a range of tissue types, including meristems, anthers/pollens, embryos, calli and even protoplasts. Cryopreservation is already reported for many medicinal plants like Rauvolfia serpentina, Datura spp., Atropa, Hyoscyamus spp. etc. Protoplast fusion or somatic hybridization has been used to bypass the sexual process.

The objective is to transfer important genes which can not be transferred through sexual means due to the operation of incompatibility systems. Somatic hybrids between Atropa belladona and Datura innoxia were reported which showed higher amounts of tropane alkaloids. Biotransformation of psychotrine cephaeline to emetine production from cell cultures of Ipecac needs to be shown economically viable when compared with synthetic process of production of emetine. Plant cell culture is of importance of improvement of medicinal plants. Complete plants have been regenerated from callus cultures, excised anthers and isolated protoplasts of many medicinal and aromatic plants. Many of the regenerated plants showed somaclonal variation and selections were made for high active principle yielding cell lines. Protoplast fusion has been plant is regenerated, microprorpagation techniques can be used to multiply and clone the desired species. Gene transfer is possible from wild and related species to desired cultivars through wide hybridization including embryo rescue systems. Thus, to sum up, various components of the application of tissue culture technology would be:

- Micropropagation
- Conservation through cryopreservation
- Bioproduction of value added secondary metabolites
- Biotransformation of bioactive molecules
- Genetic upgradation for improvement
- Somatic hybridization
- Somaclonal variations
- Transgenic plants.

The only limiting factor in commercialization of large number of medicinal plants has been the cost of cultivation. As for other annual/biennial crops per acre requirement of planting material is very large, cost of propagule is of major concern. Tissue culture can thus be adopted for species which are:

- Difficult to regenerate by conventional methods and the only way to save them from extinction is to propagate them by tissue culture;
- Species where population has decreased due to over exploitation and thus initial bulking of the stock can be taken up by tissue culture
- Species which show lot of variability in terms of the active principles

with medicinal properties. Tissue culture of selected clones will help in sustainable harvest and fetching better prices both in the domestic and international market.

- Trees with medicinal properties or elites can be identified based on their potential of yielding higher amount of active principle.

Tissue culture protocols have been developed for several plants but there are many more species which are over exploited and need conservation through in vitro techniques. Also there are large number of species for which limiting factor in expanding the area under the cultivation is the scarcity of planting material.

Choosing Priorities

It is necessary to priotise the thrust areas to obtain the output of research efforts and other resources. Several factors help in determining the priorities. These include the distribution of flora, national or regional disease pattern, availability of modern health care etc. In addition we have to keep in mind the global priorities in developing new drugs so as to get a good financial return.

The disease pattern and the priorities have national characteristics but there are several diseases which are common to tropical areas and in fact to most developing countries. These include protozoal and helminthic infections like malaria, filaria, onchocerciasis etc. Many of these diseases do not exist in developed countries and large pharmaceutical houses, therefore, do not give high priority to develop new drugs for such conditions. There is a gross mismatch between the health needs of the developing countries and the interests of the pharmaceutical industry. These should, therefore, receive priority in national/regional plans. The above examples are only illustrative but we have to evolve our own list of priority for communicable diseases.

Primary health care usually requires comparatively milder medication and the acceptability of herbal medicines for such conditions is also much more. The main considerations should be adequate availability or possible cultivation on required scale, lack of toxicity and ease of formulation.

The global thrust areas for drugs from natural sources include disease conditions whose incidence is increasing and where the modern drugs are either unavailable or unsatisfactory. Some examples of such maladies may be summarised as follows:

- Tropical diseases; antimalarial, anti-filarials and anti-leishmaniasis
- Chronic conditions: anti-arthritic agents, anti-rheumatic agents
- Immunomodulators, immunostimulants, adaptogens
- Hepatoprotectors
- Rapid wounds and ulcer healing agents

- Central stimulating or sedating agents
- Alzheimers disease: prospective agents
- Memory enhancers
- Analgesics
- Sedatives.

In considering the validation of the claims of ethnomedical therapies and derived preparations for introduction into the health-care systems, following deserve consideration:

(a) The inadequacy of animal models to serve as adequate systems to assess biological activities that can be extrapolated to the human situation. This is particularly so in some of the disease conditions for which no satisfactory modern therapy exists.

(b) The minimizing of toxicity tests needed to introduce the drug into a health care system. This is particularly necessary when the drug has been in long human use, toxic manifestations could be assessed by studying its long term effect on patients already undergoing treatment in the traditional milieu and the mode of industrial processing does not significantly vary from the ethnomedical methods. Product comparisons by modern instrumental parameters can also be made as between processed product and ethnomedical preparation.

(c) Clinical trials conducted under the supervision of competent authorities (*e.g.* WHO) must be a necessary prerequisite.

(d) Stimulation of traditional processing methods, as well as adherence to ethnomedical regiments will be most helpful in not missing the activitiy present in an ethnomedical preparation. This will also stimulate examination of ethnomedical theories of disease with a view to interpretation of these, if at all possible, within modern concepts. (The idea particularly refers to long standing and well documented systems such as Ayurveda, Unani and the Chinese systems).

(e) The Selection of the appropriate dosage form and mode of administration should be recently based on economic parameters as well as shelf-life potential in the situations prevailing in the developing world.

(f) There is some concrete evidence that pure compound need not necessarily be the best drugs. But on economic ground as well as on the therapeutic grounds it will serve all interests well if the most appropriate processing methodology of a plant or combination of plants is examined in this light (This would also give rise to interesting researches on the synergistic and/or detoxificant effects of other constituents in the medicinal plants or non medicinal plants that are found often added to polyprescriptions used in traditional systems).

REVIVAL OF TRADITIONAL MEDICINE

Today we find a renewed interest in traditional medicine. During the past decade there have been an ever increasing demand especially from developed countries for more and more drugs from plant sources.

This revival of interest in plant derived drugs is mainly due to the current widespread belief that `green medicine' is safe and more dependable than the costly synthetic drug many of which have adverse side effects. This resurgence of interest in the plant based drugs have necessitated an increased demand of medicinal plants leading to over-exploitation, unsustainable harvesting and finally to the virtual decimation of several valuable plant species in the wild.

Moreover, the habitat degradation due to increased human activities (human settlements, agriculture and other developmental programmes), illegal trade in rare and endangered medicinal plants, and loss of regeneration potential of the degraded forests have further accelerated the current rate of extinction of plants particularly the medicinal plants.

Medicinal Plants Wealth of India

India is rich in medicinal plant diversity. All known types of agroclimatic, ecologic and edaphis conditions are met within India. The biogeographic position of India is so unique that all known types of ecosystems ranging from coldest place like the Nubra Valley with - 570 C, dry cold deserts of Ladakh, temperate and Alpine and subtropical regions of the North-West and trans-Himalayas, rain forests with the world's highest rainfall in Cheerapunji in Meghalaya, wet evergreen humid tropics of Western Ghats, arid and semi-arid conditions of Peninsular India, dry desert conditions of Rajasthan and Gujarat to the tidal mangroves of the Sunderban.

India is rich in all the three levels of biodiversity-such as species diversity, genetic diversity and habitat diversity. There are about 426 biomes representing different habitat diversity that gave rise to one of the richest centres in the world for plant genetic resources. The total number of flowering plant species although only 17,000, the intraspecific variability found in them make it one of the highest in the world. Out of 17,000 plants, the classic systems of medicines like Ayurveda, Siddha and Unani make use of only about 2000 plants in various formulations.

The classical traditions were prevalent in the past particularly in the urban elite society. The rural people who constitute 70 to 75% of the Indian populations live in about 5,76,000 villages located in different agroclimatic conditions. The village people have their own diverse systems of health management. While most of the common ailments were managed in the house by home remedies which included many species and condiments like pepper, ginger, turmeric, coriander, cumins, tamarind, fenagree, tulsi, etc., more complicated cases were attended by the traditional physicians who use a large number of plants from the ambient vegetations and some products of animal or mineral origin to deal with the local diseases and ailments.

These are indeed community managed systems independent of official or government system and are generally known as Local Health Tradition (LHT). The traditional village physicians of India are using about 4500 to 5000 species of plants for medicinal purpose. There is however no systematic, inventory and documentation about the folk remedies of India. There is urgent need to document this fast disappearing precious knowledge system. The oral traditions of the villagers use about 5000 plant for medicinal purposes. India is also inhabited by a large number of tribal communities who also posses a precious and unique knowledge about the use of wild plants for treating human ailments. A survey conducted by the All India Coordinated Research Project on Ethnobiology (AICRPE) during the last decade recorded over 8000 species of wild plants used by the tribals and other traditional communities in India for treating various health problems. Some interesting observations made in the study is the use of the same species found in different regions for the same ailments while some other species are used differentially.

Strategies & Priorities

The world conservation strategy (IUCN, UNEP & WWF, 1980) defines conservations as "the management of human use of the biodiversity so that it may yield the greatest sustainable benefit to present generation while maintaining its potential to meet the needs and aspirations of future generations". The above definition invokes two complementary components "conservation" and "sustainability". The primary goals of biodiversity conservation as envisaged in the World Conservation Strategy can be summarised as follows:

1. Maintenance of essential ecological processes and life support systems on which human survival and economic activities depend,
2. Preservation of species and genetic diversity and
3. Sustainable use of species and ecosystems which support millions of rural communities as well as major industries.

Medicinal plants are potential renewable natural resources. Therefore, the conservation and sustainable utilisation of medicinal plants must necessarily involve a long term, integrated, scientifically oriented action programme. This should involve the pertinent aspects of protection, preservation, maintenance, exploitation, conservation and sustainable utilization. A holistic and systematic approach envisaging interaction between social, economic and ecological systems will be a more desirable one. The most widely accepted scientific technologies of biodiversity conservation are the in-situ and ex-situ methods.

In-situ Conservation

In has been well established that the best and cost-effective way of protecting the existing biological and genetic diversity is the 'in-situ' or on the site conservation wherein a wild species or stock of a biological community is protected and preserved in its natural habitat. The prospect of such a 'ecocentric', rather than a species centred approach is that it should prevent species from becoming endangered by human activities and reduce the need for human intervention to prevent premature extinctions. Establishment of biosphere reserves, national parks, wild life sanctuaries, sacred groves and other protected areas forms examples of 'in-situ' methods of conservation.

The idea of establishing protected area network has taken a central place in all policy decision process related to biodiversity conservation at national, international and global level.

In India 4.5% of its total geographical area constitute protected area network, comprising 8 designated biospheres, 87, national parks, 447 wild life sanctuaries.

This network encompasses various biogeographic zones and biomes rich in biotic diversity, including medicinal and aromatic plants. In addition to these there area number of sacred groves in different parts of the country particularly in South, West and Eastern parts which are also active centres on in-situ conservation of medicinal plants. Such conservation area network can attribute significantly towards the conservation and sustainable management of biological resources of our country.

However, experiences have amply demonstrated that in a densely populated developing country like India, where a sizeable population are living in close proximity to forests, declaring protected areas will not entirely be sufficient to ensure conservation on the fast eroding biological diversity. The success of any conservation programme vests solely on the efficient management of protected areas.

The involvement of local communities in conservation activities has now been increasingly realised. A people nature-oriented approach thus become highly imperative. This will help to generate a sense of responsibility among the local people about the values of biodiversity and the need to use it sustainably for their own prosperity and the maintenance of ecosystem resilience.

In-situ conservation of medicinal plants in India can be accomplished through the active support and participation of people who dwell in or near and around the protected forest areas. Involving the local mass in all phases of conservation programmes, such as planning, policy-decision process, implementation etc. will be a significant component in achieving efficient management and utilization of medicinal plant resources. A few such in-situ conservation areas have been marked and declared as medicinal plant in-situ conservation areas on the forests of three Southern States of Kerala, Tamil Nadu and Karnataka by the joint efforts of the forest departments of these States and FRLHT, Bangalore.

Ex-situ Conservation

Conservation of medicinal plants can be accomplished by the ex-situ *i.e.* outside natural habitat by cultivating and maintaining plants in botanic gardens parks, other suitable sites, and through long term preservation of plant propagules in gene banks (seed bank, pollen bank, DNA libraries, etc.) and in plant tissue culture repositories and by cryopreservation).

Botanical gardens can play a key role in ex-situ conservation of plants, especially those facing imminent threat of extinction. Several gardens in the world are specialised in cultivation and study of medicinal plants, while some contain a special medicinal plant garden or harbour special collection of medicinal plants.

India has a network of about 140 botanical gardens which include 33 botanical gardens attached to 33 universities botany departments. But hardly 30 botanical gardens have any active programme on conservation. Tropical Botanical Gardens & Research Institute (TGBRI), located in a degraded forest region of Western Ghat mountains in Kerala has an excellent example in ex-situ conservation of plant diversity in India.

The field gene bank programme launched by TBGRI from 1992-1999 is now well acclaimed as a very effective method of conservation of medicinal and aromatic plant genetic resources. This field gene bank of medicinal and aromatic plants at TBGRI, Thiruvananthapuram is essentially a blend of the ex-situ and in-situ situations.

Field Gene Bank of Medicinal Plants: The concept of establishing field gene banks of plants provide ample options for long term preservation of the genetic variability (inter-specific) of species. Field gene banks are better established in a degraded forests where efforts could be made to reforest/restock the missing species complexes, trees, shrubs, herbs, climber etc. It is indeed a recreation of a forest or rather simulation of a typical forest. Before attempting to establish such a field gene bank it is essential to have a clear understanding of the natural ecosystem such as the spatial distribution, pattern of association *i.e.*, structure and functional dynamics of the species in question. After undertaking a in depth study on the natural distribution pattern of the medicinal plants and the associated floristic elements - including their microecological niche, a well planned action programme of recreating the same in a degraded forest area or place close to the species found in nature can be attempted. TBGRI has accomplished this task of simulating the nature while establishing the field gene bank of medicinal and aromatic plants under the G-15-GBMAP sponsored by DBT, Government of India. TBGRI experience now provide ample opportunity to repeat the same elsewhere in the country.

Identification of the keystone species and umbrella species are very important in this methods. After planting the keystone and umbrella species, other species complex which include the medicinal aromatic plants in question have to be introduced. The sampling and selection of samples for introduction have to be highly knowledge and science intensive. To capture the maximum possible genetic diversity of the target species it is extremely important to collect all valuable information such as morphological variants, chemical variants or genetic variants or chemical screening of the population of the targeted species by using the latest methods and tools. The field gene bank of TBGRI has covered 30,000 accessions of 250 medicinal and aromatic plant species which include 100 endemic, rare and endangered medicinal and aromatic plants of the tropical region of India. A broad spectrum of the genetic diversity of these species were captured and introduced in this gene bank which covered morphotypes, cytotypes and chemotype and the number of samples from each species varied from 50-1000 plants.

MEDICINAL PLANTS AS A PART OF CULTURE

It is evident that the Indian people have a tremendous passion for medicinal plants and use them for a wide range of health related applications from a common cold to memory improvement and treatment of poisonous snake bites to a cure for muscular distrophy and the enhancement of body's general immunity. In the oral traditions local communities in every ecosystem from the trans himalayas down to the coastal plains have discovered the medical uses of thousands of plants found locally in their ecosystem.

India has one of the richest plant medical culture in the world. It is a culture that is of tremendous contemporary relevance because it can on one hand ensure health security to millions of people and on the other hand it can provide new and safe herbal drugs to the entire world. There are estimated to be around 25000 effective plant based formulations are available in the indigenous medical texts formulations used in folk medicine and known to rural communities all over India and around 10000 designed.

Distribution

Macro analysis of the distribution of medicinal plants show that they are distributed across diverse habitats and landscape elements. Around 70% of

India's medicinal plants are found in tropical areas mostly in the various forest types spread across the Western and Eastern ghats, the Vindhyas, Chotta Nagpur plateau, Aravalis & Himalayas.

Although less than 30% of the medicinal plants are found in the temperate and alpine areas and higher altitudes they include species of high medicinal value. Macro studies show that a larger percentage of the known medicinal plant occur in the dry and moist deciduous vegetation as compared to the evergreen or temperate habitats.

Analysis of habits of medicinal plants indicate that they are distributed across various habitats. One third are trees and an equal portion shrubs and the remaining one third herbs, grasses and climbers. A very small proportion of the medicinal plants are lower plants like lichens, ferns algae, etc. Majority of the medicinal plant are higher flowering plants.

Distribution of Medicinal Plants by Habits

Of the 386 families and 2200 genera in which medicinal plants are recorded, the families Asteraceae. Euphorbiacae. Laminaceae, Fabaceae, Rubiaceae., Poaceae, Acanthaceae, Rosaceae and Apiaceae share the larger proportion of medicinal plant species with the highest number of species (419) falling under Asteraceae.

About 90% of medicinal plant used by the industries are collected from the wild. While over 800 species are used in production by industry, less than 20 species of plants are under commercial cultivation. Over 70% of the plant collections involve destructive harvesting because of the use of parts like roots, bark, wood, stem and the whole plant in case of herbs. This poses a definite threat to the genetic stocks and to the diversity of medicinal plants if biodiversity is not sustainably used.

INTERNATIONAL TRADE IN MEDICINAL PLANTS

It has been said that as many as 35 000-70 000 species of plants have been used at one time or another for medicinal purposes (Farnsworth & Soejarto 1991). By far the greater number of species is employed in herbal medicine and is used in unrefined or semi-processed form, often in mixtures which sometimes also contain non-botanical ingredients. A few species are the sources of defined compounds used in the pharmaceutical industry. The overall quantities of plants used medically, in one way or another, are large. Farnsworth and Soejarto (1991), quoting other papers by Farnsworth, state that approximately one-quarter of all prescriptions dispensed from community pharmacies in the USA contain one or more ingredients derived from higher plants.

In many tropical and sub-tropical countries, as in Africa and South and East Asia, the majority of people resort to herbal medicine for the majority of their primary healthcare needs. There are also strong traditions of herbal medicine in parts of Europe, such as Germany, France and eastern Europe generally. The herbal sector is growing fast, increasing by 12-15% by value per year in the UK, USA and Italy (Abrahams 1992). According to a review of a recent consultancy report by McAlpine Thorpe and Warrier (1992), there are more than 2000 herbal medical companies in Europe and more than 220 in the USA; this review states that Germany is the largest market in the world for herbal medicines, with annual sales of $1.2 billion representing nearly 25% of the national pharmaceutical market. The USA is the next largest market with sales of $480 million.

It is difficult to obtain precise information about the structure and scale of the international trade in medicinal plants. Anna Lewington, who recently carried out a short-term study on behalf of WWF of the importation of medicinal plants into Europe and attendant conservation problems, found trade statistics and customs records to be very inadequate, and the industry as a whole not particularly forthcoming about its activities (Lewington 1992a). A complication in some cases is that there can be no clear distinction between medicinal, food, spice and aromatic plants.

The most recent report available to the general public dealing with European imports appears to be by the International Trade Centre, Geneva, in 1982. This report states that 8 countries then belonging to the EEC imported 80 738 tons of 'vegetation plant materials used in pharmacy' in 1980, the biggest importer being Germany with 31 452 tons, followed by France. Quantities will certainly be larger now, as it is widely acknowledged that the trade has grown. Lewington (1992a) estimates that 500, and possibly as many as 600, species of medicinal plants are traded through Hamburg, Germany, which lies at the heart of the import business in Europe. In 1980 India was the biggest exporter of medicinal plants to Europe (10 055 tons out of the 80 738 imported). Eastern Europe is another important source of supply.

Major international trade in medicinal plants is not only from developing to urban-industrial countries. For instance, there is major trade from the Himalayas, including Nepal, to India and beyond, mostly for use in herbal medicine (notably ayurvedic medicine). The volume of this trade is unknown, because it is believed that the greater part of it passes through unofficial channels. Unregulated harvesting of medicinal plants in the Himalayas is a cause for conservation concern.

The majority of conservation problems that result from existing trade in medicinal plants arise if the plants are 'wild' collected, as opposed to being cultivated. Lewington (1992a) reports that it is very difficult to determine the precise origin of medicinal plants currently imported into Europe, a complicating factor being that some species which are cultivated are also collected to some extent from the wild. Judging by Lewington (1992a) and various articles in Akerele et al. (1991), only a few species, required in large quantities, are cultivated to any significant extent. The great majority of species in international trade, certainly most of those which are used in herbal medicine, are harvested in the wild.

MEDICINAL PLANTS OF WESTERN GHATS

The earth is home to a rich and diverse array of living organisms, whose genetic diversity and relationships with one another and with their physical environment constitutes biodiversity (variability among living organisms from all sources and the ecological complexes of which they are part, which includes within species, between species and of ecosystems). This biodiversity is the natural biological capital of the earth, and its conservation and sustainable management presents important opportunities for all nations, especially India.

Over the centuries, people in India have had a fascination and respect for the natural heritage, traditional plant ethics and tried to conserve it in varied ways possible. The sacred grooves (considering certain flora or biotic elements as divine) is an unique tradition which has been responsible for preserving pockets of biodiversity in various parts of the country (Khan T. I, 2001). India, while following the path of development, has been sensitive to the needs of conservation. India's strategies for conservation and sustainable utilization of biodiversity in the past have comprised of providing special status and protection to biodiversity rich areas by declaring them as national parks, biosphere reserves, ecological fragile and sensitive areas. One such area is the Western Ghats which runs majestically parallel to the west coast of India. Conservation of the rich biological wealth of Western Ghats turns out to be a priority. And, the richness of the Western Ghats is further increased by the exclusive varieties of medicinal plants that the Ghats has to its credit.

Western Ghats

India is endowed with a variety of natural resources. All along the west coast the Western Ghats are sprawling. The entire Western Ghats is known for its biodiversity, richness and endemism of different species.

The Western Ghats is richly credited with varied kind of vegetation and unimaginable topographical features. Biogeographically, the hill chain of the Western Ghats constitutes the Malabar province of the Oriental realm, running parallel to the west coast of India from 8° N to 21° N latitudes, 73° E to 77° E longitudes for around 1600 km. Rising up from a relatively narrow strip of coast at its western border, the hills reach up to a height of 2800 m before they merge to the east with the Deccan plateau at an altitude of 500-600 m. The average width of this mountain range is about 100 km. This bioregion is highly species rich and under constant threat due to human pressure, and is considered one of the 18 biodiversity hot spots of the world. With its complex, heterogeneous landscapes and high levels of biodiversity, it forms an ideal ground for the testing and elaboration.

The tropical climate complimented by heavy precipitation from southwest monsoon and favourable edaphic factors create an ideal condition for the luxuriant growth of plant life, which can be seen only in few parts of the world. With its rainfall regime, the western slopes of the Ghats have a natural cover of evergreen forest, which changes to moist and then dry deciduous type as one comes to the eastern slopes. The vegetation reaches its highest development towards the southern tip in Kerala with rich tropical rain forests.

The Western Ghats presents a whole range of gradients, both altitudinal as well as latitudinal in climatic factors, such as total annual rainfall, maximum temperatures. This tremendous environmental heterogeneity found across the Ghats, of topography, soils, rainfall, number of dry months per year and temperature, makes for an extremely environmentally heterogeneous biogeographic area, with a tremendous amount of diversity, both plant and animal.

Species Diversity: Spatial Distribution

The plant species known to be from the Western Ghats is about 4500 species out of which 35 percent are endemic. Levels of endemism in this area are high – nearly 2000 species of higher plants, 84 species of fishes, 87 species of amphibians, 89 species of reptiles, 15 species of birds and 12 species of mammals are endemic to the Western Ghats. Three major gradients in the distribution of this diversity, especially for flowering plants, have been recognized. The first and major one occurs along the north-south direction, species diversity increases as one travels from north to south direction along the Ghats. Southward increase of number of rainy days can be related to this phenomenon. The decrease in rainfall, relates to the decrease in diversity from west to east. The third known gradient is an increase in number of plant species found with the increase in temperature, as one goes from higher elevation hills to lower coastal plains. This heterogeneous condition, which is affluent all along the ranges and regions of the Western Ghats makes it an ideal ground for the luxurious growth of plants with therapeutic value. But since the region is being uncontrollably invaded by urban development and human settlements, life of such valuable medicinal wealth is at stake. And with the patronage of herbal medicines and their products increasing, there is an urgent need to conserve the endemic diversity in the medicinal plants before it is wiped out from nature. Therefore, collection and cultivation of such species and the conservation of their genetic traits by genetic engineering and tissue culture techniques is the present day call for conservationists.

Medicinal Plants

Plants have been used as healers and health rejuvenators since time immemorial. Even now, WHO recognizes that medicinal plants plays an important role in the health care of about 80 percent of World population in developing countries and depend largely on traditional medicines, of which herbal medicines constitutes the most prominent part. The rest of the 20 percent also depend substantially on the plant-based medicines.

Among the rich and varied plants of Indian forests the medicinal plants constitute an important source, the use of which for human and veterinary health care has probably continued, in an unbroken tradition for well over 2 millenium. Many people have defined medicinal plants in many ways, out of which the accepted definition given by the Agricultural and Natural Resource Development is,

" Plants that are recognized by people to have reliable and effective medicinal values, are commonly used in treating and preventing specific ailments and diseases, and play an essential role in health care. "

The number of medicinal plants in India, both indigenous and introduced has been estimated to be between 3, 000 to 3, 500 species of higher plants. The Glossary of Indian Medicinal Plants has listed around 3, 000 plants. Two thousand five hundred plants have been reported to be used in ethno-medicine (Jain, 1991). The number of plants listed in Ayurvedic Materia Nighantu is 560 in Bhav Prakash Nighantu (Kumar 2000). The Ayurvedic Drug Formulary prepared by Department of Indian System of Medicine, lists 387 plants (Sarin, 1996). The Unani system of medicine describes 440 plants (Said, 1969) out of which 360 are common to other systems practiced in the country. The number of plants having confirmed therapeutic properties or yielding a clinically useful chemical compound thus lies around 700 species. The occurrence of these medicinal plants and availability of raw materials from them is as follows:

- Plants occurring wild in forests, grasslands, aquatic and desert ecosystems, associated with other forms of natural vegetation.
- Plants growing as weed.
- Plants cultivated as ornamentals or as cereal, fruit, vegetable, spice, oil seed, essential oil or other cash crop.
- Plants cultivated as medicinal crop.

In addition, almost 25% of the entire compounds of current prescription drugs were derived originally from plant sources. Of the estimated 25, 000 flowering plant species in the world today, only about 10% have been scientifically examined for their medical application, mostly in rudimentary way. Undoubtedly, many more plant-derived medicinal substances await discovery. The information on the medical wealth of these examined 10% of plant species is scattered in different sources. The Western Ghats is very rich in its medicinal wealth. The forests and hills of this region is a treasure house of about 700 medicinal plants. Out of which some are used for traditional and folk medicinal practices. Many are exploited commercially for their active enzymes and their commercial value.

Medicinal plant species of Western Ghats represent a variety of life form ranging from lichen, algae, herbs, shrubs, climber and trees, which are annuals to perennials.

Moreover these species are distributed from canopy to understorey and are characterized seasonally. The auto-ecology and syn-ecology of medicinal plant species is complex and their proper understanding requires a sound knowledge of the ecology, taxonomy and ethno-botany for these species. Western Ghats with its species diversity is a treasure house of different kinds medicinal plants.

The limited knowledge on the varied use of the medicinal plants, their availability and extent of distribution weakens the ways to utilize these resources efficiently. Therefore, it is required to bring the information in various sources into one roof.

Importance of medicinal plants

- Medicinal plants are used at the household level by women to improve the health of the family members.
- At the village level by medicine men or tribals
- By the practitioners of classical traditional systems of medicine such as Ayurveda, Chinese medicine, or the Japanese Kampo system.
- Medicinal plants are gaining importance in the fields of research, especially in the field of genetics and biotechnology.

From the trade data available, it is clear that the global market for medicinal plants has always been very large. To give an example of the extent of trade volumes even at that time, according to one report commissioned by the World Wide Fund for Nature, the total import in 1980 of "vegetable materials used in pharmacy" by the European Economic Community was 80, 738 tons (Lewington 1992).

India was the largest supplier by far, with 10. 055 tons of plants and 14 tons of vegetable alkaloid and their derivatives. It is also true that due to the rising international demand, many important medicinal plant species are becoming scarce and some are facing the prospect of extinction.

Therefore it is important to conserve the extensively traded medicinal plants in its natural environment or cultivating it in favorable environments.

Out of the large variety of species available in the Western Ghats, about 50 species hold a very high value in the folk and herbal health forms for the treatment of different forms of ailments. The most common plants like the *Mimosa pudica, Hibiscus angulosus, Leucas aspera, Phyllanthus neruri, Calotropis gigantea, Tridax procumbens, Parthenium hysterophorus* (which is considered to be a noxoious weed) are all found to have cure for many major ailments like jaundice, asthma, piles, bronchial and blood disorders.

Plants like *Anona squamosa, Buchanania lanzan, Semecarpus anacardium, Dioscorea bulbifera and Aphanamixis polystachya* are recommended for various forms of tumor. Plant parts of Pepper (fruit) and Cinnamom (bark) when mixed together make up a very strong formula for curing Migraine. Frequent doses of medicinal plant extracts of *Rhincanthus nasuta, Momordica dioica, Cinnamomum zeylanicum, Ophiorhizza mungos* relieves cancer patients. The spread of knowledge on the natural wealth is more important for a country like India, at a time when the synthetic drugs are stealing the economy rates.

Most of the medicinal plants are found to occupy forest types like deciduous forests, evergreen forests and they are found in fallow lands and wayside.

It can be noted that the plants that were very common in the area when they were first studied have got into the IUCN Red List over the years. *Rauvolfia serpentina, Saraca asoca, Gymnema sylvestre, Gloriosa superba, Strycnos nux-vomica* are included in the list which are very rich in their medicinal strength but are in the verge of extinction.

The Western Ghats also hosts many medicinal plants that are endemic to the area. Appropriate conservation strategies have to be implemented immediately to protect the fragile habitats of many such medicinal plants. The information on few of the endemic species is gathered and a region specific list is given below.

Natural Resources of Medicinal plants

- Conservation of natural resources and the capability to utilize them in sustained manner are essential for the well being and continued survival of man.
- Under the duress of over exploration and habitat degradation a number of wild plants are essentially facing a constant threat of extinction.
- Out of the 60, 000 plant species that are listed as threatened of extinction, over 20, 000 (or more) are from India alone.
- The botanical survey of India has prepared a provisional list of

threatened plants which includes a large number wild (or) wild relatives of food, horticultural, medicinal and aromatic plants.

- India is endowed with a unique wealth of biota which inlcude a large number of medicinal and aromatic plants.
- Many of these plants are rare and endemic and found only in wild sources.
- The population explosion coupled with the improved standard of living led to ruthless exploitation, resulting in the imminent danger of extinction of these plants.
- Most of these wild medicinal and aromatic plants are highly habitual specific, found only in forests and occupying highly specialized ecological niche with restricted distribution.
- There are neither biological informations nor adequate knowledge of casual factors that led to their rarity in the habital.
- There is however, now an urgent need to evolve a sound strategy for the management and conservation of these plants on a long term basis.
- To evolve suitable strategies for conservation (or) the domestication/ cultivation of medicinal plants, it is very essential to study the complete biological and ecological back ground of these species.
- Under domestication outside their normal ecological range (or) under the distributed eco-system conditions may of the wild medicinal and aromatic plants tend to behave differently.
- In some cases it becomes difficult to grow them (or) it may not even survive.
- In certain other cases if survives and grows but may not be producing the desired traits.
- A through understanding on their reproductive and growth biology as well as identification of the biological and ecological constraints leading to their reduced fitness, restricted distribution (or) even extinction etc., is therefore, necessary.
- An understanding of the biological and ecological back ground of the species in their normal habitat is also essential to understand their conservation biology as well as to predict their behaviour under artificial cultivation.

Strategies for conservation of medicinal plants:

- The conservation of the wild medicinal plants or any other such threatened species can be tackled by scientific techniques as well as social actions.
- There are basically two scientific techniques of conservation of genetic diversity of these plants.

- They are the in situ and ex situ method of conservation.

In Situ conservation:

- It is only in nature that plant diversity at the genetic, species and eco-system level can be conserved on long-term basis.
- Unless plant populations are conserved in the wild, that is in natural habitats, in viable breeding populations, they run the risk of extinction.
- It is necessary to conserve in distinct, representative biogeographic zones inter and intraspecific genetic variation.

Current status:

- In Karnataka, Kerala and Tamil nadu and more recently in Maharashtra the forest department in collaboration with FRUHT (Foundation for Rural Revitalization of Local Health Tradition) have established a network of 33 "Medicinal Plants Conservation Areas" (MPCAs) across the entire altitudinal range of south India.
- Each of these reserves is around 200 ha in size.

Regulation and wild collection:

- Regulating the harvest of medicinal plants from the wild for commercial purposes.
- Particularly those species whose harvest inevitably involves destructive collection.
- Local communities can develop a stake in sustainable harvesting of medicinal plants from the forest and village, district and state level co-operative are set up to manage collection, storage and marketing.

Current status:

- LAMP societies as they function at present neither benefit the primary tribal collectors nor provides adequate powers (or) accountability of the LAMPs with regard to protection and management of forests.
- The marketing function of LAMPs is also weak, so that collectors do not get remunerative prices through LAMP sales.

EX situ conservation

A. Ethno-medicinal plant gardens:

- Creation of a network of regional and sub-regional ethno-medicinal plant gardens which should contain accessions of all the medicinal plants known to the various ethnic communities in different regions of India.
- This chain of gardens will act as regional repositories of our cultural and ethno-medicinal history and embody the living traditions of our socity's knowledge of medicinal plants.

Current status:

- There are estimated to be around 50 such gardens in the country ranging from acre to 40 acres some of them were set up by an All India Health Network.
- More recently a network of 15 such gardens have been set up in 3 states of South India with the initiative of FRLHT. One of the gardens is located in TBGRI, (Tropical botanical garden research institute) Palode at Thiruvananthapuram.

B. Gene banks:

- While it is known that the largest proportion of local bio-diversity in all our eco-system is used for medicinal purposes, very little is known about their conservation status in the wild.
- What is likely is that a large number of medicinal plant species are under various degrees of threat.
- The precautionary principles would suggest that an immediate and country-wide exercise be taken up to deposit seeds of wild medicinal plants with a first priority to known Red listed species and endemic species.

Current status:

- The department of bio-technology, Government of India has recently taken the initiative to establish 3 gene banks in the country.
- One is with ICAR at the NBPGR (National Bureau of plant genetic Resources) Campus, the second is with CIMAPs, (Cental Institute of Medicinal and Aromatic plants) Lucknow and the third with TBFRI in Thiruvananthapuram.

C. Nursery network:

- The most urgent and primary task in order to ensure immediate availability of plants and planting materials to various user groups is to promote a nation wide network of medicinal plant nurseries, which will multiply all the regional specific plants that are used in the current practice of traditional medicine.
- These nurseries should become the primary sources of supply of plants and seed material that can be subsequently multiplied by the various users.

Current status:

- Planting material for 40 odd species of medicinal and aromatic plants is reportedly available in the ICAR and CSIR (CIMAP) network.
- In South India FRLHT has recently set up a network of 55 supply nurseries.

D. Cultivation:

- Figures projecting demand and trade in medicinal plant species globally indicate a step upward trend in the near future.
- One estimate puts the figure of world trade in medicinal plants and related products at US $ 5 trillion by A. D. 2050 (world bank report, 1996).
- The demand so far has been met mainly from wild sources.
- This can't go on for much longer; policy intervention is urgently needed to encourage and facilitate investments into commercial cultivation of medicinal plants.
- Cultivation of medicinal plants however, is inversely linked to prevalence of easy and cheap collection from the wild, lack of regulation in trade, cornering of the profits from wild collection by a vast network of traders and middlemen and absence of industry's interest in providing buy-back guarantees to growers.

Current status:

- In the Govt. sector agro-technology of 40 odd species has been developed by ICAR-Agricultural University System and CSIR (CIMAOs & RRL, Jammu and Jorhat).
- In recent years industries like Dabur, Zandu, Indian Herbs, Arya Vaidya Shala, and Arya Vaidya Pharmacy and others have made some symbolic efforts to initiate cultivation.
- Since 1984 NABARD (National Bank of Agricultural and Rural Development) has formulated schemes for financing cultivation and processing of medicinal plants.

E. Community based enterprises:

- The income generated by the traditional medicine industry benefits small section of the socity.
- This will also increase the stake of rural communities in conservation and change the skewed nature of income distribution of the industry.

Current status:

- Three community based enterprises are known in south India, one in Gandhigram Trust, (Dindigul), Preemade development Society (Peermade) Kerala and the third by VGKK in B. R. Hills, Mysore.

ENDEMIC SPECIES

Karnataka's Species Name

Aglaia elaeagnoidea(Juss.) Benth
Artocarpus hirsutus Lam.

Cayratia pedata (Lam.) Juss. Ex Gagnep
Diopyros paniculata Dalz.
Mucuna pruriens (L.) DC.
Tabernamontana heyneana Wall.

Kerala's Species Name

Artocarpus hirsutus Lam.
Cinnamomum wightii Meisner
Diopyros paniculata Dalz.
Garcinia gummi-gutta (L.) Robs.
Rhododendron arboreum (Zenk.) Tagg.

Maharashtra's Species name

Artocarpus hirsutus Lam.
Ervatamia heyneana Cooke.
Rauvolfia serpentina (L.) Benth. Ex Kurz.

The medicinal plant species of Western Ghats which are categorized by the IUCN is listed below.

Tamil Nadu's Species Name

Artocarpus hirsutus Lam.
Cinnamomum wightii Meisner
Diopyros paniculata Dalz.
Garcinia gummi-gutta (L.) Robs.
Garcinia indica Choiss
Michelia nilagrica Zenk.
Rhododendron arboreum (Zenk.) Tagg.

IUCN CATEGORIZED SPECIES

Species Name

Celastrus paniculata Willd.
Curculigo orchoides Gaertn.
Gymnema sylvestre (Retz.) R. Br. ex Schult.
Hemidesmus indicus (L.) R. Br.
Mucuna monosperma (Lam.) Taub.
Rauvolfia serpentina (L.) Benth. ex Kurz
Saraca asoca (Roxb.) Dewilde
Tylophora indica (Burm. f.) Merr
Flemingera peltata J. E. Smith

Holarrhena superba L.

Artocarpus hirsutus Lam.

The conservation of these species in specific and a search for natural alternatives to these would pave way for excavating the hidden medicinal wealth in many other widely available plants in the region. Western Ghats was and will remain an area where the therapeutics of nature can be excavated. Hence, efforts have to be taken to bring to limelight the use of nature's doctors, methods to conserve them and to sustain their existence for the future generations.

OPPORTUNITIES IN DEVELOPING THE MEDICINAL PLANTS SECTOR

For developing the 'herbal industries', the northern India possesses a rich diversity of medicinal plant species across the various forest types along an altitudinal gradient (as discussed in the use and diversity of medicinal plants). Such a high diversity of medicinal plants would be helpful for further scientific research on exploring their medical efficacy, value addition, and use in curing various old and new diseases. India has already established a reputation as a low-cost manufacturer of high quality generic drugs in the global market. This fact can be used as an important tool for the marketing of herbal products produced in India. It is expected that India's aim to build a golden triangle between traditional medicine, modern medicine, and modern science will be a boon for developing the traditional herbal medicine and the medicinal plants sector.

Existing Policies

In the National Five Year Plans of India, the medicinal plants sector has been identified as an integral part of the Indian System of Medicine and Homeopathy. In 1983, the National Health Policy recognized that the large stock of health manpower in Ayurveda, Siddha, Unani, Homeopathy and Naturopathy had not been adequately utilized; therefore, steps need to be taken to move towards a meaningful integration of the indigenous and modern systems of medicine. The Planning Commission and the National Medicinal Plants Board (NMPB) of the Government of India have prepared a policy document on the promotional and commercial aspects of the medicinal plants sector. In addition, the NMPB has prioritized 32 and Planning Commission has enlisted 24 medicinal plant species for research and development in order to meet the desired aim of the medicinal plant sector. The Biodiversity Act 2002 has framed many rules for sustainable utilization of medicinal plants and to mitigate the chances of bio-piracy.

According to Uttaranchal state action plan, the Forest Department of the state will have to identify two major areas in each Forest Division; namely the conservation area and the developmental area. The conservation areas will be selected based on their rich medicinal plants diversity and marked for in-situ conservation and complete protection in the concerned Forest Division. In the developmental areas, apart from protection of the existing bio-resources, the medicinal plant species of the neighbouring areas will also be introduced and cultivated at a large scale.

The remaining areas in the Forest Division will remain open for sustainable harvesting of the medicinal plant species. A Joint Harvesting Team, composed of medicinal plants experts, Forest Department officials and some selected local people, will be constituted, which will decide the extent of annual harvesting of the desired medicinal plant species. The various policies at national and state level and their subsequent implementation will provide an opportunity in the advancement of medicinal plants sector. This model of conservation and cultivation of the medicinal plants may be useful for generating the raw material for the 'Herbal Industries' as well as for ensuring the conservation of the rare medicinal plants.

Institutional Support

In India, many government and non-government organizations have had the focused attention on improving the medicinal plants sector. Opportunities for funding have been created to assist the person who is willing to work and to build capacity of the medicinal plants sector. According to the mandate of NMPB, the projects may be submitted for funding within two major schemes: viz., a promotional scheme and a commercial scheme. The major thrust areas within the promotional scheme are: (1) survey and inventory of medicinal plants, (2) in-situ conservation and ex-situ cultivation of selected medicinal plants, (3) production of quality planting material, (4) diffusion of knowledge through education and communication, (5) promotion of global and domestic market system, and (6) strengthening research, development and man power. Within the commercial scheme, the major thrust areas are: (i) bulk production of medicinal plants and ensuring supply of quality planting material, (ii) expansion of selected medicinal plants farming areas, (iii) value addition in harvesting, processing and marketing of medicinal plants, and (iv) developing innovative marketing mechanism. Apart from the two major themes, the role of NMPB is to co-ordinate with the different ministries, departments, organizations, state and union territory Governments in order to develop and strengthen the medicinal plant sector. One of the major roles of NMPB is to make contacts with national and international organizations devoted to similar mandates and goals. A total of 35 State Medicinal Plants

Boards have also been created by NMPB for the smooth functioning of the medicinal plants sector.

Approximately 35,000 hectares of land has been selected and brought under cultivation under the supervision of NMPB for the large-scale farming of commercially important medicinal plants. One of the schemes of NMPB is a contractual farming in which any group, institution or person that possesses at least 3 years of experience in medicinal plants sector would be eligible to receive at least 30% financial assistance of the total project cost .

Ten years before establishment of NMPB (during 1992-93 financial years), a single project was launched to study the medicinal plants of the Himalayan region. During past one decade, there has been a considerable expansion in the Himalayan medicinal plants research as it is evident that many projects have been launched exclusively on the medicinal plants during that period. Of the total 4254 projects sanctioned by NMPB over past 5 years, 732 projects have been sanctioned to 11 hill states in northern India.

All these projects are expected to strengthen the medicinal plants sector, to bridge the gaps and to meet the challenges in developing the sector. In addition to major funding organizations, the G.B. Pant Institute of Himalayan Environment and Development has sanctioned projects on the medicinal plants of northern India under the scheme of Ministry of Environment & Forests. The Council of Scientific and Industrial Research is building up a Traditional Knowledge Digital Library, which will contain > 35,000 herbal medical formulations used in Ayurvedic system of medicine .

The National Bank for Agriculture and Rural Development (NABARD) has established a policy with a viewpoint to develop a suitable environment for financial institutions by providing bankable models for some 50 medicinal and aromatic crops with the unit cost and scale of finance at the state level. Additionally, NABARD assists in supporting the capacity building of prospective entrepreneurs through Rural Entrepreneurs Development Programmes by providing 100% refinancing. NABARD has also close linkages with the NMPB and different State Medicinal Plants Boards. Attempts have been made by various organizations at different levels to establish and promote the medicinal plants sector.

Recommendations for Developing the Medicinal Plants Sector

The present worldwide interest in plant-based medicines of Indian origin needs to be harnessed by reframing a clear policy for the promotion of commercial cultivation, research and development, and for the increase in exports of medicinal plants. For the development of the medicinal plant sector, there is a need to develop the coordinated efforts at each stage (*e.g.* research, cultivation, collection, storage, processing, manufacturing and marketing), which would be supported by an appropriate policy framework.

Selection of medicinal plant species for cultivation is an initial important step for the development of the medicinal plants sector. Economic feasibility is the major rationale for a decision to bring medicinal plant species into cultivation. Apart from the priority species selected by the Planning Commission and the NMPB, the rare species banned for collection from the wild should also be taken on a priority basis for cultivation because a majority of such species are very expensive, have high demand and low supply. Cultivation may not be economical if a medicinal plant species is abundant in the wild and easily collected. Therefore, the less abundant species in the wild should be promoted for the large-scale cultivation. Farming of any medicinal plant species should be brought into practice only after the reliable cultivation technology of the concerned species is available. A large variation in climatic and soil conditions in northern India sustain a variety of medicinal plant species, which may be cultivated according to their niche.

For developing the medicinal plants sector, there is a need to: (1) document indigenous uses of medicinal plants, (2) certify raw material for quality control, (3) develop and improve the agro-technology for valuable medicinal plants, (4) officially recognize and protect the customary laws of indigenous people, (5) prepare a clear policy for granting permits for cultivation within stipulated time, (6) conduct regular research and training on better harvesting and processing techniques, (7) investigate various pathological agents infecting medicinal plants, (8) setup a community-based management of medicinal plants farming and marketing, (9) analyze the market policies, (10) monitor and evaluate the status of medicinal plants with the assistance of local communities, (11) conserve the critical habitats of rare medicinal plant species, and (12) share benefits judiciously arising from local people's knowledge on medicinal plants. These attempts may reduce dependency on wild resource base, and generate alternative income opportunities for the rural and underprivileged communities.

The medicinal plants sector can be improved if the agricultural support agencies would come forward to help strengthen the medicinal plants growers, and if research institutions would help the plant growers by improving their basic knowledge about cultivation practices. Awareness and interest of farmers, supportive government policies, assured markets, profitable price levels, access to simple and appropriate agro-techniques, and availability of trained manpower are some of the key factors for successful medicinal plants cultivation.

The diffusion of any available scientific knowledge on medicinal plants should be made operational by a network structure of communication.

Currently there are number of herbs which are used in curing diseases but are not documented in details due to a lack of communication and relatively low frequency of their uses. The traditional uses of low profile and lesser-known medicinal plants should also be documented to disseminate their therapeutic efficacy by preparing well acceptable medicines and also to reduce the pressure on over-exploited species.

Apart from the more than 9992 licensed pharmacies with 717319 registered practitioners of Ayurveda, Siddha, Unani and Homeopathy in India, there are many unregistered herbal practitioners in India who prepare their own traditional herbal formulations for curing different diseases, and the available herbal formulations should be standardized for their efficacy. Such scientifically prepared medicine will place herbal medicine in a proper perspective and help in getting a broad global market. Some people do try to take advantage through the introduction of less effective medicinal plants in the name of well-established high-value medicinal plants.

Such attempts must be discouraged. To discourage such malpractices, the certification of raw material should be done for quality control by using the modern tools such as thin layer chromatography and high performance thin layer chromatography. In addition, high performance liquid chromatography (HPLC), volumetric analysis, gas chromatography, column chromatography, and gravimetric determinations may be used for standardization and for quality control. Various factors relating to pathological agents (*e.g.* bacteria, virus, fungi and nematodes) and infected medicinal plants should be investigated by identifying the various symptoms of diseases such as mildew, rust, necrosis, spots, blight, rot, wilt, galls, curl and canker to produce the healthy farming of medicinal plants.

On many occasions, the collection of planting material, especially of rare and endangered medicinal plant species from natural habitats for various experimental purposes by researchers, also poses a threat on their natural populations in wild. The researchers must be aware on the germination potential, seedlings and rhizomes survival strategies of the desired species collected from wild for scientific experiments. Researchers must plant a similar number of individuals back in nature after completion of research work on the collected species. There is also a communication problem between researchers and farmers. This communication problem limits a researcher's capability to deal with the farmers' problems. Hence, communication links between researchers, extension services of institutions, and farmers should be strengthened.

The majorities of current research programmes on the medicinal plants conservation are being shifted from ecosystems to species levels. Although there are protected areas across the Himalaya, most of the protected areas have a focused attention on the preservation of faunal diversity except for a few protected areas such as the Valley of Flowers in North West Himalaya and the Tipi Orchid Sanctuary in North East Himalaya. There is not a single protected area focusing on the conservation of medicinal plants.

Thus, there is an urgent need for identification and notification of areas for the conservation of medicinal plants on a priority basis. Most of the documentation and research on indigenous uses of medicinal plants is focused on the human aspect. Animal husbandry is the backbone of economy in a majority of indigenous societies. Maintaining the good health of livestock will benefit these indigenous societies. Since there are many medicinal plant species used in curing the various animal related disorders and diseases, the research work also needs to be done on the uses of medicinal plants for curing livestock diseases.

Being a part of tradition, there are many other social issues attached with medicinal plants sector. The indigenous knowledge on harvesting, storage and usage of medicinal plants built over centuries needs to be taken into account for improving the sector and allocating scare resources among the competing demands. Development of medicinal plants farming, encouragement of traditional herbal use and herbal healers, establishing medicinal plants conservation areas, establishing the Social Capital Trust for herbal healers, establishment of linkages among various stake-holders, etc., are among some of the social issues that need to be honored and addressed properly. The folklore on several medicinal plants and the formulation developed by using them is well recognized in different ethnic communities living in northern India. These folklores should be brought into laboratory for validation.

IDENTIFICATION AND CONSERVATION OF MEDICINAL PLANTS

As a global community, we are now in the midst of a crisis in loss of biological and cultural diversity. The current ongoing loss of biodiversity is the greatest contraction of life since the end of the Mesozoic Era sixty-five million years ago — a wave of extinctions that extinguished the dinosaurs (Wilson 1992). Although prehistoric extinction spasms tended to claim mostly animals, plants too are now threatened with extinction on a large scale. One-fourth of all tropical plants may be wiped out in the next 30 years. Outside the tropics, the greatest concentration of threatened plants is found in southern Africa, where 13% of endemic plants are threatened. In southwestern Australia, two-thirds of plant species are endangered by a fungal disease carried by humans walking or driving through the bush. In the US nearly 1 in 8 native species is in danger. According to the 1997 IUCN Red List of Threatened Plants compiled by the World Conservation Union, worldwide 13.8% of vascular plants are imperiled. In addition, much of earth's biodiversity is clustered in tropical regions. Many of these "hotspots" of diversity are populated by indigenous peoples. Today most of the world's indigenous peoples are as imperiled as their homelands, threatened by loss of habitat and westernization.

The World Health Organization (WHO) estimates that 3.5 billion people in developing countries rely on plant-based medicine for their primary health care. In Africa, which is home to 28.1 million of the world's 40 million people living with HIV-AIDS, traditional healers are a crucial component of the health care system, and may be the only source of care and treatment for the poor and disenfrachised (Green 2002). Herbal therapies are growing rapidly in popularity in industrial countries as well. The FAO estimates that between 4000 and 6000 species of medicinal plants are traded internationally, with China accounting for about 30% of exports.

In 1992, the U.S. retail market for herbal remedies reached $1.5 billion, and the European market is considerably larger. But the success of plant-based medicines is not without its cost. Some plant species are rapidly disappearing from the wild due to overcollection.

Until about 1960, only a single plant species was known to have been rendered extinct by the actions of humans. The first exterminated species was known as silphion, and flourished in the sixth century B.C. in a Greek colony in present-day Libya. It was a medicinal plant used for a variety of conditions ranging from hemorrhoids to facilitating uterine contractions. It grew wild and was never cultivated, and a concentrated extract of its stem was worth its weight in silver. As a result, it became scarce, then extinct, due entirely to human overcollection for medicinal use.

Wise use and management of our natural resources is crucial to the welfare of the people who depend on these natural sources of medical treatment.

Fewer than 1-2% of the world's 250,000 flowering plants have been analysed for medicinal value, yet in some tropical regions species are disappearing faster than they can be identified, let alone studied for medical efficacy. The current rate of species extinction is now thought to be 100 to 1,000 times higher than "background" levels (Stork 1997). Wild medicinal plant collection can contribute to habitat destruction and can cause an immediate problem for local or indigenous peoples who may rely on a plant for their health needs, as the case of the African cherry tree illustrates.

The bark of Prunus africana, the African cherry tree, is highly esteemed by traditional healers in central and west Africa, but it is also popular among European doctors for treating prostate disorders.

In recent years Cameroon has been the leading supplier to Europe, resulting in clearance of the tree's montane forest habitat and destruction of cherry stands, whilst also making it scarce for local healers to harvest (Tuxill 1999). Clearly a balance between harvesting and replanting this resource is badly needed.

Ethnobotanical Research Yields Substantial Return on Investment

After decades of decline in natural products research, the systematic examination of nature's resources is once again on the rise. A number of university and government research institutes and pharmaceutical companies are actively pursuing the development of new medicinal compounds from plants.

Conservationists and large pharmaceutical companies are now allies, a movement spearheaded by the well-publicized joint venture between Merck and Costa Rica's INBio — a bold effort to catalogue and protect the tiny Central American country's biodiversity by proving the value of intact ecosystems through quantifiable natural product isolation and production.

The benefits to be gained by screening plants for potential medical efficacy are substantial, both economically and socially. A number of promising compounds are currently being investigated. For example, the NCI is studying four species having anti-HIV activity including *Ancistrocladus korupensis* from Cameroon, *Calophyllum sp.* from Malaysia, *Conospermum sp.* from Australia, and *Homolanthus sp.* from Western Samoa. The *Ancistrocladus* also shows promise as a new antimalarial agent.

Additional efforts to discover new medicinal compounds involve working with local and indigenous peoples throughout the developing world. There is little doubt that some of the great diversity of chemical compounds found in nature could be developed as therapeutic agents, with the help of these peoples. This would be of great value to global health, provided that the development and benefits gained from new molecular entitites derived from biodiversity are equally distributed both to people who need the medication and to the countries and regions from which they have been discovered. This is a part of the social justice that must go hand in hand with attempts to develop products based on the indigenous knowledge systems.

It is imperative that local and indigenous peoples are the beneficiaries of efforts to capitalize on their traditional knowledge and remain the guardians of the forest and their ancestral lands.

Maintaining biological and cultural diversity requires acknowledging the value of indigenous knowledge systems, including the "specialist" knowledge of traditional healers (*curanderos, shamans, etc.*), as well as the "common" medicinal plant knowledge of community members. It is also crucial to acknowledge the importance of traditional medicine to these peoples. After all, the same medicinal plants that we are researching for "new" pharmacological activity have, in many cases, been used for hundreds to thousands of years within a traditional system of medicine that includes information about safety, efficacy and effectiveness that is not dependant on our concepts of value. Given the dependence of many of the world's peoples on traditional plant-based medicines, efforts to conserve biological and cultural diversity, and to develop "new" compounds, should not undermine these traditional knowledge systems.

WORLD HEALTH ORGANIZATION PROGRAM

About ten years ago, the World Health Organization launched its program of 'Health for all by the year 2000.' Right from the outset of the program, WHO realized that any program adopted in any of the minimally industrialized countries would have no impact if it did not take into consideration the development and integration of traditional medicine into the primary health care programs of these countries.

WHO has estimated conservatively that between 60 and 90 percent of the population of the non-industrialized countries rely on medicinal plants to meet their health care needs, either totally or partially. With the scarcity of doctors and paucity of hospitals and clinics, the large majorities of these populations have to rely on sources other than allopathic medicine for their health care. For example, in Ghana there is one traditional doctor for approximately every 400 people, while the ratio of allopathic doctors to patients is 1 for 12,000.3

Various reports from the United Nations (UNCTAD and GATT) have indicated that 33 percent of drug products in the highly industrialized countries are derived directly from higher plants; most of these are tropical plants growing in equatorial countries. Lower plants and microbes produce another 27 percent of drugs found on the market. Indeed, more than 67 percent of the world's plant species — at least 35,000 of which have potential medicinal value — originate in non-industrialized countries of the 'South'. The market for plant-based drugs is growing every year throughout the world. These drugs now account for over $US 50 billion of the total worldwide drug market now totaling over $US 173 billion.

The estimated manufacturer's price value of medicinal materials derived from plants obtained from the developing countries of the South is expected to reach between 35 and 47 billion US dollars by the year 2000.6 Of the total world pharmaceutical sales of $US 172.56 billion, as of 1989, Africa accounted for only 2.1 billion US dollars. In fact, the highly industrialized countries — which constitute only 20 percent of the total world population of now over 5 billion — consume 80 percent of all pharmaceuticals produced in the world. So, how do Africa's 500 million people, for instance, take care of their health if their total share in world pharmaceutical consumption is only 1.2 percent (US$ 2.142 billion)? Indeed, the total for all developing countries is only 15 percent of worldwide pharmaceutical purchasing. Whatever means or method used by this section of the world's population ought to be fully recognized in any formulation of health policies or programs aimed at 'health for all' by the year 2000.7 The international community has a clear duty to ensure the full conservation of whatever alternative sources of health care are currently available to the remaining 80 percent of the world's population normally classified as belonging to the 'South'.

Right from the beginning of the WHO's program, the organization recognized the peculiar circumstances that obtain in less industrialized countries with respect to traditional medicine and health care delivery. Both WHO and UNICEF recognized that in view of the widespread use and acceptability of traditional medical practice, no impact will be made on Africa's overall health care status without due recognition, development and integration of traditional medicine into the primary health care delivery system of each country or region. This recognition led to the WHO/UNICEF 1978 conference in Alma Ata, USSR, at which the participants resolved and specifically urged member states to:

(i) initiate comprehensive programs for the identification, evaluation, cultivation and conservation of medicinal plants used in traditional medicine;

(ii) ensure quality control of drugs developed from traditional plant remedies by using modern techniques and applying suitable standards and good manufacturing practices.

This conference was followed in 1988 by another in Thailand, at which the Chiang Mai declaration to 'save plants that save lives' was made. This declaration formally brought the rational and sustainable use and conservation of medicinal plants into the arena of public health policy.

The Alma Ata declaration of 1978 was followed subsequently by various policy decisions of the Inter-African Committee on Medicinal Plants and African Traditional Medicines of the Organization of African Unity (OAU). These policy decisions were aimed at implementing WHO's recommendations. Several African countries including Ghana have initiated programs aimed at maximizing the contribution of herbal medicine to their primary health care delivery nationwide. These programs have raised some very pertinent questions and problems of considerable importance for Africa particularly, and for the 'Third World' in general. These include questions that are socioeconomic, ethical, legal and environmental.

Development of medicinal plants relies very heavily on the knowledge carried by indigenous peoples and rural societies. In recent times this has raised concerns about equitable sharing of the benefits of such knowledge and the intellectual property ('IP') rights of these indigenous rural communities. Securing such rights and protections entails specific dilemmas and policy implications, which I will examine throughout the rest of this essay.

Socioeconomic Considerations

World trade in medicinal plants accounts for about 30 percent of the total drug market. This percentage excludes plants used as raw material sources for the essential oils required to manufacture cosmetics, food additives and for other non-medicinal purposes. Most of these medicinal plants come from less industrialized countries that supply them as cheap raw materials to the multinational pharmaceutical manufacturers in the more industrialized countries. Of 76 compounds obtained from higher plants that are present in US prescriptions, only 7 percent are commercially produced by total synthesis. In 1976, imports of medicinal plants worldwide were estimated to be $US 355 million. This rose to $US 551 million by 1980 — an increase of over 60 percent within four years. But when these medicinal plants are processed into suitable dosage forms as safe and efficacious drugs, they are sold to the public at prices far beyond the affordable range for the majority of people in the relatively poor countries. Yet it is the botanic resources of these same countries that make possible the manufacture of these drugs for commercial markets.

A typical example is the Madagascar rosy periwinkle *Catharanthus Roseus*, a plant indigenous to Africa that has been used for several years in East Africa for the treatment of cancer and diabetes. Research on this plant yielded two very important anti-cancer drugs: *vinblastine* and *vincristine*. Although the plant is native to Madagascar, it was the US pharmaceutical firm Eli Lilly that commercialized the drugs from germplasm obtained from the Philippines and Jamaica. Vincristine is now the drug of choice for the treatment of childhood leukemia, and it has an annual retail value of over $US 150 million. Vinblastine is used for treating Hodgkin's disease, a serious ailment of unknown origin resulting in enlarged lymph glands, increased numbers of lymphoid tissue cells (*hyperplasia*) in the spleen, liver and other organs, as well as anemia. Before the discovery of vincristine, the survival rate of children with leukemia was about 20 percent. Now the success rate for this drug is over 80 percent. But a 5mg ampoule of vincristine sulfate injection costs about $US 80, making the drug virtually inaccessible to most leukemia children outside the industrialized world.

Maytansine belongs to a class of compounds called the ANSA Macrolides, first discovered from microbes and now found to occur in higher plants. It was first isolated by Kupchan in the US from the plant *Maytenus serrata* obtained from Ethiopia. Maytansine showed promising clinical results as a potential antileukemic drug, but died of cancer before his work could be published. Later, higher yields of the compound were found in a Kenyan species, *Maytenus buchananii*, and a South African plant *Putterlickia verrucosa*. The compound is active against various strains of lymphocytic leukemia and melanoma, and has been on clinical trials for some time.

It is interesting to note that one of the *Maytenus* species has been in popular use for almost 50 years in a South African herbal mixture for carcinoma and sarcoma. But alas, as in the case with vincristine, if maytansine finally gets on the market neither Ethiopia, Kenya nor South Africa will get the millions of dollars accruing from its sales. (Nor is it likely that an average citizen needing the drug in any of these source countries will be able to afford it). Plants are not patentable; but synthetic routes or isolation methods are. Similar examples abound.

Unfortunately, even though our herbalists can continue to provide some relief for cancer patients by administering the crude plant extracts of *Maytenus* and *Catharanthus*, their knowledge, which originally led to the discovery of the landmark drugs just described, cannot be rewarded in the same way as multinational drug companies get their rewards and profits.

This means that the non-industrialized countries are not deriving any economic benefit from the exploitation of their nations' medicinal plant resources. Moreover, as noted already, the approach adopted by the Western world for production and distribution of drugs from plants is far from satisfactory for the majorities living where these essential resources exist. Therefore, in formulating policies for the exploitation of our medicinal plants, policy makers will have to consider how best to manage our natural resources for the full benefit of our citizenry.

MEDICINES REGULATION BENEFIT OF PUBLIC HEALTH

Medicines have the potential for benefit to individuals who use them and to the public health. But all effective medicines may be associated with adverse effects. The law recognises that medicines should not be treated as an ordinary general commodity by placing specific restrictions on them.

There is a specific licensing system for medicines, operated in the UK by the Medicines and Healthcare products Regulatory Agency (MHRA). The MHRA is the Government agency which is responsible for ensuring that medicines and medical devices work, and are acceptably safe. Its work is underpinned by robust and fact-based judgements to ensure that the benefits to patients and the public justify the risks. Its licensing schemes cover the whole range of medicines for human use, from registration for herbal and homeopathic remedies to marketing authorisation for the latest innovative advanced technology medicinal products. This guide uses the general term 'licence' to refer to all these schemes.

The MHRA also contributes to the work of licensing medicines in the European Union (EU), co-ordinated by the European Medicines Agency (EMA). The EMA operates a centralised procedure for the scientific review of applications for innovative medicines, leading to a marketing authorisation from the European Commission that is valid across the EU.

The basis of the licence for any medicine is the Summary of Product Characteristics (SPC). This sets out the details of what the product is licensed for, how it should be administered and warnings and side effects. The SPC sets the boundaries for what can be claimed in advertising for the product. The licence also determines how the product may be supplied. This may be on prescription only or non-prescription, either through pharmacies under the supervision of a pharmacist or on general sale. This in turn determines to whom the product may be advertised.

Special Requirements for Traditional Herbal Medicinal Products (THMs)

All advertisements for herbal medicinal products with a traditional herbal registration of the Regulations should include the following additional statement:

"Traditional herbal medicinal product for use in[specify one or more indications for the product consistent with the terms of the registration] *exclusively based upon long-standing use as a traditional remedy"*. The words "as a traditional remedy" have been added to the statement required by law to ensure that consumers are not misled as to the length of time they need to use the product. This wording has been agreed with advertising regulatory bodies and the industry's Herbal Forum.

Care should be taken in devising advertising for these products to ensure that claims are in line with the approved indication for the product and do not mislead as to the efficacy of the product. Where the indication states "traditionally used for ..." or similar wording, this information should be stated in advertising materials. Claims such as "clinically proven" or "effective in ..." are not acceptable for THMs since the registration is based exclusively on long-standing use. Claims that a product is "organic" may only be made for products that have been certified by an approved Certification Body as meeting organic standards applicable to the production of herbal medicines.

Special Requirements for Homeopathic Medicines

Advertising for homeopathic medicinal products is also subject to the requirements set out in this Guide. The MHRA has developed specific guidance for the advertising of homeopathic medicinal products. A copy of the guidance can be found at Appendix 2. There are two current licensing schemes under which homeopathic medicines may be licensed in the UK and the requirements for advertising are specific to the licensing scheme used.

For products granted a certificate of registration under Part 6 of the Regulations read with Schedule 10 (the Simplified Scheme), only the information specified on the labelling may be used in advertising. No mention of a specific indication may be made. For products granted a marketing authorisation under Part 5 of the Regulations (the National Rules Scheme), the indication is based upon UK homeopathic practitioners' traditional homeopathic use of the product, and product claims and advertising must be clearly set in the context of traditional homeopathic use. Advertising that implies that a product's efficacy is based on clinical trial data or the use of wording to imply that efficacy has been demonstrated, such as 'effective for' or 'works fast to relieve', is not acceptable.

Medicines Suitable for Advertising to the Public

Advertising to the public is permitted for medicines legally classified pharmacy sale (P) or General Sale List (GSL), subject to compliance with the Regulations. The Regulations prohibit the issue of any advertisement wholly or mainly directed to the general public which is likely to lead to the use of a prescription only medicine (POM). Government controlled vaccination campaigns that have been approved by Health Ministers are exempt from this prohibition.

The Cancer Act 1939 ("the Cancer Act") prohibits any advertisement to the public that contains an offer to treat any person for cancer, or to prescribe any remedy for its treatment, or to give any advice in connection with the treatment of the condition. The Cancer Act is administered and enforced by the Trading Standards Service. Medicines which contain psychotropic or narcotic substances cannot be advertised to the general public, with the exception of products listed in Schedule III to the Narcotic Drugs Convention 1961 as amended (Cm 2631, available from The Stationery Office) or exempted under paragraphs 2 and 3 of Article 3 of the Psychotropic Drugs Convention 1971 (Cm 7330) (those products containing narcotic or psychotropic substances in such quantities as to be exempt from the stringent controls of the Conventions).

Provision of Medical or Pharmaceutical Education, Goods and Services

Schemes which are launched by the pharmaceutical industry offering sponsorship of research posts, study visits and suchlike may well be acceptable provided that there is no element of promotion of individual products associated with them. The provision of goods or services to hospitals and health care units for the benefit of patients should not be dependent upon, or subject to, the prescription or supply of medicinal products and should not refer to them by name.

Disease Awareness and Health Education Campaigns

Campaigns relating to human health directed at the general public with a view to providing information, promoting awareness or educating the public about a particular condition or disease are encouraged. Care must be taken to ensure that the information provided does not make product claims for the material to remain outside the definition of an "advertisement" under the Regulations. In particular, use of brand names, restricting the range of treatments described in the campaign or drawing attention to the campaign by advertising which is likely to lead to the use of a specific prescription only medicine or medicines can all lead to a potential breach of the Regulations.

The MHRA has developed supplementary guidance to help ensure that information provided by pharmaceutical companies and others on health and disease does not fall within the advertising legislation by promoting prescription only medicinal products to the public, and to promote good practice.

Patient Support Materials

Companies may also provide non-promotional information to support patients who have been prescribed a particular medicine. This is sometimes required as part of a risk management plan. Any such programme should provide a demonstrable benefit to the patient. Materials are usually provided to health professionals to give to their patients.Support materials may include alert cards for patients to carry, leaflets about the disease and the treatment or additional advice on how to take the medicine, for example a video showing how the product is prepared and administered. The material should be factual and promotional claims must not be included. Consideration should always be given to whether this information can be included in the patient information leaflet which accompanies all medicines.

Copies of these materials may also be made available on a company internet site for reference purposes. If a website provides both information for the general public and copies of materials aimed at patients prescribed the product, the sections for each target audience should be clearly separated and clearly marked for the target audience. Adequate non-promotional information must be provided for general members of the public so that individuals do not need to access sections designed for patients unless they choose to seek further detailed information. Members of the public should not be encouraged to access information which is not intended for them.

MEDICINAL PLANTS : PREPRATION OF DRUGS

At present, the medicinal plants have been used as a basic raw material for the preparation of drugs in a number of traditional system including folk herbal tradition, Ayurvedic system, Unani system and Homeopathy as well as in the Modern or Allopathy System. Records of early Hindu civilization reveal that a considerable number of drugs used in modern medicine were in use even in the ancient times. Medicinal plants discovered by the traditional societies are proving to be an important source of potentially therapeutic drugs (Cox and Ballick, 1994). Worldwide, at least 122 prescribed drugs are based on substances found in plants (Rijal, 1997). Around 21,000 species of plants are reported to have medicinal uses around the world (Shrestha et. al., 2000). In Nepal, more than 700 species of medicinal plants used in traditional medicine practices were recorded in the past, and now 1403 species have been reported which represents about 20% of the total estimated flowering plants of Nepal (Tiwari, 1999). Most of the species are wild, while few are exotic, naturalized or cultivated since long.

Nepal is a multi---ethnic nation with diverse languages, religions and cultural traditions. There are more than 100 caste/ethnic groups speaking 92 languages and 124 dialects (CBS, 2001). The entire ethnic groups have their own culture, tradition and way of living. So, the traditional healing practices differ from one ethnic group to another, since it highly depends upon its culture, myths, rituals, economic and social costs, distance, convenience, time, traditional beliefs, fame of specific cures and like, and on knowledge regarding the utilization and availability of the plant resources of the surrounding areas. Even within the same ethnic group, the healing system differs from one district to another due to geographical, cultural, religious, and social differences. In the alpine and sub-alpine region, the traditional practice is highly influenced by Tibetan medicine because of common social, cultural, religion, language and ethnicity in Tibet and the northern religion of Nepal, and the healers are known as Amchis. While in the temperate region, the task is performed by Shamans (Traditional healers) known as Dhami-Jhankri, Guni-Ojha, or Janne in general, and in tropical region by healers known as Guruwa, Bharra and Gurau. (Rajbhandary, 2001).

There are many unexplored places in Nepal where people are still using the traditional method for healing purposes. The documentation and analysis of such knowledge is lagging, and thus such knowledge of local people is on the verge of extinction. So, there is an urgent need for the protection and revival of traditional medicinal knowledge and practices in the ethnic community that can be important means of providing affordable and sustainable health care. So, the present research works in an effort to document such knowledge in Magar ethnic community of Salija VDC of Parbat District.

Magars are the third most populated ethnic/caste group of Nepal comprising 7.1% of the total population (CBS, 2001). They are one of the aborigines of Nepal. The regions that the magar inhabits are the districts of Palpa, Gulmi, Argakhanchi, Syangja, Baglung, Parbat, Myagdi, Tanahun, Gorkha, Nawalparasi, Rupandehi in the western region, Rolpa, Rukum, Dolpa, Dailekh, Jajarkot, Pyuthan in the mid-western region, and Illam, Taplejung, Dhankuta, Sunsari, Sarlahi, Okhaldhunga in the eastern region.

Besides these areas, there are small pockets of Magars spread out in the region of the hot Terai, both east and west, and also in the hills and the areas around the Central Region of Nepal.. On the basis of language, customs and geographical distributions, the Magars are divided into Barha Magarant-Magar, Atha Magarant-Magar, High Mountain-Magar, Chhantyal and other Magars. However, these groups do not differ in their original traditions and their social affairs.

CONSISTS OF TRADITIONAL MEDICINE

Traditional medicine consists of those beliefs and practices relating to diseases which are products of indigenous cultural development and are not explicitly derived from the conceptual framework of the modern medicine (Mishra et. al., 2006).

Most of the times, the type, preparation, and uses of traditional medicines are largely influenced by folklore customs and the cultural habits, social practices, religious beliefs and superstitions of the people who prescribe or use them. Because of their origin in the remote past and the fact that most of them are still practiced almost in the same way as in the past maintaining the tradition, they are collectively called as traditional medicine.

It involves the use of both material and non-material components. The material components invariably comprise parts or organs of plants, animals and their products as well as minerals and other natural substances. The non-material components, which constitute important items of religious and spiritual medicines, include torture, magic, incantations, amulets and rituals like sacrifices, appeasement of evil spirits, etc. Diagnosis of diseases is based mainly on physical and psychological symptoms. Rural people preferred traditional medicine because of easy accessibility, low cost and cultural acceptability, elaborate patient-healer relationship, long term family association and friendly attitude of healers.

Skills and techniques on the traditional utilization of natural resources

Historically, Magar people inhabit the area near the forest, forest patches, and forest boundary, and they are more concentrated on the rural hilly areas of Nepal. So, they must have rich knowledge, skills and techniques on the traditional utilization of natural resources, especially the locally found plant species for traditional healing purposes, as the traditional medicine play a key role in the primary health care of rural people. However, there has not been serious attempt undertaken to properly document such traditional medicine. In addition, such traditional remedies are much less practiced in recent years, and are on the verge of extinction. It may be due to plants which are getting lost or becoming less available because of habitat destruction, deforestation, population growth, lack of conservation knowledge etc. or new generation do not care for it through affected by the modernization. It is, therefore, important that before the oral folklore about the use of plant and animal is lost forever, it must be preserved and properly documented, since such knowledge bear prospects for many valuable discoveries. Thus, the present study is initiated to document the plant and animal species used by the Magar communities for traditional healing purposes.

Rationale of the Site Selection

Salija VDC of Parbat district was the study site that was selected for the present research work that lies in the Western Development Region of Nepal.

Since the research work was focused on the investigation and documentation of indigenous knowledge and techniques on the use of medicinal plants in the Magar community, this area has been chosen for the study site as the area was important for the medicinal plant resources as well as remote from the city area with large percentage of Magars inhabitants (i.e. 61.94%) still using traditional herbal healing practices.

Nature and Sources of Data

The present research work was based on both the primary and secondary data. Primary data has been collected from the field study, and the secondary data from the relevant textbooks, research paper and publications, journals etc.

Sampling Method and Sample Size

By using purposive or judgement (non-probability) sampling method, the researcher selected the sample of 27 resource persons that includes local healers (*Dhami/Jhankri*), knowledgeable elder people, community leader, VDC chairperson, forest ranger, medicinal plant collectors, school teacher as well as youth and local people from the study area in order to fulfill the intended objectives of the present research work as well as to get the research questions answered.

PRIMARY DATA COLLECTION TECHNIQUES

Key Informant Interview

This method was used in order to obtain the detail information about the plants used in herbal medicine as well as to explore the local illness, and indigenous knowledge system and techniques on the utilization of medicinal plants for curing those diseases among the Magars of study area.

So, the interview was taken using checklist with the following key informants for the present research work:

Group Interview

Unstructured interview with small groups of people that comprises from youth, local people to elderly persons was conducted that helped to obtain the general information on various subjects like perception of local people, especially youth, on traditional medicine and modern medicine, sources of medicinal plants and their local condition, the problems faced by the traditional healers etc. that has supported to fulfill the intended objectives of present study.

Focus Group Discussion

Focus group discussion with 6-8 respondents was conducted during the research period that included local healers, elder people, forest ranger, community leader, school teacher, VDC chairperson and other knowledgeable people of the community.

Participant Observation

The study area was personally observed in order to understand its physical and cultural settings. The researcher also observed the events like preparation of herbal medicine, treatment of local patients etc. directly. Similarly, the actual condition of medicinal plants in the forests, the different sources and the local management practices of medicinal plants has been observed and recorded.

Informal Discussion

Informal discussions with local people like farmer, youths, elder persons as well as with knowledgeable people of the community has been helpful for obtaining the relevant and necessary information.

Specimen Collection

The medicinal plants used for traditional healing practices were collected from the study area for their identification and classification.

The plant specimens was collected and preserved as herbarium by standard a technique which was later identified in Kathmandu by the help of Botanist. The plants were taxonomically classified into division, family, genera and species.

MEDICINAL PLANT SPECIES

The major findings on the documentation of plant species used in traditional medicine by the local Magars of the Salija VDC, Parbat. It also discusses on the division and habit of recorded medicinal plant species as well as different plant parts used for the folk medicine. It is oragnized into several sub-headings i.e. Plant Species Used in Traditional Medicine, Diversity of the Medicinal Plants and Plant Parts Used.

Plant Species Used in Traditional Medicine

The present finding reveals that the Magar people of the study area have sound knowledge on the use of different medicinal plant species for their own local health care system. It was found that they make use of some 85 species of medicinal plants belonging to 52 families and 80 genera with 2 unidentified species for curing different ailments/diseases by using their own indigenous knowledge system.

Diversity of the Medicinal Plants

Among the total 85 medicinal plant species found to be used in the folk medicine in the study area, 63 species were Dicotyledon that comprises of 74.11% of total species, 13 species were Monocotyledon (15.29%), 2 species were Gymnosperm (5.88%), 5 species were Pteridophytes (2.33%), and 1 species was Lichene and Mycophyta comprising 1.17% each. Based on the life form of those species, 17 species were Trees, 11 species were Shrubs, 45 species were Herbs, 5 species were Climbers, 4 species were Ferns, and 1 species was Grass, Lichen and fungus each. So, herbs were the primary source of medicinal plants in terms of the number of species followed by trees (20%), shrubs (12.94%), climbers (5.88%), ferns (4.70%), and grass, lichen and fungus each comprising 1.17% of total species.

Plant Parts Used

Different plant parts such as roots, leaves, seeds, bark, rhizome, stem, bulb, flower, young shoots, thallus, latex and sporocarp were used either in the raw form or through processing to extract important drugs out of them in the folk medicine by the local Magars of the study area. In some cases, the whole plant including the root was utilized. The most frequently utilized plant part was the root (22 medical remedies) followed by the leaf (14 medical remedies) and seed (10 medical remedies). Similarly, the whole plant was used for 13 medical remedies.

INDIGENOUS KNOWLEDE ON MEDICINAL PLANTS

This chapter reports the different diseases or ailments treated by using the medicinal plants among the local Magars of study area. It also presents the detail on the indigenous knowledge of using such medicinal plants such as their mode of preparation, form of medication, route of administration as well as discusses on the present status of such knowledge in the study area. It is organized into several sub-headings i.e. Diseases/Ailments Treated, Forms of Medication, Route of Administration, Details on the Uses of Medicinal Plants and Status of Traditional Medicine in the Study Area.

Diseases/Ailments Treated

The recorded 85 medicinal plant species have been found to be used for the treatment of 49 different ailments/diseases by the local Magars of the study area by using their own indigenous knowledge system. Respiratory tract infections (fever, *kufat*, headache, sinusitis, cough/cold etc.), gastro-intestinal ailments (mouth ulcer, cholera, stomach pain, *ganogola*, indigestion, constipation, diarhea, dysentery, intestinal worm and gastric), skeleto-muscular problems (swelling, body pain, back pain, dislocated bone/fracture, rheumatism) and dermatological infections (scabies, skin disease, boils, herpes zoaster, *khatira*) were the most frequent ailments or diseases treated with the medicinal plants. The largest numbers of remedies i.e. 20.40% of all remedies were used to treat gastro-intestinal ailments by using 29 medicinal plant species. 12.24% remedies were used to cure respiratory tract infections using 20 plant species while 10.20% were used for skeleto-muscular problems and dermatological infections each using 12 and 11 medicinal herbs respectively. Similarly, 4.08% remedies were used for ENT problems such as tonsilitis, ear pain etc. using 3 medicinal plant species, and to a lesser extent for cuts and wound (8 species), overheat (6 species), garmi dhatu (3 species), skin burn (3 species), blood pressure (3 species), diabetes (2 species), *chetibeti lageko* (2 species), *begar pareko* (2 species), menstrual disorder (2 species), dental problem (4 species) and hair tonic, insomnia, lizard stings, dog bite *nasa chudeko, hilole Khako, galphudo, bikh pareko*, fish bone pricks and agalactia, each of them, by utilizing1 medicinal plant species.

Forms of Medication

The plant species used in the traditional medicine were used in different forms like juice, decoction, infusion, paste, powder, diluted drugs and smoke in the study area. Sometimes, the fresh or dried plant parts were used in their raw or natural form.

Mortar and pestle made of local stone were used for crushing, pounding and grinding the required plant parts or whole plants at home to extract important drugs out of them in required form. The crushed part of a plant was squeezed in a thin cloth to obtain the juice. Likewise, a paste was prepared by pounding the plant part with some water.

For a decoction, the plant parts or whole plants were boiled with water until the liquid was reduced to about half the amount. The dried medicinal plant part was grounded to obtain the powder. Infusion was prepared by soaking the plant parts in the water for certain duration, generally overnight. These forms of medication were diluted in water to form diluted drug.

The juice was the most used forms of medication that comprises of 33.05% of plant species followed by decoction (15.24%), paste (14.40%), raw (13.55%), powder (12.71%), infusion (5.08%), diluted drug (4.23%) and smoke (1.69%), the least used form.

Route of Administration

Medical administration included inhalation, instillation, oral absorbtion which are internal medication, and poultice/applying and rubbing/massage which are external medication. Most of the medication were administrated orally (32 remedies) and poultice/applying (17 remedies) followed by massage (4 remedies), inhalation (3 remedies) and instillation (1 remedies).

Status of Traditional Medicine in the Study Area

The present findings reveal that almost all the people of study area have little or more knowledge on the medicinal properties of plant species and their uses. However, local healers (Dhami/Jhankri) were the most popular one in the village for practicing the folk medicine. The investigation reveals that there were some 15-20 local healers in the study area, some were still active, some very old and some were new learners. Besides them, the other knowledgeable groups, like women and elders, also practice home remedy.

According to the local healers of the study area, they acquired the knowledge about the medicinal uses of plant species from their Guru (God) who taught them in their dream. Also during *Jhankri basne* period, the healer identify the illness of their patient, and treat them accordingly by giving local drug extracted from the plants, and also involves rituals such as incantations, amulets, magic, sacrifices, charms, religious verses etc. Besides Dhami/Jhankri, the other knowledgeable groups learned about the uses of medicinal plant species from those family members who practiced such healing system in the past as well as from other knowledgeable groups.

Generally, the patients were examined in the morning or evening in particular days like Tuesday, Saturday and others that depend on healers. The healers both visit the patients' house and even stay at night if necessary or the patient comes to the healers. Food grains, local brewed alcohol, vegetables, chicken etc. were some items of fees paid to the healers. Money was paid only by few patients. Thus the treatment was affordable and easily available to the local people.

Some of the local healers were reluctant in sharing their knowledge about medicinal plants and their properties. They strongly believe that, if such knowledge is shared then their guru gets angry, and they will lose their knowledge forever which was the punishment for them. They told that, if they disclose about the medicinal plants and their properties, then their healing properties would be lost. Even if the incantations and charms are taught to other, they become invalid. However, other healers and knowledgeable people don't believe such things, and they freely shared their knowledge.

The traditional home remedy was much less practiced now in comparison to the past few years in the study area. The study revealed that some of the local people prefer the facility of Health Post, located at the Salija village, and go for the modern medicine instead of going to local healers, especially those who are exposed to outside world or who are rich enough to afford allopathic medicine. But still some prefer *Dhami/Jhankri* system at first hand, and only if it doesn't work go for other alternatives. So most of the people use both the traditional healing system and allopathic system simultaneously, first traditional medicine and then allopathic system or vice-versa. The local healers also recommend their patients to the hospital when the case is not in their hand. However, simple common ailments like cough and cold, cut and wound, low fever etc. were treated at home by the villagers themselves. It was found that local people have not fully depended upon the modern medicine for the primary health care services.

Some of the folk remedies in the study area include the use of plant and animal species in combination. For example, for the treatment of back pain *Anethum sowa, Lepidium sativum, Bergenia ciliata* and *Curcuma caesia* was used together with *Anadenus sps.* Similarly, honey of *Apis cerana* was mixed with the juice of *Amomum zingiber* to cure cough. The paste made from the shit of *Rattus rattus* and young shoot of *Urtica doica* was used in the wound of dog bite. The mixture of honey of *Apis cerana,* blood of *Gallusgallus domesticus* or *Capra hircus,* juice of *Citrus aurantifolia* and powder of *Curcuma longa* was used for the treatment of menstrual disorder.

The medicinal plant species reported to have folk medical utility in the present study area are also supported by the findings of other researchers. For example, the flower of *Woodfordia fruticosa* was reported to be used in curing dysentery in the present study. Manandhar (1990), Acharya (1996), Manandhar (1992), Karki (2001) and Oli et.al., (2005) also reported similar use in their study. But Manandhar (1998) reported the use of its bark to treat boils on the tongue and to relieve angular stomatitis, Joshi et.al., (2000) reported to treat scabies and vomiting, and Gurung (2002) reported its use in diarrhoea. *Berberis asiatica* and *Mahonia napaulensis* was used for opthalmological uses in the present study which was supported by the study of Subedi (1998), Karki (2001), Gurung (2002) and Shrestha et.al., (2003) while Joshi et.al., (2000) reported the use of *Berberis asiatica* for muscular pain and blood purification. The use of *Rhododendron arboreum* for fish bone prick and dysentery in the present study is similar to the study of Subedi (1998), Karki (2001), Gurung (2002) and Shrestha et.al., (2003). The root of *Potentilla fulgens* was reported to be used in dental problem in the present study similar to the study conducted by Manandhar (1995), Subedi (1998) and Joshi et.al., (2000), while Rai (2003) reported its use in diarrhoea and gastric trouble. Subedi (1998), Karki (2001), Gurung (2002) and Rai (2003) reported the use of *Lyonia ovalifolia* for curing skin diseases like scabies similar to the present findings. Similarly, the root, fruit and young shoot of *Rubus ellipticus* was used for curing gastric, fever, kufat and cough in the present study. Subedi (1998), Karki (2001), Gurung (2002), Rai (2003) and Shrestha et.al., (2003) also reported its similar use in their research. Joshi et.al., (2003) reported the similar use of *Ageratina adenophora, Myrica esculenta, Acorus calamus, Rhus semialata, Drymaria cordata, Cuscuta reflexa* var *reflexa, Asparagus racemosus, Fragaria nubicola, Zanthozylum armatum* and *Solanum capsicoides* as in the present study for the treatment of cuts and wounds, rheumatism, cough and cold, dysentery, sinusitis, jaundice, agalactia, tonsilitis, stomach disorder and dental problem respectively.

ORGANIZATION SYSTEM OF MEDICINAL PLANTS

The study area was very rich in medicinal plants resources. About 120 medicinal plants were identified from different sources like forest, home garden, cropland, and village periphery. The villagers were quite aware about the importance of the medicinal plant species, and have been actively involve in their management and conservation.

There was a separate nursery of medicinal plant species, along with the nursery of tree species, managed by the local people where important medicinal plant species like Sugandhawal, Raklamol, Bajradanti, Pakhanved, Butkesh, Jethimadhu, Chiraito, Padamchalnu etc. was grown. These medicinal plants were later cultivated in the community forest of the village. Some of the villagers even bought these species in order to cultivate them at their home garden or cropland.

Among the 10 community forest in the VDC, two of them namely, Hampal Community Forest and Juddhabir Community Forest have been identified by the villagers to be rich in medicinal plant resources. So, the grazing on such area has been stopped, and sometimes only limited grazing has been allowed. The forest ranger and some villagers carried out periodic patrolling of these forests in order to avoid the illegal harvesting of medicinal plants.

Some of the villagers were planting or cultivating the demanded medicinal plant species in their home garden and cropland for their local use. Some were even actively involved in harvesting of those medicinal plants from cultivated area, make ayurvedic medicine and supply to other places, even to India. Only the organic manure was used in the cultivated area with periodic weeding, and mostly the cultivation was done in wet areas.

Local healers and the knowledgeable groups were the one who mostly make the use of medicinal plant species for folk remedy. These groups have their own collection guidelines that, directly or indirectly, contribute in the sustainable use of plant species. They collect the medicinal plants only when needed in certain days like Sunday, Tuesday and full moon day. Some of healers believed that the medicinal plants of nearby home will not work as, according to them, the plants were unpurified by domestic animals, people etc. and that the plants lost their healing properties. Thus, the forest becomes the main source of medicinal plants for them. But other practitioners collect them from any area that is accessible and abundant.

Certain guidelines for collecting medicinal plants were followed by the collectors, which help in the sustainable use of those species. For e.g. when the roots or rhizome of plants has to be collected, then only the required amounts was collected, and keep some of them in their original places for their regeneration. Thus, only the needed parts and amount of medicinal plants were collected that ultimately contribute in their sustainability and proper management.

3

Ayurvedic Medicine

Ayurveda Ayurvedic medicine is a system of traditional medicine native to the Indian subcontinent and practiced in other parts of the world as a form of alternative medicine. In Sanskrit, the word *ayurveda* consists of the words *âyus*, meaning "longevity", and *veda*, meaning "related to knowledge" or "science". Evolving throughout its history, ayurveda remains an influential system of medicine in South Asia. The earliest literature on Indian medical practice appeared during the Vedic period in India. The *Sucœruta Sanhitâ* and the *Charaka Sanhitâ* were influential works on traditional medicine during this era. Over the following centuries, Ayurvedic practitioners developed a number of medicinal preparations and surgical procedures for the treatment of various ailments and diseases.

In Western medicine, Ayurveda is classified as a system of complementary and alternative medicine (CAM) that is used to complement, rather than replace, the treatment regimen and relationship that exists between a patient and their existing physician.

Overview

Ayurveda is grounded in a metaphysics of the "five great elements"—all of which compose the Universe, including the human body. Chyle or plasma (called *rasa dhatu*), blood (*rakta dhatu*), flesh (*mamsa dhatu*), fat (*medha dhatu*), bone (*asthi dhatu*), marrow (*majja dhatu*), and semen or female reproductive tissue (*shukra dhatu*) are held to be the seven primary constituent elements—saptadhatu of the body. Ayurveda deals elaborately with measures of healthful living during the entire span of life and its various phases. Ayurveda stresses a balance of three elemental energies or humors: *vata* (air & space – "wind"), *pitta* (fire & water– "bile") and *kapha* (water & earth – "phlegm"). According to ayurveda, these three regulatory principles— *Doshas* —are important for health, because when they are in balanced state, the body is healthy, and when imbalanced, the body has diseases. Ayurveda holds that each human possesses a unique combination of *Doshas*. In ayurveda, the human body perceives attributes of experiences as 20 *Guna*. Surgery and surgical instruments are employed. It is believed that building a healthy metabolic system, attaining good digestion, and proper excretion leads to vitality. Ayurveda also focuses on exercise, yoga, meditation, and massage. Thus, body, mind, and spirit/ consciousness need to be addressed both individually and in unison for health to ensue.

The practice of *Panchakarma* is believed to eliminate toxic elements from the body. Eight disciplines of ayurveda treatment, called *ashtangas*, are given below:

- Internal medicine (*Kaaya-chikitsa*)
- Paediatrics (*Kaumarabhrtyam*)
- Surgery (*Shalya-chikitsa*)
- Eye and ENT (Shalakya tantra)
- Demonic possession (*Bhuta vidya*) : *Bhuta vidya* has been called psychiatry.
- Toxicology (*Agadatantram*)
- Prevention diseases and improving immunity and rejuvenation (*rasayana*)
- Aphrodisiacs and improving health of progeny (*Vajikaranam*)

In Hindu mythology, the origin of Ayurveda medicine is attributed to the physician of the gods, Dhanvantari.

PRACTICES OF AYURVEDIC MEDICINE

Balance

Hinduism and Buddhism have been an influence on the development of many of ayurveda's central ideas — particularly its fascination with balance, known in Buddhism as *Mâdhyamaka*. Balance is emphasized; suppressing natural urges is seen to be unhealthy, and doing so may almost certainly lead to illness. However, people are cautioned to stay within the limits of reasonable balance and measure. For example, emphasis is placed on moderation of food intake, sleep, sexual intercourse, and the intake of medicine.

Diagnosis

The *Charaka Samhita* recommends a tenfold examination of the patient. The qualities to be judged are:

- constitution
- abnormality
- essence

- stability
- body measurements
- diet suitability
- psychic strength
- digestive capacity
- physical fitness
- age.

In addition, Chopra (2003) identifies five influential criteria for diagnosis:

- origin of the disease
- prodrominal (precursory) symptoms
- typical symptoms of the fully developed disease
- observing the effect of therapeutic procedures
- the pathological process'.

Ayurvedic practitioners approach diagnosis by using all five senses. Hearing is used to observe the condition of breathing and speech. The study of the vital pressure points or *marma* is of special importance.

Hygiene

Hygiene is an Indian cultural value and a central practice of Ayurvedic medicine. Hygienic living involves regular bathing, cleansing of teeth, skin care, and eye washing. Occasional anointing of the body with oil is also prescribed.

Treatments

Ayurveda stresses the use of plant-based medicines and treatments. Hundreds of plant-based medicines are employed, including cardamom and cinnamon. Some animal products may also be used, for example milk, bones, and gallstones. In addition, fats are used both for consumption and for external use. Minerals, including sulfur, arsenic, lead, copper sulfate and gold are also consumed as prescribed. This practice of adding minerals to herbal medicine is known as *rasa shastra*.

In some cases, alcohol is used as a narcotic for the patient undergoing an operation. The advent of Islam introduced opium as a narcotic. Both oil and tar are used to stop bleeding. Traumatic bleeding is said to be stopped by four different methods ligation of the blood vessel; cauterisation by heat; using different herbal or animal preparations locally which facilitate clotting; and different medical preparations which constrict the bleeding or oozing vessels. Different oils may be used in a number of ways including regular consumption as a part of food, anointing, smearing, *head massage*, and prescribed application to infected areas.

Shrotas

Ensuring the proper functions of channels (shrotas) that transport fluids from one point to another is a vital goal of Ayurvedic medicine, because the lack of healthy shrotas is thought to cause rheumatism, epilepsy, paralysis, convulsions, and insanity. Practitioners induce sweating and prescribe steam-based treatments as a means to open up the channels and dilute the Doshas that cause the blockages and lead to disease.

History

Around 1500 BC, ayurveda's fundamental and applied principles got organised and enunciated. Ayurveda traces its origins to the Vedas, *Atharvaveda* in particular, and is connected to Hindu religion. *Atharvaveda* (one of the four most ancient books of Indian knowledge, wisdom and culture) contains 114 hymns or formulations for the treatment of diseases. Ayurveda originated in and developed from these hymns. In this sense, ayurveda is considered by some to have divine origin. Indian medicine has a long history, and is one of the oldest organised systems of medicine. Its earliest concepts are set out in the sacred writings called the Vedas, especially in the metrical passages of the Atharvaveda, which may possibly date as far back as the 2nd millennium BC. According to a later writer, the system of medicine was received by a man named Dhanvantari from Brahma, and Dhanvantari was deified as the god of medicine. In later times his status was gradually reduced, until he was credited with having been an earthly king. The *Sushruta Samhita* of Sushruta appeared during the 1st millennium BC. Dwivedi & Dwivedi (2007) – on the work of the surgeon Sushruta – write:

"The main vehicle of the transmission of knowledge during that period was by oral method. The language used was Sanskrit — the vedic language of that period (2000–500 BC). The most authentic compilation of his teachings and work is presently available in a treatise called *Sushruta Samhita*. This contains 184 chapters and description of 1, 120 illnesses, 700 medicinal plants, 64 preparations from mineral sources and 57 preparations based on animal sources. "

Underwood & Rhodes (2008) hold that this early phase of traditional Indian medicine identified 'fever (takman), cough, consumption, diarrhea, dropsy, abscesses, seizures, tumours, and skin diseases (including leprosy)'. Treatment of complex ailments, including angina pectoris, diabetes, hypertension, and stones, also ensued during this period. Plastic surgery, cataract surgery, puncturing to release fluids in the abdomen, extraction of foreign elements, treatment of anal fistulas, treating fractures, amputations, cesarean sections, and stitching of wounds were known. The use of herbs and surgical instruments became widespread. The *Charaka Samhita* text is arguably the principal classic reference. It gives emphasis to the triune nature of each person: body care, mental regulation, and spiritual/consciousness refinement.

Other early works of ayurveda include the *Charaka Samhita*, attributed to Charaka. The earliest surviving excavated written material which contains the works of Sushruta is the *Bower Manuscript*, dated to the 4th century AD. The Bower manuscript quotes directly from Sushruta and is of special interest to historians due to the presence of Indian medicine and its concepts in Central Asia. Vagbhata, the son of a senior doctor by the name of Simhagupta, also compiled his works on traditional medicine. Early ayurveda had a school of physicians and a school of surgeons. Tradition holds that the text *Agnivesh tantra*, written by the sage Agnivesh, a student of the sage Bharadwaja, influenced the writings of ayurveda.

The Chinese pilgrim Fa Hsien (ca. 337–422 AD) wrote about the health care system of the Gupta empire (320–550) and described the institutional approach of Indian medicine, also visible in the works of Charaka, who mentions a clinic and how it should be equipped. Madhava (fl. 700), Sarngadhara (fl. 1300), and Bhavamisra (fl. 1500) compiled works on Indian medicine. The medical works of both Sushruta and Charaka were translated into the Arabic language during the Abbasid Caliphate (ca. 750). These Arabic works made their way into Europe via intermediaries. In Italy, the Branca family of Sicily and Gaspare Tagliacozzi (Bologna) became familiar with the techniques of Sushruta. British physicians traveled to India to see rhinoplasty being performed by native methods. Reports on Indian rhinoplasty were published in the *Gentleman's Magazine* in 1794. Joseph Constantine Carpue spent 20 years in India studying local plastic surgery methods. Carpue was able to perform the first major surgery in the western world in 1815. Instruments described in the *Sushruta Samhita* were further modified in the Western World.

CURRENT STATUS OF AYURVEDIC MEDICINE

Within India

In 1970, the Indian Medical Central Council Act which aims to standardize qualifications for ayurveda and provide accredited institutions for its study and research was passed by the Parliament of India. In India, over 100 colleges offer degrees in traditional ayurvedic medicine. The Indian government supports research and teaching in ayurveda through many channels at both the national and state levels, and helps institutionalize traditional medicine so that it can be studied in major towns and cities. The state-sponsored Central Council for Research in Ayurveda and Siddha (CCRAS) is the premier institution for promotion of traditional medicine in India. The studies conducted by this institution encompass clinical, drug, literary, and family welfare research. To fight biopiracy and unethical patents, the Government of India, in 2001, set up the Traditional Knowledge Digital Library as repository of 1200 formulations of various systems of Indian medicine, such as Ayurveda, Unani and Siddha. The library also has 50 traditional Ayurveda books digitized and available online.

Central Council of Indian Medicine (CCIM) a statutory body established in 1971, under Department of Ayurveda, Yoga and Naturopathy, Unani, Siddha and Homoeopathy (AYUSH), Ministry of Health and Family Welfare, Government of India, monitors higher education in Ayurveda. The Bachelor of Ayurveda, Medicine and Surgery (BAMS) degree is the basic five-and-a-half year course of graduation. It includes eighteen different subjects comprising courses on anatomy with cadaver dissections, physiology, pharmacology, pathology, modern clinical medicine & clinical surgery, pediatrics, along with subjects on ayurveda like *Charaka Samhita*, history and evolution of ayurveda, identification and usage of herbs (*dravyaguna*), and ayurvedic philosophy in diagnostics and treatment. Many clinics in urban and rural areas are run by professionals who qualify from these institutes. Mukherjee & Wahile cite World Health Organization statistics to demonstrate the popularity of traditional medicine as the primary system of health care.

Outside India

Academic institutions related to traditional medicine in India have contributed to ayurveda's international visibility. Kurup (2003) comments on the role of Gujarat Ayurved University:

Several international and national initiatives have been formed to legitimize the practice of Ayurvedic medicine as CAM in countries outside India:

- WHO policy of traditional medicine practice
- The US National Centre for Complementary and Alternative Medicine
- The National Ayurvedic Medical Association
- The European Federation for Complementary and Alternative Medicine
- The European Ayurveda Association

In 2009, the United States of America National Centre for Complementary and Alternative Medicine (NCCAM) of the National Institutes of Health expended $1. 2 million of its $123 million annual budget on ayurvedic medicine-related research.

Due to different laws and medical regulations in the rest of the world, the unregulated practice and commercialization of Ayurvedic medicine has raised ethical and legal issues; in some cases, this damages the reputation of Ayurvedic medicine outside India.

Journals

A variety of peer reviewed journals focus on the topic of ayurvedic medicine:

- Ancient Science of Life
- Theoretical and Experimental Journal of Ayurveda and Siddha
- Journal of Research & Education in Indian Medicine (*JREIM),*
- AYU
- The International Journal for Ayurveda Research.

None of the journals except IJAR are PubMed indexed. The first subspeciality journal for the field of Ayurvedic medicine was launched in July 2010. It's focus is rheumatology and it is titled the Journal of Clinical Rheumatology in Ayurveda.

Patents

In December 1993, the University of Mississippi Medical Centre had a patent issued to them by United States Patent and Trademark Office on the use of turmeric for healing.

The patent was contested by India's industrial research organization, Council for Scientific and Industrial Research (CSIR), on the grounds that traditional ayurvedic practitioners were already aware of the healing properties of the substance for centuries, and that this prior art made the patent a case of bio-piracy. The Government of India had become involved in promoting traditional medicine by 1997. R A Mashelkar, director-general of the Indian Council of Scientific and Industrial Research, made the following observation: "This is a significant development of far-reaching consequences for the protection of the traditional knowledge base in the public domain, which has been an emotional issue for not only the people of India but also for the other third world countries."

Scientific Evidence

As a traditional medicine, many ayurveda products have not been tested in rigorous scientific studies and clinical trials. In India, research in ayurveda is largely undertaken by the statutory body of the Central Government, the Central Council for Research in Ayurveda and Siddha (CCRAS), through a national network of research institutes.

A systematic review of ayurveda treatments for rheumatoid arthritis concluded that there was insufficient evidence, as most of the trials were not done properly, and the one high-quality trial showed no benefits.

A review of ayurveda and cardiovascular disease concluded that while the herbal evidence is not yet convincing, the spices are appropriate, some herbs are promising, and yoga is also a promising complementary treatment.

Some ayurvedic products, mainly herbs used for phytotherapy, have been tested with promising results. Studies suggest that Turmeric and its derivative curcumin are antioxidants. *Tinspora cordifolia* has been tested.

Among the medhya *rasayanas* (intellect rejuvenation), two varieties of *Salvia* have been tested in small trials; one trial provided evidence that *Salvia lavandulifolia* (Spanish sage) may improve word recall in young adults, and another provided evidence that *Salvia officinalis* (Common sage) may improve symptoms in Alzheimer's patients.

In some cases, ayurvedic medicine may provide clues to therapeutic compounds. For example, derivatives of snake venom have various therapeutic properties. Many plants used as *rasayana* (rejuvenation) medications are potent antioxidants. Neem appears to have beneficial pharmacological properties.

Mitra & Rangesh (2003) hold that cardamom and cinnamon stimulate digestive enzymes that break down polymeric macromolecules in the human body. Research suggests that *T. arjuna* is useful in alleviating the of angina pectoris and in treating heart failure and coronary artery disease. *T. arjuna* may also be useful in treating hypercholesterolemia.

Safety

Rasa shastra, *the practice of adding metals, minerals or gems to herbs, is a source of toxic heavy metals such as lead, mercury and arsenic. Adverse reactions to herbs due to their pharmacology are described in traditional ayurvedic texts, but ayurvedic practitioners are reluctant to admit that herbs could be toxic and the reliable information on herbal toxicity is not readily available.*

A 2004 study found such toxic metals in 20% of ayurvedic preparations that were made in South Asia for sale around Boston and extrapolated the data to the United States more broadly. It concluded that excess consumption of these products could cause health risks. A 2008 study of more than 230 products found that approximately 20% of remedies (and 40% of *rasa shastra* medicines) purchased over the Internet from both US and Indian suppliers contained lead, mercury or arsenic.

Traditionally the toxicity of these materials are believed to be reduced through purification processes such as *samskaras* or *shodhanas* (for metals), which is similar to the Chinese *pao zhi*, although the ayurvedic technique is more complex and may involve prayers as well as physical pharmacy techniques. One medical journal reported:

"Crude aconite is an extremely lethal substance, yet ayurveda looks upon it as a therapeutic entity. Crude aconite is always processed, i.e. it undergoes 'samskaras' before being utilised in the Ayurvedic formulations. This study was undertaken in mice, to ascertain whether "processed" aconite is less toxic as compared to the crude or unprocessed one. It was seen that crude aconite was significantly toxic to mice (100% mortality at a dose of 2. 6 mg/mouse) whereas the fully processed aconite was absolutely non-toxic (no mortality at a dose even 8 times as high as that of crude aconite). Further, all the steps in the processing were essential for complete detoxification. "

Following concerns about metal toxicity, the Government of India ruled that ayurvedic products must specify their metallic content directly on the labels of the product. The harmful effects of the samples is attributed in part to the adulterated raw material and lack of workers trained in traditional medicine. In a letter to the Indian Academy of Sciences, director of the Interdisciplinary School of Health Sciences, University of Pune Patwardhan Bhushan stated that the metal adulteration is due to contamination and carelessness during the much faster modern manufacturing processes, and does not occur with traditional methods of preparation.

METHOD OF AYURVEDIC MEDICINE

Ayurveda has, for several years, exalted the virtues of the vegetarian diet emphasizing on the benefits of green leafy vegetables. Although greens, like spinach have gained universal acceptance through the vastly popular Popeye, they have always been part of the staple diet recommended by Ayurvedic physicians. Greens are rich in fibre and antioxidants and contain natural pigments like lutein that keep several diseases, such as macular degeneration, at bay. Ayurveda recommends that greens be included as part of every individual's daily diet to cure diseases and to keep them at bay.

The Ayurvedic method of cooking these vegetables is simple and easy to digest. Separate the edible leaves from the weeds and grass. Wash well. Chop and cook by adding ghee and a small amount of rock salt. Add a pinch of pepper powder for taste. Cook for 5–7 minutes only. If the leaves lack taste or have a bitter, astringent taste, cooked green gram (peeled) may be added towards the end and mixed well. Adding coconut to the greens makes them heavy to digest. It may be added only when the person has very good digestion (Agni).

The methods of preparing the following green leaves is detailed below-

Drumstick Leaves

Indications:

- Balances all the three doshas (Tridosha)
- Relieves:

- Loss of appetite
- Internal body heat
- Heat of head
- Giddiness
- Eye diseases

- It is an aphrodisiac
- Relieves constipation
- Helps in downward movement of air and faeces

Preparation:

Ingredients:

Drumstick Leaves – 2 bunches

Mung dhal – 1

Mustard – 1 tsp

Asafoetida – 1 pinch

Cumin seeds – 1 tsp

Ghee – 2 tsp

Rock salt – according to taste

Method

Separate the leaves, wash and chop them. Cook mung dhal well in water. When mung dhal is fully cooked, add the chopped leaves and cook for few minutes till the leaves become tender. Season it with asafoetida, mustard and cumin seeds fried in ghee.

Hummingbird Tree Leaves

Indications:

- Balances pitta and kapha
- Bitter in taste
- Has to be taken occasionally
- It is not advised during medication as it has the potency to reduce the power of medicine
- Antidote for poisons
- It is cooling
- Good for fever
- It is a laxative
- Helps in digestion
- It is a tonic
- Cures insanity
- It is a considered as a satvic food

Preparation
Ingredients:
Hummingbird Tree Leaves – 2 bunches
Mung dhal – 1 spoon
Mustard – 1 tsp
Asafoetida – 1 pinch
Cumin seeds – 1 tsp
Red chilly – 1
Ghee – 2 tsp
Grated coconut – 3 spoons full
Rock salt – according to taste.

Method

Add ghee in a deep pan and heat. Season mustard, asafetida, cumin seeds and red chilly. Now add the chopped leaves and mung dhal. Add little rock salt. Stir occasionally and cook till done. Finally add grated coconut and mix well.

Radish Leaves

Indications:

- Balances kapha
- Relives tumours
- It is an aphrodisiac
- Helps in elimination of urine
- It is a laxative
- Relieves flatulence
- Strengthens the stomach
- It is a stimulant
- It is antiscorbutic - Relieves scurvy

It is suggested in the treatment of-

- Stomach disorders
- Piles
- Urinary disorders
- Syphilis
- Lung diseases
- Jaundice
- Rheumatism
- Difficulty in urination
- Anemia

- Scurvy
- Tuberculosis
- It causes burning sensation in chest.

Preparation

Ingredients:

Radish Leaves – 2 bunches

Mung dhal – 1

Mustard – 1 tsp

Asafoetida – 1 pinch

Cumin seeds – 1 tsp

Ghee – 2 tsp

Rock salt - according to taste.

Method

Separate the leaves. Wash and chop them. Cook the mung dhal well in water. When mung dhal is cooked, add the chopped leaves and cook for few more minutes till the leaves become tender. Season with asafetida, mustard and cumin, using ghee.

Spinach

Indications:

- Balances vata and pitta
- Increases Kapha
- Very tasty
- Aphrodisiac
- Reduces excessive thirst
- Reduces burning sensation and heat
- It is a laxative
- It is soothing and bland – demulcent Reduces inflammation
- It is cooling - refrigerant
- Reduces fever
- It is a diuretic
- Suggested in the treatment of

— Dropsy

— Venereal diseases

— Urinary diseases

— Dandruff

Preparation

Ingredients:

Spinach – 2 bunches Mung dhal – 1
Mustard – 1 tsp
Asafoetida – 1 pinch
Cumin seeds – 1 tsp
Ghee – 2 tsp
Rock salt - according to taste.

Method

Separate the leaves. Wash and chop them. Cook the mung dhal well in water. When mung dhal is fully cooked, add the chopped leaves and cook for few minutes till the leaves become tender. Season with asafoetida, mustard and cumin seeds using ghee.

Indian Spinach

Indications:

- Balances all the three doshas (Tridosha)
- Soothing and bland
- Allays irritation and inflammation
- It is cooling
- It is a diuretic and a laxative
- Used in treatment of

— Dropsy
— Gonorrhea
— Catarrh
— Urinary disorders
— Stomach troubles
— Difficulty in urination
— Burning sensation
— Leucorrhoea
— Anorexia
— Vomiting
— Diabetes.

Preparation

Ingredients:
Indian Spinach – 2 bunches
Mung dhal – 1
Mustard – 1 tsp
Asafoetida – 1 pinch

Cumin seeds – 1 tsp
Ghee – 2 tsp
Rock salt – according to taste.

Method

Separate the leaves. Wash and chop them. Cook the mung dhal well in water. Add the chopped leaves to the cooked mung dhal, along with a little rock salt and cook for a few minutes, till the leaves become tender. Season with asafoetida, mustard and cumin seeds using ghee.

Mint Leaves

Indications:

- Balances vata and kapha
- It is a good appetizer
- Causes contraction on skin application and reduces swelling
- It is cooling - refrigerant
- Strengthens the stomach
- It is a diuretic
- It is a stimulant
- Relieves flatulence - carminative
- Relieves spasms
- It is an aphrodisiac
- Restores the normal tone of tissues - tonic
- Promotes the oral ejection of mucus by spitting (Expectorant)
- Found to be effective in the treatment of

— Digestive disorders
— Liver disorders
— Gall bladder disorders
— Anorexia
— Vomiting
— Poor digestion (manda Agni)
— Bleeding diseases
— Diarrhea.

Preparation

Ingredients:
Mint leaves – 2 bunches
Black gram (urud dal) – 3 spoons full
Ginger – 1 small piece
Ghee – 10 ml

Pepper – 1
Rock salt – according to taste.

Method

It is usually prepared as chutney. Separate the leaves. Wash and sauté them in ghee for two minutes. Along with sautéed black gram, ginger, rock salt, and pepper, put it into a mixer and grind it into a smooth paste. The chutney is now ready.

Little Hogweed Leaves

Indications:

- Reduces Pitta
- Increases the secretion of breast milk
- It strengthens the stomach
- It is a refrigerant, a tonic and a diuretic It is soothing and bland
- Allays irritation and inflammation (Demulcent)
- Smoothens and protects the mucus membranes
- Gradually induces change and restores healthy functions without evacuations.
- Used in the treatment of -

— Urinary disorders
— Bleeding disorders
— Gonorrhea
— Bitta diseases
— Dysentery
— Body heat

Preparation

Ingredients:
Hogweed leaves – 2 bunches
Mung dhal – 1
Mustard – 1 tsp
Asafoetida – 1 pinch
Cumin seeds – 1 tsp
Ghee – 2 tsp
Rock salt – according to taste.

Method

Separate the leaves. Wash and chop them. Cook the mung dhal well in water. When mung dhal is cooked, add the chopped leaves, add little rock salt and cook for few minutes till the leaves become tender. Season with asafoetida, mustard and cumin seeds using ghee.

Amaranthus

Indications:

- Reduces vata and pitta
- Good for children, adult and the aged
- It is very tasty and is an appetizer
- Relieves cough and fever
- The white and red varieties have similar properties.

Preparation

Ingredients:
Amaranthus leaves – 1 bunch
Ghee – 10 ml
Urud dal – 1 spoon full
Mustard – 1tsp
Pepper powder – 1 pinch
Asafoetida – 1 pinch
Rock salt – 1 pinch.

Method

Separate the leaves from the weeds and grass. Wash it well. Chop it and cook using very little rock salt.

Add a pinch of pepper powder for taste. Cook for 5-7 minutes only.

Season with asafoetida, mustard, urud dal and cumin seeds using ghee.

Green Amaranthus

Indications:

- Balances vata and pitta
- Improves Agni (Digestive power)
- Helps in making gold bhasma (gold powder).

Preparation

Ingredients:
Green Amaranth leaves – 1 bunch
Ghee – 10 ml
Urud dal – 1 spoon full
Mustard – 1tsp
Pepper powder – 1 pinch

Asafoetida – 1 pinch
Rock salt – 1 pinch

Method

Separate the leaves from the weeds and grass. Wash it well. Chop it and cook using very little rock salt. Add a pinch of pepper powder for taste.

Cook for 5-7 minutes only. Season with asafoetida, mustard, urud dal and cumin seeds using ghee.

Tropical Amaranth

Indications:

- Balances vata and kapha
- Leaves are slightly sweet in taste
- Improves beauty
- Tender leaves are to be used
- Effective antidote against drug poison
- It is very effective in the treatments of-

— Eye diseases
— Cough
— Catarrh
— Ulcers
— Difficulty in urination
— Swelling
— Poisoning

Preparation

Ingredients:
Tropical Amaranth leaves – 1 bunch
Ghee – 10 ml
Urad dal – 1 spoon full
Mustard – 1tsp
Pepper powder – 1 pinch
Asafoetida – 1 pinch
Rock salt – 1 pinch

Method

Separate the leaves from the weeds and grass. Wash it well. Chop it and cook using very little rock salt. Add a pinch of pepper powder for taste. Cook for 5-7 minutes only. Season with asafoetida, mustard, urad dal and cumin using ghee.

Spleen Amaranth

Indications:

- Pacifies the 3 Doshas (tridoshas)
- It is a stimulant and an aphrodisiac
- Strengthens the tissues (Dhatu) of the body
- It is a rejuvenator (rasayana)
- Useful in the treatment of

— Fevers
— Cough
— Rheumatism
— Paralysis
— Tremors
— Kapha and Vata disorders
— Many other diseases.

Preparation

Ingredients:
Spleen Amaranth leaves – 1 bunch
Ghee – 10 ml
Urud dal – 1 spoon full
Mustard – 1tsp
Pepper powder – 1 pinch
Asafoetida – 1 pinch
Rock salt – 1 pinch

Method

Separate the leaves from the weeds and grass. Wash it well. Chop and cook it using very little rock salt. Add a pinch of pepper powder for taste. Cook for 5-7 minutes only. Season with asafoetida, mustard, urud dal and cumin seeds using ghee.

Spleen Amaranth

Indications:

- Pacifies the 3 Doshas (tridoshas)
- It is a stimulant and an aphrodisiac
- Strengthens the tissues (Dhatu) of the body
- It is a rejuvenator (rasayana)
- Useful in the treatment of

— Fevers

— Cough
— Rheumatism
— Paralysis
— Tremors
— Kapha and Vata disorders
— Many other diseases

Preparation

Ingredients:
Spleen Amaranth leaves – 1 bunch
Ghee – 10 ml
Urud dal – 1 spoon full
Mustard – 1tsp
Pepper powder – 1 pinch
Asafoetida – 1 pinch
Rock salt – 1 pinch

Method

Separate the leaves from the weeds and grass. Wash it well. Chop and cook it using very little rock salt. Add a pinch of pepper powder for taste. Cook for 5-7 minutes only. Season with asafoetida, mustard, urud dal and cumin seeds using ghee.

Marsilea Leaves

Indications:
- It is cooling
- Tonic – it produces and restores the normal tone of the tissues It is also a brain tonic
- Improves memory
- Has good taste
- Specially indicated for -

— Liver diseases
— Spleen diseases
— Diabetes
— Insanity
— Diabetes with Pitta predominance.

Preparation

Ingredients:
Marsilea Leaves– 2 bunches

Black gram (urud dal) – 3 spoons full
Ginger – 1 small piece
Ghee – 10 ml
Pepper – 1
Rock salt – according to taste.

Method

It is prepared as chutney. Take the leaves separately, wash and sauté using ghee for 2 minutes. Then put it into a mixer along with sautéed black gram, ginger, rock salt, and pepper to make the chutney.

AYURVEDA IN INDIA

Ayurveda in India—the science of life, the origin of most forms of natural and alternative medicine—has its mention in one of the oldest (about 6, 000 years) philosophical texts of the world, the Rig Veda. The Sutrasthana of Charaka Samhita, a much referred ayurvedic text, says; "The three—body, mind and soul—are like a tripod, the world stand by their combination; in them everything abides. It is the subject matter of ayurveda for which the teachings of ayurveda have been revealed. "

In its broader scope, ayurveda in India has always sought to prepare mankind for the realization of the full potential of its self through a psychosomatic integration. A comprehensive health care is what this natural and alternative medicine prescribes for the ultimate self-realization.

"Life (ayu) is the combination (samyoga) of body, senses, mind and reincarnating soul. Ayurveda is the most sacred science of life, beneficial to humans both in this world and the world beyond. " —Charaka Samhita, Sutrasthana, 1. 42-43.

The verses of Rig Veda, the earliest source of ayurveda, refer to panchamahabhut (five basic elements of the entire creation), and the three doshas or primary forces of prana or vata (air), agni or pitta (fire) and soma or kapha (water and earth) as comprising the basic principles of ayurveda. One branch of Indian philosophy—Sankhya states that there are 24 elements, all of which constitute the foundation of the gross world: earth, water, fire, air and ether.

These five elements in different combinations constitute the three body types/doshas—vata dosha (air and ether), pitta dosha (fire) and kapha dosha (earth and water). The panchamahabhut and the dosha theories are the guiding factors of ayurveda as a therapeutic science. The Rig Veda also mentions organ transplants and herbal remedies called soma with properties of elixir.

This science or knowledge of healing, as mentioned in the Rig Veda, was revealed to Rishi Bharadvaja from the great Cosmic Intelligence. The knowledge consists of three aspects known as the Tri-Sutras of ayurveda, which are—etiology or the science of the causes of disease, symptomatology or the study and interpretation of symptoms and medication and herbal remedies. Approximately, during 4, 000 to 3, 000 BC, Sam Veda and Yajur Veda, the second and third Vedas came into being.

Chanting of mantras and performance of rituals were, respectively, dealt in these two Vedas. And, during 3, 000 to 2, 000 BC Atharva the fourth Veda was authored, of which ayurveda is an upaveda (subsection).

Though it had been practiced all along, it was around this time that ayurveda in India, was codified from the oral tradition to book form, as an independent science. It enlists eight branches/divisions of ayurveda: Kayachikitsa (Internal Medicine), Shalakya Tantra (surgery and treatment of head and neck, Ophthalmology and Otolaryngology), Shalya Tantra (Surgery), Agada Tantra (Toxicology), Bhuta Vidya (Psychiatry), Kaumarabhritya (Pediatrics), Rasayana (science of rejuvenation or anti-aging), and Vajikarana (the science of fertility). The oldest treatise available on this codified version is Atreya Samhita.

The most fascinating aspect of ayurveda is, it was using almost all methods of healing like lifestyle regimen, yoga, aroma, meditation, gems, amulets, herbs, diet, jyotishi (astrology), colour and surgery etc. in treating patients. Though ayurveda came into being as an independent upaveda of Atharva Veda, it has close links with other Vedas also. The Yajur Veda, which recommends rituals to pacify the panchamahabhuts in a view to heal both the Cosmic Being and the individual soul, is related to ayurveda in its principles and regulations of lifestyle. The upaveda called Dhanur Veda or the martial arts and ayurveda both refer to each other in the treatment of marmas or sensitive points in the body. Ayurveda recommends specific ayurvedic massages, exercises and bodywork for this purpose.

Around 15, 00 BC ayurveda was delineated into to two distinct schools: Atreya—The School of Physicians, and Dhanvantari—The School of Surgeons. This made ayurveda a more systematically classified medical science, hereafter. Dhanvantari, who is considered to be a reincarnation of Lord Vishnu, was the guiding sage of ayurveda. He made this science of health and longevity popular and widely acceptable. In fact, these two schools of thought led to the writing of two major books on ayurveda—Charaka Samhita and Susruta Samhita.

These two Samhitas were written in the early part of 1000 BC. The great sage-physician Charaka authored Charaka Samhita revising and supplementing the text written by Atreya, which has remained the most referred ayurvedic text on internal medicine till date. Susruta, following the Dhanvantari School of Thought, wrote Susruta Samhita, comprising the knowledge about prosthetic surgery to replace limbs, cosmetic surgery, caesarian operations and even brain surgery. He is famed for his innovation of cosmetic surgery on nose or rhinoplasty. Around 500 AD, Vagbhatt compiled the third major treatise on ayurveda, Astanga Hridaya. It contained knowledge comprising the two schools of ayurveda.

From 500 AD to 1900 AD, sixteen major Nighantus or supplementary texts on ayurveda like Dhanvantari Bhavaprakasha, Raja and Shaligram among others were written incorporating new drugs, expansion in applications, discarding of old drugs and identification of substitutes. These texts mention about 1814 varieties of plants in vogue.

Evidences show that ayurveda had nurtured almost all the medical systems of the world. The Egyptians learnt about ayurveda long before the invasion of Alexander in the 4th century BC through their sea-trade with India. Greeks and Romans come to know about it after the famous invasion. The Unani form of medical tradition came out of this interaction. In the early part of the first millennium ayurveda spread to the East through Buddhism and greatly influenced the Tibetan and Chinese system of medicine and herbology. Around 323 BC, Nagarjuna, the great monastic of Mahayana Buddhism and an authority on ayurveda had written a review on Susruta Samhita. In 800 AD ayurveda was translated into Arabic. The two Islamic physicians Avicenna and Razi Serapion, who helped form the European tradition of medicine, strictly followed ayurveda. Even, Paracelsus, considered to be the father of the modern western medicine toed the line of ayurveda, as well.

In the postmodern age, the popularity of this vibrant tradition of ayurveda lies in its, subtle yet scientific, approach to heal a person in its totality. It aims, not only at healing the body, but also the mind and spirit, at one go. Its unique understanding of the similarities of natural law and the working of human body, as well as its holistic treatment methods, help it to strike a balance between the two. This gives ayurveda an edge over other healing systems. Perhaps that's the reason behind ayurveda being the longest unbroken medical tradition in the world, today.

Charaka Samhita

Charaka Samhita is considered to be the most ancient and authoritative writing on ayurveda available today. It also explains the logic and philosophy on which this system of medicine is based. The detailed biography of the composer of this treatise—that is, sage Charaka—is not known to the posterity. Interestingly, it is not an original writing of a single person rather like all Vedic knowledge it is a continuation and renewal of that ancient knowledge system.

In fact, Charaka had redacted the Agnivesa Samhita (an edited version of Atreya Samhita). The available form of Charaka Samhita was again worked upon by Drdhabala (living in about 400 AD) long after sage Charaka.

According to Charaka, science is dependent upon yukti—a quality of the intellect that enables it to perceive phenomena brought into existence by a multiplicity of causes. Thus, it's not surprising that much of the treatise of Charaka Samhita is in the form of a symposium wherein groups of ayurvedic scholars take up a series of topics for discussion. This gives indication that the science of ayurveda is a product of constant verification, fine-tuning and authentication by an active community of physicians. The samhita mentions about the gradual development of the fetus within the womb in minutes that equals the modern medical version in accuracy.

The language is Sanskrit and is written in verse form. The style is in keeping with the Vedic oral tradition of conserving knowledge. The samhita contains 8, 400 metrical verses.

Charaka followed the Atreya School of Physicians, which predominantly deals with treatments through internal and external application of medicine. Though the samhita contains all the theoretical knowledge of ayurveda it's focus is on healing the body, mind and soul of a patient in the minimum invasive manner that's Kayachikitsa. Hence, he placed great emphasis on the diagnostic part of the treatment. So much so that he classified everything from solar calendar to topography to the timing of the birth of a child. He identified eight stages of a disease from its inception to the culmination. Charaka also laid great emphasis on the timing and manner of the collection of medicinal plants.

Charaka sought to correct the element of fire or the digestive function in a body. It sought to alter the chemical processes in the cells by purification methods and medicinal application. From a greater perspective Charaka laid emphasis for health and longevity to strike a balance between one's corporeal and spiritual being. That is the reason why Charaka went so detail into the diagnosis of a disease's origin.

Susruta Samhita

Susruta wrote his samhita, the most authentic text on the practice of ayurvedic surgery around the sixth century BC Susruta is, also, renowned as the father of plastic surgery. He represents the Dhanvantari School of surgeons. His samhita discussed in minute details on how to perform prosthetic surgery to replace limbs, cosmetic surgery on nose and on other parts of the body, cesarean operations, setting of compound fractures, and even brain surgery. Susruta's original work seems to have been revised and supplemented by Nagarjuna between the third and fourth centuries AD.

This branch of medicine is believed to have arisen in part from the exigencies of dealing with the effects of war. Epic Ramayana, mentions remarkable feats of surgery having taken place in the past. We have reference to the transplantation of an eyeball and a head in epics. The style Susruta Samhita is both prose and poetry with poetry being the greater portion. This work, also, is said to be a redaction of oral material passed down verbally from generation to generation.

This work is unique in that it discusses blood in terms of the fourth doshic principle. This work is the first to enumerate and discuss the pitta subtypes. Susruta details about 125 surgical instruments used by him mostly made of stones, wood and other such natural materials. The Susruta Samhita presents many innovations in ayurvedic surgery. Use of shalaka—meaning foreign body (here, rods or a probe etc.) is mentioned by Susruta. Some of the classifications found in the Susruta Samhita are not even traced by the modern medical science. It described five types of pterygium, and the prognosis it made about glaucoma has not been improved since. In fact he is the first surgeon in medical history who systematically and elaborately dealt with anatomical structure of eye.

Susruta has discussed about 72 diseases of the eye. He has stipulated drug therapy for various types of conjunctivitis and glaucoma along with surgical procedures of the removal of cataract, pterygium, diseases of ear, nose and throat.

The Susruta Samhita, besides being the most authentic text on practice and theory of surgery, is also the most commonly quoted text on health.

Astanga Hridaya

Astanga Hridaya is accepted as the third major treatise on ayurveda. Around 500 AD, Vagbhatt compiled this samhita. It contained knowledge comprising the two schools of ayurveda—the school of surgery and the school of physicians.

There is another similar work called the Astanga Sangraha belonging to the same period. It is slightly bigger in size than the Astanga Hridaya, and is written in verse form whereas the later text was in prose form. It is believed either there are two works by a person or two persons with the same name. However, both the works came into being after the Charaka and Susruta Samhitas. The Astanga Hridaya primarily deals with kayachikitsa besides, discussing in detail about various surgical treatments. The kapha subtypes are first listed and described in this samhita, completing exhaustive explanation of vata, pitta, kapha with their five subtypes.

Astanga Hridaya seems to emphasize on the physiological aspect of the body rather than the spiritual aspects of it like its counterparts—Charaka and

Susruta Samhitas. Despite that, the quality and range of its discussions about ayurveda makes it a work to reckon with.

YOGA/NATUROPATHY/UNANI/SIDDHA AND HOMOEOPATHY

Unani or Yunani means "Greek", and has its origins in the Greek word Iônía or Iôníe, a placename given to a Greek populated coastal region of Anatolia. Unani, part of the trio Indian medicines – ayurveda, siddha and unani. It is used to refer to Graeco-Arabic or Unani medicine, also called "Unani-tibb", which is based on the teachings of Hippocrates, Galen, and Avicenna, and the concepts of the four humours: Phlegm (Balgham), Blood (Dam), Yellow bile (bafrâ') and Black bile (Saudâ').

Unani medicine – Though the threads which comprise Unani healing can be traced all the way back to Claudius Galenus of Pergamum, who lived in the second century of the Christian Era, the basic knowledge of Unani medicine as a healing system was developed by Hakim Ibn Sina (known as Avicenna in the west) in his medical encyclopedia The Canon of Medicine. The time of origin is thus dated at circa 1025 AD, when Avicenna wrote The Canon of Medicine in Persia. While he was primarily influenced by Greek and Islamic medicine, he was also influenced by the Indian medical teachings of Sushruta and Charaka.

IHBT is constantly striving to generate new knowledge to fulfill its mission of sustainable management of Bioresources in the himalayan region by adopting a multidisciplinary approach in R & D activities. The Institute has five Divisions engaged in research of high scientific impact.

The importance of medicinal plants in traditional healthcare practices, providing clues to new areas of research and in biodiversity conservation is now well recognized. However, information on the uses for plants for medicine is lacking from many interior areas of Himalaya. Keeping this in view the present study was initiated in a tribal dominated hinterland of western Himalaya.

The study aimed to look into the diversity of plant resources that are used by local people for curing various ailments. Questionnaire surveys, participatory observations and field visits were planned to illicit information on the uses of various plants. It was found that 35 plant species are commonly used by local people for curing various diseases. In most of the cases (45%) under ground part of the plant was used. New medicinal uses of Ranunculus hirtellus and Anemone rupicola are reported from this area. Similarly, preparation of "sik" a traditional recipe served as a nutritious diet to pregnant women is also not documented elsewhere. Implication of developmental activities and changing socio-economic conditions on the traditional knowledge are also discussed.

Background

Out of the total 4, 22, 000 flowering plants reported from the world, more then 50,000 are used for medicinal purposes. In India, more than 43% of the total flowering plants are reported to be of medicinal importance. Utilization of plants for medicinal purposes in India has been documented long back in ancient literature. However, organized studies in this direction were initiated in 1956 and off late such studies are gaining recognition and popularity due to loss of traditional knowledge and declining plant population. Right from its beginning, the documentation of traditional knowledge especially on the medicinal uses of plants, has provided many important drugs of modern day.

Even today this area holds much more hidden treasure as almost 80% of the human population in developing countries is dependant on plant resources for healthcare.

In the interior areas of western Himalaya plants become the only source of medicine and well being. However, information on the uses of plants as traditional medicines has not been documented from various interior areas of western Himalaya such as Chhota Bhangal. Due to its remoteness and lack of modern health facilities dependence on plants for medicine is very high. Ironically, information on the uses of plants for medicine from this area is completely lacking.

At the same time, the area is undergoing rapid transformations due to its recognition as an ideal paragliding site and is therefore becoming more market oriented. This can be seen in the changed cropping patterns of the local people. The role of market economy in depletion of traditional knowledge has been well documented in many parts of Himalaya. Thus many important leads to drug discovery may be lost in absence of proper documentation.

Keeping this in view, the present study was initiated, with an aim to identify knowledgeable resource persons and document their knowledge of on the utilization of medicinal plants in Chhota Bhangal area of western Himalaya.

Land and People

Chhota Bhangal represents one of the most interior areas of western Himalaya and is located in the hill state of Himachal Pradesh (HP). More than 3500 flowering plants have been reported from HP, of which almost 500 plants are believed to be of medicinal importance. Located between 45 N lat to 45 7.772 N and 45 452 E long to 45 53.832 Chhota Bhangal is a pristine area with good vegetation. The area is rich in forests that comprises mainly of moist Himalayan temperate forests with one or the other species of oak (Quercus spp.) in dominance. In some areas, dry Himalayan temperate forests dominate the vegetation.

They mainly consist of Cedrus deodara intermingled with other tree species such as Abies pindrow and Picea smithiana. Rhododendron campanulatum and Betula utilis form the tree line in the area. The dominating under canopy flora includes Berberis lycium, Prinsepia utilis, Viburnum nervosum and a diversity of herbs and grasses. These forests form the catchment area of the Uhl river that flows through the region and forms the life support system of the Bhangalis. Bhangalis represent a tribal community of the Himalaya that are very God fearing and follow Hinduism. Though they can easily understand and speak Hindi (which is the national language of India), amongst themselves they communicate in pahari dialect. They are mainly agropastoralists and rear sheep and goats. During summer season (June to September) they migrate to their temporary settlements at higher regions (>3500 m) and during winters they return to their lower altitude settlements at 1800 m. In addition to livestock rearing, agriculture is the main occupation of Bhangalis. Wheat forms the main agricultural crop. However, under the influence of market, recently the cultivation of potato and French beans has increased in the area at the cost of indigenous crops.

Bhangalis are a repository of traditional knowledge especially on the utilization of plants for medicinal purposes. This can be easily understood from the following local sayings which are very popular in the area.

"Bana, basuti te bare jethi houan thethi manu kian more" meaning a man cannot die of disease in an area where Vitex negundo (bana), Adhatoda vasica (basuti) and Acorus calamus (bare) are found, provided that he knows how to use them. Similarly another verse that is common in the area is "Harad, bahera amla bich payi giloye, jithonye char chijan utho admi kyon moye".

It means that a person will not succumb to disease in an area where Terminalia chebula (harad), T. bellerica (bahera), Emblica officinalis (amla) and Tinospora cordifolia (giloye) plants are available. Recently the area has come up on the world tourism map because of its recognition as an ideal paragliding site. In addition to paragliding thousands of tourists visit the area for its scenic beauty and high peaks & passes.

Results

The study reveals that in absence of modern health facility people in the area depend on plants for medicinal purposes. Based on the initial reconnaissance survey and group discussions where emphasis was on identification of knowledgeable resource persons it was found that, information on the medicinal uses of plants now seems to be confined to elder people (above 40 years of age) only. Younger generation is ignorant about the vast medicinal resources available in their surroundings and is more inclined towards market resources. All the resource persons identified were in the age group of 40–55 years and all of them were familiar with the medicinal plants growing in their vicinity. It was also found that men knew comparatively more then females. Their could be many reasons for this, females have more household working pressure in western Himalaya and so they had limited time and secondly they could have been little hesitant while talking to us as we were an all male team. In all, the people use 35 different plants for curing various ailments, out of which 25 were herbs, 5 trees, 4 shrubs and one climber. In most of the cases (45%), underground parts were used for curing ailment followed by leaves and aerial parts. Stem and flowers were the least used plant parts. The specimen number of the plant that has been deposited in the herbarium (PLP) of IHBT has also been provided. The plants are arranged in alphabetic order.

Locally used medicinal plants – These plants were used for curing a total of 21 diseases ranging from simple stomach-ache to highly complicated male and female disorders. Even jaundice and kidney stones were treated by them.

Maximum number of plants were used for curing female disorders and fever followed by joint pain, gastric problems and nasal bleeding. It was also found that a single plant may be used for curing many ailments such as, Artemisia sieversiana that is used both as an abortifacient and also for joints pains. Similarly Parthenocissus semicordata is used against leucorrhoea and piles.

Though, majority of the plants are available in the vicinity of village forests, however, for some, that are found in the alpine regions, people have to cover long distances on foot sometimes more than 20 km. Aconitum heterophyllum that occurs above 3500 m in the alpine regions of Chhota Bhangal is used for curing stomach ache and fever and is one of the highly traded species. Its tuber are sold at a rate of Rs. 1500/kg in the area. Another important plant of the alpine region is Picrorhiza kurrooa. It is used by Bhangalis for curing joint pains and fever and the dried rhizomes of the plant are sold at a rate of Rs. 60/kg. Rheum australe also occurs in the alpine zone, the roots of which are used by Bhangalis for curing joint pains and swellings. The plant is traded from the area and the dried roots fetch a price of Rs 55/kg. Few plant species, such as Berberis asiatica, B. lycium, Prinsepia utilis and Rubus niveus are very common in the village surroundings. Berberis asiatica is used for curing jaundice while B. lycium is used against eye disorders.

The root of both these plants also yields a yellow dye while the fruits are eaten. Prinsepia utilis also occurs in the open areas around villages and its roots are used for wound healing and as an antidote to poison. The roots of Rubus niveus are used for curing excessive bleeding during menses. All these four species are presently not traded from the area. A very common plant that occurs on rocks and boulders in Chhota Bhangal is Bergenia ciliata. It has very long and stout roots which are used for curing kidney stones. Cirsium wallichii and Rumex nepalensis are common around the temporary settlements of Bhangalis and are used by them. C. wallichii is used for curing gastric troubles while R. nepalensis is used as anti allergic. Ranunculs hirtellus that occurs in moist areas along water channels is used for curing swelling in testes.

Anemone rupicola is also found in moist areas and is use against ear problems. In addition, five commonly occurring tree species namely, Aesculus indica, Grewia optiva, Pinus roxburghii, Prunus cerasoides and Rhododendron arboreum, are also used by the Bhangalis for curing various ailments. The fruits of A. indica are used in preparation of a nutritious recipe called "sik". For this, after removing the seed coat, the fruit is washed and kept for drying. It is then powdered and roasted with ghee (clarified butter) till it becomes brown. Later sugar and water are added to it. It can be stored for 2 to 3 days.

It is a pre-and post-pregnancy food for ladies. It is also used for curing excessive bleeding and pain during menses. The beautiful red flowers of R. arboreum in addition to being eaten raw as salad are used for curing nasal bleeding. Young leaves of the plant are considered to be poisonous. G. optiva and P. cerasiodes are used for curing joint pains. Oil is also extracted from the fruits of P. cerasiodes. Pinus roxburghii is used as diuretic.

Number of plants used for treating various diseases. – It was also found that people are hesitant to disclose their knowledge. It is this knowledge that provides them recognition in the society and hence they do not want to share it. In most of the cases, it was found that this knowledge has been orally transferred from one generation to other and at each level a bit of it has been lost. The people themselves say that, compared to them their forefathers knew much more. It was also found that the local people are concerned about the degradation of medicinal plants in wild. Due to recent shift towards herbal medicines the pressures on the resources have increased and the market is fast expanding. It is to be noted that nearly 130 medicinal plants are in heavy demand from Himachal Pradesh and as already mentioned many important plants are traded from Chhota Bhangal.

Discussion

Many of the plants that are used by the local people in Chhota Bhangal find mention in ancient medicinal literature and are also used in different medicines systems such as, the Ayurveda and Unani.

Aconitum heterophyllum that is used by the Bhangalis for curing stomach ache finds mention in Ayurveda for curing stomach ache and fever. It is one of the main ingredients of "Ativishadi churna", "Chandraprabha vati" and "Amritarishta" ayurvedic medicines. In Unani system of medicine it is an important ingredient of "Sufuf habib" which is used for curing piles and also of "Ma'jun jograj guggal" that is used against arthiritis. Similarly Picrorhiza kurrooa which Bhangalis use for joint pains is used for curing fever, jaundice, asthma, and leucoderma in Ayurveda. In Unani it is used for curing leucoderma and piles.

It forms an important ingredient of medicine "Arogyawardhini" which is used for treating hepatobiliary disorders and of "Hepax" which is useful in pregnancy anaemia.

The overexploitation of A. heterophyllum and P. kurrooa for trade has lead to a drastic decline in their population and now both are endangered. Rheum australe is another important plant especially in the Unani medicine system where it is an important constituent of "Itrifal Mulayyin" used for curing constipation; "Hab Shabyar" used for curing headache, "Haba Shafa" used against cough and cold and "Roughan aqrab" used for piles. The plant also finds mention for curing diarrohea amongst livestock. Due to high extraction pressure and declining population, the plant has been designated as vulnerable. Berberis asiatica and B. lycium are used in Ayurveda and Unani for treating eye disorders incidentally the Bhangalis also use them for eye disorders. Similarly, Bergenia ciliata that is used by Bhangalis for curing kidney stones is used for curing urinary disorders, splenic enlargement, ulcers and dysentery in ayurveda. In Unani it is used against hydrophobia, splenic enlargement, mennorrhgia and liver disorders. It is one of the main ingredients of "Cystose" drug that is used for cleaning urinary tract infections. During the surveys, it was observed that a large number of plants are used for curing female disorders compared to males. This can be attributed to the fact that unlike men, women are shyer and therefore find treatment in the community itself. The work load on them is also comparatively higher and hence they hardly find time to visit market places for treatment.

Unani medicine, like Western medicine (which also arose from the Greek background) owes its origination to Hippocrates (460-377 B.C.) and his numerous followers. Other Greek medical masters, such as Dioscorides and Galen, who we recognize as the forerunners of Western herbal medicine, are also considered founders of Unani medicine.

The adoption of Greek medicine into the Islamic culture was depicted by Husain F. Nagamia MD, Chairman International Institute of Islamic Medicine, and former President of the Islamic Medical Association, as arising in the ancient city of Jundishapur (near Baghdad). The timing of events is described in relation to rule of caliphs, the civil and religious leaders of Muslim states, who are considered to be successors of Mohammed.

In Pakistan, India, Bangladesh and other countries, there are hundreds of Unani Medical Colleges where Unani System of medicine is taught, in five and half year courses and the graduates are awarded BUMS (Bachelor of Unani Medicine and Surgery) or other degrees. There are about 10 Unani medical Colleges where a Postgraduate degree is being awarded to BUMS Doctors. all these colleges are affiliated to reputed universities and recognized by the Governments. It is interesting to note that use of Ranunculus hirtellus, Rubus niveus and Anemone rupicola for the described medicinal purposes seems to be restricted to this area, as use of these plants for the said diseases could not be found in the literature perused for the western Himalaya. Similarly, preparation of "sik" has not been documented in the literature for the western Himalaya.

It can be concluded from the study that Bhangalis inherit a rich traditional knowledge and documentation of this knowledge has provided novel information from the area. They still depend on the plants for medicinal purposes and are very much concerned about their degradation in wild as they now have to travel even more far to collect these plants. The incoming of roads and coming up of the area as an important tourist destination has allured the younger generation towards market economy, this certainly will have larger implications. Thus, the present documentation of traditional knowledge from an area where novel information has been generated will not only provide recognition to this knowledge but will also help in its conservation vis-à-vis providing pharmacological leads for the betterment of human society.

4

Ethnobotany

Ethnobotany is considered as a branch of ethnobiology, the study of past and present interrelationships between human cultures and the plants, animals, and other organisms in their environment. Like its parent field, ethnobotany makes apparent the connection between human cultural practices and the sub-disciplines of biology. Ethnobotanical studies range across space and time, from archaeological investigations of the role of plants in ancient civilizations to the bioengineering of new crops. Furthermore, ethnobotany is not limited to nonindustrialized or nonurbanized societies. In fact, co-adaptation of plants and human cultures has changed and perhaps intensified in the context of urbanization and globalization in the twentieth and twenty-first centuries. Nonetheless, indigenous, non-Westernized cultures play a crucial role in ethnobotany, as they possess a previously undervalued knowledge of local ecology gained through centuries or even millennia of interaction with their biotic (living) environment.

The significance of ethnobotany is manifold. The study of indigenous food production and local medicinal knowledge may have practical implications for developing sustainable agriculture and discovering new medicines. Ethnobotany also encourages an awareness of the link between biodiversity and cultural diversity, as well as a sophisticated understanding of the mutual influence (both beneficial and destructive) of plants and humans. In this unit, we will discuss the historic roots of ethnobotany and a brief knowledge about different areas associated with it. The unit intends to highlight the role that local people's knowledge and cultural perspectives can play in resource management and conservation.

INTRICATE RELATIONSHIP BETWEEN CULTURE, PLANTS, HUMANS AND OUR ENVIRONMENT

The main objective of this unit is to expand awareness about the intricate relationship between culture, plants, humans, and our environment. After going through this unit you will be able to-

1 Define the ethnobotany and discuss the scope of the subject area covered by this descipline.
2 Discuss the historic roots of ethnobotany and the role that human/plant interactions have had in managing natural resources, and the influence of human on the evolution, distribution and utilization of major food and medicinal plants.
3 Understand and discuss the broad spectrum of terminology of ethnobotany that is often associated with it.
4 Discuss the role, importance and contribution of ethnomedicine, ethnopharmacology, ethnoecology, ethnogynaecology, ethnomycology, etc., in our modern civilization.
5 Discuss the people-plant relations focusing upon impacts of plant conservation and opportunities for sustainable use.

MEANING AND SCOPE OF ETHNOBOTANY

Since the beginning of civilization, people have used plants to provide them food, shelter, medicines, as well as the materials for construction and the manufacture of crafts and tools and many other products like fuel, paints, poison, etc.

Plants often have ritual characters and are used because of their variety of properties. Nowadays their chemical and genetic characters are increasingly explored for human benefits. It had been possible due to ethnobotanical studies that have provided us a plenty of information data about plants either useful or harmful.

Ethnobotany is the study of how people of a particular culture and region make the use of indigenous plants. Ethnobotanists explore how plants are used for such things as food, shelter, medicine, clothing, hunting, and religious ceremonies. These plants are known as ethnobotanicals.

The term *ethnobotany* was suggested by John Harshberger in 1896 to delimit a specific field of botany and to describe plant uses. It was defined as *"the use of plants by aboriginal peoples"*. Its scope was much elaborated by Ford (1978) and Faulks (1958). Prior to this term (ethnobotany), many botanists were already including the use of plants by people within their study.

However, it was Harshberger who proposed that *discipline of ethnobotany* might be developed with its own definition, scope, objectives and methodologies.

Although Harshberger's definition still provide the root of the ethnobotany, but to describe the field in broader sense ethnobotanists have given their definitions time to time. Let us look at the slight changes in emphasis through a review of current definitions.

- Ethnobotany is considered to encompass all studies which concern the mutual relationship between plants and traditional peoples (Cotton, 1996).
- In broad terms, ethnobotany is the study of the interrelationship between plants and people. The two major parts of ethnobotany are encapsulated in the word itself; ethno, 'the study of people', and botany, 'the study of plants'. However, the field is limited on both sides. On the botanical sides of the field, few ethnobotanical studies are concerned with plants that have no connection to people. On the ethno side, most studies are concerned with the ways indigenous peoples use and view plants. And those uses and those views can provide deep insights into the human conditions.
- According to Ford 1994, ethnobotany is concerned with a wide range of interest of plants in cultural and ecological context.
- According to Martin 1995, ethnobotany is the part of ethnoecology which concerns plants.
- Turner 1996 has given an appropriate definition that is "the science of people's interaction with plants".

So, from the above recent definitions, it may be said that the ethnobotany has become a broader discipline, which is interested in all studies about the relationship between people and plants.

TERMS OF ETHNOBOTANY

Let us recall what we have discussed so far. The term 'Ethnobotany' was first coined by Harshberger in 1895. Ethnobotany deals with the direct relationship between plants and human. A number of terms are used in varied areas of ethnobotanical research, such as ethnotaxonomy, ethnomedicine, ethnopharmacology, ethnomycology, ethnoecology, etc.

Though it was Harshberger who first mentioned the ethnobotany as a descipline, but its history begins long before that. Many known scientists had already referred important plants and their various uses in their published records.

In India, it was Dr. S. K. Jain who made pioneering investigations on ethnobotany and affectionately known as "Father of Indian Ethnobotany".

Archaeoethnobotany deals with the study of identification of materials from archaeological sites for studies on migration of human cultures, dispersal and domestication of crops, etc. while paleoethnobotany deals with the identification of fossilized plant materials and remains for studies an ancient plant economy, paleobotanical history of crops and changing patterns of the use of plant life by human cultures.

Ethnoecology is the field of study of the past and present interrelationships between human societies, and their living and non-living environment. The importance of ethnoecological research is now increasing by the fact that indigenous system could usefully be incorporated into the sustainable development of modern civilization and its management.

Ethnopharmacology is an interdesciplinary science which deals with the identification, description, observations and experimental investigations of the ingredients used in various recipes prepared by aborigines and the effects of indigenous drugs on animals and human.

While ethnomedicine, ethnogynaecology, ethnoophthalmology, ethnoorthopaedics are specific study branches as their name suggests and are linked with ethnopharmacology to some extent. Ethnomusicology deals with the study of music of tribals and aborigins, its documentations, forms and content. Ethnolinguistic is the study of relationship between language and culture in different ethnic groups.

The study of use of toxic plants as fish poisons, arrow poisons in human societies is known as ethnotoxicology and the use of narcotics in ancient culture is considered under ethnonarcotics. After a thorough study, now we are well familier with the fact that *Ethnobotany* is a field on rise nowadays. It is a field of research of great value and have gaines much interest of botanists, chemists, socialists, etc. because of its large study areas. It is possible now to conserve and maintain the biodiversity and indigenous culture with the help of ethnobotanical studies.

ETHNOPHARMACY

Ethnopharmacy is the interdisciplinary science that investigates the perception and use of pharmaceuticals (especially traditional medicines, but not only), within a given human society. It deals with the study of the pharmaceutical means considered in relation to the cultural contexts of their use, e.g. the study of the cultural determinants that characterise the uses of these means within a culture.

It involves studies of the:

1. identification and ethnotaxonomy (cognitive categorisation) of the (eventual) natural material, from which the remedy will be produced (medical ethnobiology: ethnobotany or ethnomycologyor ethnozoology);
2. traditional preparation of the pharmaceutical forms (ethnopharmaceutics);
3. bio-evaluation of the pharmacological action of such preparations (ethnopharmacology);

4. their clinical effectiveness (clinical ethnopharmacy);
5. socio-medical aspects implied in the uses of these pharmaceuticals (medical anthropology/ethnomedicine).
6. public health and pharmacy practice-related issues concerning the public use and/or the re-evaluation of these drugs.

Ethnopharmacy is often erroneously associated with ethnopharmacology, which is instead "only" focused on the bio-pharmacological evaluation of traditional medicines.

Ethnopharmacy shares instead a common terrain with medical anthropology and anthropology of pharmaceuticals.

INFORMATION ON THE ECONOMIC ASPECTS OF PLANTS

The study of plants in the service of mankind has been a part of human civilization since ages. Information on the economic aspects of plants has been passed from one generation to the next generation. With the knowledge of the traditional practices botanists of world examined the practical uses of plants either reported or unreported. And in the light, a new branch of botany was emerged and termed as *ethnobotany*.

Though the term "ethnobotany" was not coined until 1895 by the US botanist John William Harshberger, the history of the field begins long before that. In AD 77, the Greek surgeon Dioscorides published "*De Materia Medica*", which was a catalogue of about 600 plants in the Mediterranean. It also included information on how the Greeks used the plants, especially for medicinal purposes. This illustrated herbal contained information on how and when each plant was gathered, whether or not it was poisonous, its actual use, and whether or not it was edible (it even provided recipes). Dioscorides stressed the economic potential of plants. For generations, scholars learned from this herbal, but did not actually venture into the field until after the Middle Ages.

In 1542 Leonhart Fuchs, a Renaissance artist, led the way back into the field. His "*De Historia Stirpium*" cataloged 400 plants native to Germany and Austria. John Ray (1686-1704) provided the first definition of "species" in his "*Historia Plantarum*": a species is a set of individuals who give rise through reproduction to new individuals similar to themselves.

In 1753 Carl Linnaeus wrote "*Species Plantarum*", which included information on about 5,900 plants. Linnaeus is famous for inventing the binomial method of nomenclature, in which all species get a two part name (genus, species).

The 19th century saw the peak of botanical exploration. Alexander von Humboldt collected data from the new world, and the famous Captain Cook brought back information on plants from the South Pacific. At this time major botanical gardens were started, for instance the Royal Botanic Gardens, Kew. Edward Palmer collected artifacts and botanical specimens from peoples in the North American West (Great Basin) and Mexico from the 1860s to the 1890s.

Once enough data existed, the field of "aboriginal botany" was founded. Aboriginal botany is the study of all forms of the vegetable world which aboriginal peoples use for food, medicine, textiles, ornaments, etc. The first individual to study the emic perspective of the plant world was a German physician working in Sarajevo at the end of 19th Century: Leopold Glueck. His published work on traditional medicinal uses of plants done by rural people in Bosnia (1896) has to be considered the first modern ethnobotanical work.

The term "ethnobotany" was first used by a botanist named John W. Harshberger in 1895 while he was teaching at the University of Pennsylvania. Although the term was not used until 1895, practical interests in ethnobotany go back to the beginning of civilization when people relied on plants as a way of survival.

Other scholars analysed uses of plants under an indigenous/local perspective in the 20th century: e.g. Matilda Coxe Stevenson, Zuni plants (1915); Frank Cushing, Zuni foods (1920); Keewaydinoquay Peschel, Anishinaabe fungii (1998), and the team approach of Wilfred Robbins, JP Harrington, and Barbara Freire-Marreco, Tewa pueblo plants (1916).

In the beginning, ethonobotanical specimens and studies were not very reliable and sometimes not helpful. This is because the botanists and the anthropologists did not come together on their work. The botanists focused on identifying species and how the plants were used instead of including how plants fit into people's lives. On the other hand, anthropologists were interested in the cultural role of plants and not the scientific aspect. Therefore, early ethnobotanical data does not really include both sides. In the early twentieth century, botanists and anthropologists finally collaborated and the collection of reliable, detailed data began.

Beginning in the twentieth century, the field of ethnobotany experienced a shift from the raw compilation of data to a greater methodological and conceptual reorientation. Today, the practice of ethnobotany requires a variety of skills:

1 *Botanical training* for the identification and preservation of plant specimens

2 *Anthropological training* to understand the cultural concepts around the perception of plants

3 *Linguistic training* to transcribe local terms and understand native morphology, syntax, and semantics.

Ethnobotanists engage in a broad array of research questions and practices, which do not lend themselves to easy categorization. However, the following headings attempt to describe some of the key areas of modern ethnobotanical study.

Archaeoethnobotany

Archaeoethnobotany is the study of the ethnobotany of identification of the plant materials from archaeological sites for studies on migration of human cultures, and origin, dispersal and domestification of crops etc.

It is closely linked to ethnobotany, as it is difficult to understand the ecology of modern environments without considering the environmental history that often involves prehistoric human interventions. There are a large number of examples from archaeological remains, among them few are mentioned here.

Kalpa Vraksha in stone sculptures denotes *Adansonia digitata* basically a semi arid zone species. They grow in semi dry areas where there is scanty vegetation. This plant has augmental and vegetable component besides ensured additional income to villagers derived from its fruit whose water is tonic and nutritive. The stem fibre is used as cordage. Branches and leaves are considered as a cattle feed and flowers are used in medicine.

The history of the domestication of the cereal grain maize (commonly known as "corn") is of particular interest to archaeoethnobotanists. The process is thought by some to have started 7,500 to 12,000 years ago. Recent genetic evidence suggests that maize domestication occurred 9000 years ago in central Mexico, perhaps in the highlands between Oaxaca and Jalisco. Archaeological remains of early maize cobs, found at Guila Naquitz Cave in the Oaxaca Valley, date back roughly 6,250 years; the oldest cobs from caves near Tehuacan, Puebla, have been dated to approximately 2750 B.C.

Ethnoecology

Ethnoecology is the scientific study of the way different groups of people in different locations understand ecosystems around them; the environments in which they live; and their relationship with these. It seeks valid, reliable understanding of how we as humans have interacted with the environment and how these intricate relationships have been sustained over time.

The "ethno" (see ethology) prefix in ethnoecology indicates a localized study of a people, and in conjunction with ecology, signifies people's understanding and experience of ecologies around them. A few definitions of ethnoecology are given below:

Definition 1- " Ethnoecology encompasses all studies which describes local peoples interaction with the natural environment including subdisciplines such as ethnobiology, ethnobotany, ethnoentomology and ethnozoology" (Martin 1995).

Definition 2- " Ethnoecology is the sciences of how people unerstand the relationship between human, animals, plants and physical elements of local environment".

Thus, ethnoeology is a multidisciplinary field that intregates techniques from biology, anthropology, ethnology, linguistics, economy and other fields. Ethnoecologists do not only work in primary forests, they are also interested in a broad range of vegetation types which have been altered by people, ranging from homegardens to mature secondary forests, where the majority of plants are found. Research focuses on the ecological knowledge of the indigenous people and of traditional agriculturists. Ethnoecologists address theoretical questions about the relationship between human and their environment and the answers contribute to rural development poverty alleviation, healthcare and conservation (Martin 1995). Thus ethnoecology is not limited to pure science, it can help to understand the dynamic relations between biodiversity and social and cultural systems.

Ethnomedicine

Ethnomedicine is a sub-field of medical anthropology that deals with the study of traditional medicines—not only those with relevant written sources (e.g., Traditional Chinese Medicine and Ayurveda), but also those whose knowledge and practices have been orally transmitted over the centuries. While the focus of ethnomedical studies is often the indigenous perception and use of traditional medicines, another stimulus for this type of research is drug discovery and development. Major pharmaceuticals such as digoxin, morphine, and atropine have been traced to foxglove, opium, and belladonna, respectively. Ethnomedical investigations in this century have led to the development of important drugs such as reserpine (a treatment for hypertension), podophyllotoxin (the base of an important anti-cancer drug), and vinblastine (used in the treatment of certain cancers).

In the scientific arena, ethnomedical studies are generally characterized by a strong anthropological approach, or by a strong biomedical approach, particularly in drug discovery programs. The focus of anthropological studies is the perception and context of use of traditional medicines, while biomedical approaches often focus on discovering therapeutic molecules, such as the anti HIV/AID molecule prostratin.

Ethnogynaecology

Ethnogynaecology is the study which deals with various diseases among women in tribal societies, related to sterility, conception, abortion, etc., and the use of abortifacients.

The drugs obtained from the plants to treat certain gynaecological problems have been reported to be useful and safe. *Santalum album, Terminalia arjuna, Rauvolfia serpentina, Aloe vera, Lawsonia innermis, Ocimum sanctum* are some examples of the plants which have been proved beneficial in treating gynaecological problems. *Withania somnifera, Lawsonia innermis* were used as abortifacient by local peoples since ages.

Ethnomusicology

Ethnomusicology is defined as "the study and cultural aspects of music and dance in local and global contexts." Formed from the Greek words *ethnos* (natio) of music. Jeff Todd Titon has called it the study of "people making music." Although it is often thought of as a study of non-Western musics, ethnomusicology also includes the study of Western music from an anthropological or sociological perspective. Bruno Nettl (1983) believes it is a product of Western thinking, proclaiming "ethnomusicology as western culture knows it is actually a western phenomenon." Nettl believes that there are limits to extraction of meaning from an indigenous culture's music due to perceptual distance of the Western observer from the culture. However, the growing prevalence of scholars who study their own musical traditions, and an increasing range of different theoretical frameworks and research methodologies has done much to address criticisms such as Nettl's.

While musicology's traditional subject has been the history and literature of Western art music, ethnomusicologists study all music as a human social and cultural phenomenon. The primary precursor to ethnomusicology, comparative musicology, emerged in the late 19th century and early 20th century through the practice of people such as Bela Bartok, Zoltan Kodaly, Constantin Brailoiu, Vinko Zganec, Franjo Ksaver, Carl Stumpf, Erich von Hornbostel, Curt Sachs and Alexander J. Ellis. Comparative musicology and early ethnomusicology tended to focus on non-Western music that was transmitted through oral traditions. But, in more recent years, the field has expanded to embrace all musical styles from all parts of the world.

The Society for Ethnomusicology has been the primary academic organization for the discipline of ethnomusicology since its inception in 1955. Ethnomusicologists often apply theories and methods from cultural anthropology, cultural studies and sociology as well as other disciplines in the social sciences and humanities. Though some ethnomusicologists primarily conduct historical studies, the majority are involved in long-term participant observation. Therefore, ethnomusicological work can be characterized as featuring a substantial, intensive ethnographic component.

Some ethnomusicological works are created not necessarily by 'ethnomusicologists' proper, but instead by anthropologists examining music as an aspect of a culture. A well-known example of such work is Colin Turnbull's study of the Mbuti pygmies. Another is Jaime de Angulo, a linguist who intensively studied the music of the natives of Northern California. Additionally, Anthony Seeger, professor at the University of California, Los Angeles, studied the music and society of the Suya people in Mato Grosso, Brazil.

Ethnomycology

Ethnomycology is the study of the historical uses and sociological impact of fungi ("fungi lore"), and can be considered a subfield of ethnobotany or ethnobiology. Although in theory the term includes fungi used for such purposes as tinder, medicine and food (including yeast), it is often used in the context of the study of psychoactive mushrooms such as psilocybin-containing mushrooms, Ergot and *Amanita muscaria*. By analogy to the term entheogen the term "entheomycology" (entheos meaning literally "god within", more freely translated "inspired") has been suggested for the study of psychoactive mushrooms used for spiritual purposes.

The researcher Robert Gordon Wasson rekindled interest in this field of study in the late 1920s, inspiring later (sometimes non-academic) researchers such as Terence McKenna, Carl Ruck, Giorgio Samorini, Keewaydinoquay Peschel, Richard Evans Schultes, John Allegro, Clark Heinrich, Dan Merkur, and James Arthur.

Besides mycological determination in the field ethnomycology depends to a large extent on anthropology and philology. One of the major debates among ethnomycologists is Wasson's theory that the Soma mentioned in the Rigveda of the Indo-Aryans was the *Amanita muscaria* mushroom. Following his example similar attempts have been made to identify psychoactive mushroom usage in many other (mostly) ancient cultures, with varying degrees of crediblity. Another much written about topic is the content of the Kykeon, the sacrament used during the Eleusinian mysteries in ancient Greece between approximately 1500 BC and 396 BC. Although not an ethnomycologist as such, philologist John Allegro has made an important contribution suggesting, in a book controversial enough to have his academic career destroyed, that *Amanita muscaria* was not only consumed as a sacrament but was the main focus of worship in the more esoteric sects of Sumerian religion, Judaism and early Christianity. Clark Heinrich claims that *Amanita muscaria* use in Europe was not completely wiped out by orthodox Christianity but continued to be used (either consumed or merely symbolically) by individuals and small groups such as medieval Holy Grail myth makers, alchemists and Renaissance artists.

While Wasson views historical mushroom use primarily as a facilitator for the shamanic or spiritual experiences core to these rites and traditions, McKenna takes this further, positioning that the ingestion of psilocybin was perhaps primary in the formation of language and culture and identifying psychedelic mushrooms as the original "Tree of Knowledge". There is indeed some research supporting the theory that psilocybin ingestion temporarily increases neurochemical activity in the language centers of the brain and, though this is hardly enough to substantiate McKenna's ambitious claim, it does indicate a need for more research into the uses of psychoactive plants and fungi in human history.

Ethnonarcotics

This is the study of the use of narcotics, snuffs, hallucinogens, etc., in primitive human societies. Opioid drugs, also called opiates or narcotics, have been used since the beginning of recorded history. Opium is derived from a white liquid produced by the poppy plant, first cultivated in the Middle East and Asia.

It was used therapeutically in ancient cultures to induce calm and to relieve pain, and recreationally to induce euphoric dream states. Tobacco (*Nicotiana tabacum*), one of the main narcotics is used for smoking and chewing. Tobacco smoking was made known to Europeans, about the year 1492, having been observed by followers of Columbus when visiting the West Indian island. The tobacco plant was first introduced into India by the Portuguese about the year 1605 during the later part of the reign of Akbar.

Ethnopharmacology

Ethnopharmacology is the scientific study correlating ethnic groups, their health, and how it relates to their physical habits and methodology in creating and using medicines. As an amalgamation of the social science of ethology and the medical science of pharmacology, ethnopharmacology studies the pharmacological aspects of a culture's medical treatment as well as its social appeal, including taste, symbology, and religious context. Through this, a culture's exposure to pharmacological substances can be determined.

Ethnopharmacology is related to botany in that many pharmaceuticals are delivered through plants. It is also often associated with ethnopharmacy, but while the aim of ethnopharmacology is the bio-evaluation of the effectiveness of traditional medicines, the former deals instead with much broader trans-disciplinary aspects related to the study of perception, use and management of pharmaceuticals (not necessarily traditional medicines) within a given human societies.

When investigating a natural products used by a certain culture as a medicine, it is important that the method of collection, extraction, preparation are the same or similar to those by the ethnic group as it is these processes which have allowed safe usage of the substance and give its safety records.

Ethnotaxonomy

The term *ethnotaxonomy* refers either to that subdiscipline within ethnology which studies the taxonomic systems defined and used by individual ethnic groups, or to the operative individual taxonomy itself, which is the object of the ethnologist's immediate study. For example, in many West African languages, the perceptual world of color is classified into the principal categories "Red," "White," and "Black" (finer gradations being secondary). The range of wavelengths that an English-speaker calls *blue* would be a subcategory of "Black."

The set of categories of family relationships evinced by the ethnic group's kinship system is another ethnotaxonomy. An example of this might be the Hawaiian kinship system, where all members of a generation of the same sex are referred to by a single term. Both the relationships termed *mother* and *aunt* in English fall into the same taxon "Mother-Aunt". This does not mean that the users of this taxonomy are confused about the concept "Birth-Mother," only that it is a subcategory.

Conversely, an ethnotaxonomy such as the Sudanese kinship system or that used in ancient Rome, where no two relationships have the same denotation, may show much more granularity than the English system. Thus the relationship called *aunt* in English is not fundamental in Latin, but either *amita* "Father's Sister" or *matertera* "Mother's Sister" must be chosen. Latin and Sudanese are called a "descriptive systems," and Hawaiian is called a "classificatory" system, but it is obvious that this terminology is English-centred, the difference being one of degree, rather than kind.

Categories of plants, "Useful" and "Harmful," etc., are yet another well-known example. Indeed, in recent years there has been a vogue usage of the term ethnotaxonomy limiting it to ethnobotany and ethnopharmacology, because of the "rediscovery" of the medicinal and commercial value of plants disclosed by examining the botanical ethnotaxonomies of lesser-known cultures.

Ethnotoxicology

Ethnotoxicology deals with various toxic plants used as fish poison, arrow poison etc., and these studies are mostly concerned with tribal people. Poisonous plants contain powerful toxic ingredients (phyto-chemicals) which if introduced into the body of any animal system, may be of relatively smaller quantity, will affect deleteriously and may be fatal at times. These toxic substances injure the basic life principles that is the protoplasm and the harmful effects produced, may be immediate or accumulative, the later may appear after a period of time when the poison reaches upto a specific concentration due to repeated administration. *Aloe barbedensis, Datura stramonium, Euphorbia pulcherrima, Jatropha curcas, Lantana camara, Ricinus communis,* etc., are some examples of toxic plants which have been used by ancient people from time immemorial.

Paleoethnobotany

Paleoethnobotany, is the archaeological sub-field that studies plant remains from archaeological sites. Major research themes are recovery and identification of plant remains, the use of wild plants, the origins of agriculture and domestication, and the co-evolution of human-plant interactions. Paleoethnobotanists use a variety of methods to identify and recover plant remains. One method used to recover macroremains is to sieve excavated material manually in a water bath in order to allow the organic material to float on the surface.

This method is known as *flotation.* The matrix (the soil from a suspected archaeological feature) is slowly added to agitated water. The soil, sand, and other heavy material, known as *heavy fraction,* will sink to the bottom. The less dense organic material such as charred seeds, wood and bone will tend to float to the surface. The material that floats to the top, called *light fraction,* is gathered with a sieve. The organic light fraction is then available for examination. Samples of the heavy fraction are also gathered for later analysis. Other types flotation processes include machine-assisted flotation and froth flotation. A paleoethnobotanist may also find concentrated remains of plants that typically are only grown through active cultivation (such as corn, beans, and squash). At the same site, an archaeologist might identify features such as stone walls surrounding enclosures arrayed in a pattern, and deep, layered middens with concentrations of domesticated animal remains such as goats or pigs. An analysis of the site, set within the context of the archaeological features and animal and plant remains, would suggest a settled agrarian community.

Paleoethnobotanists also recover and analyse microremains phytoliths, pollen palynology, human paleofeces (sometimes called coprolite), and impressions in ceramic sherds (such as the imprint of grains in mixing bowl). Palynology is a mature and distinct scientific discipline that studies pollen, typically in the context of reconstructing past environments. Dendrochronology, the study of growth rings on trees relating to study of past environments, is another scientific discipline useful to paleoethnobotanical study.

Ethnocosmetics Cosmetics

Ethnocosmetics deals with the study of cosmetics of ancient past which were used by ladies to make their self beautiful. Ethnobotanical studies revealed the fact that certain plants were used as cosmetics by ancient people to look themselves much better. Like *Rosa chinensis, R. centifolia, R. damascena,* these varities of rose are still used for making cosmetics and perfumes. Earlier *Itra* were used to scent themselves and were made by pure extraction of the essential oils from the fragrent plants. *Lawsonia innermis* has long been used in India and Middle East countries for colouring palms of hands, soles of feet and finger nails. *Atropa belladonna* has long been used in Italy by ladies to dilate their pupils in a time when it was believed that the dreamy, intoxicated stare thus produced was the height of fetching beauty; an extract of belladonna was used as eye drops as part of their makeup preparations.

Ethnolinguistics Linguistic Anthropology

Ethnolinguistics is a field of linguistic anthropology which studies the language of a particular ethnic group. Ethnolinguistics is frequently associated with minority linguistic groups within a larger population, such as the Native American languages or the languages of immigrants. In these cases, ethnolinguistics studies the use of a minority language within the context of the majority population, and it also studies the perception of the language by the majority population.

More generally, ethnolinguistics studies the relationship between language and culture, and the way different ethnic groups perceive the world. A well-known (but controversial) ethnolinguistic subject is the Sapir-Whorf Hypothesis, which states that perception is limited by what can be described in one's own language.

Ethnolinguists study the way perception and conceptualization influences language, and show how this is linked to different cultures and societies. An example is the way spatial orientation is expressed in various cultures. In many societies, words for the cardinal directions East and West are derived from terms for sunrise/sunset. The nomenclature for cardinal directions of Eskimo speakers of Greenland, however, is based on geographical landmarks such as the river system and one's position on the coast. Similarly, the Yurok lack the idea of cardinal directions; they orient themselves with respect to their principal geographic feature, the Klamath River.

Ethnoorthopaedics Surgery Concerned

Ethnoorthopaedics is the study which deals with the surgery concerned with acute, chronic, traumatic, and overuse injuries and the other disorders of the musculoskeletal system by different cultures. There are not much records about the orthopaedics of ancient times. However, it was found in the literature that Edwin Smith Papyrus, an Egytian, dealed extensively with the setting of bones, traumatic injury such as dislocation of jaw, arm or shoulders, bruises, various fractures which include those of the limbs, ribs, nose, and skull.

Ethnoophthalmology Visual Pathways

It is the study which deals with the ophthalmology (surgery of the visual pathways i.e. eyes) in primitive human societies. Since ages *Atropa belladona, Emblica officinalis, Butea monoseprma, Terminallia bellerica* has been used in ophthalmology. Sushruta wrote *Sushruta Samhita* in about fifth Century B.C. in India. He described about 72 ocular diseases as well as several ophthalmological surgical instruments and techniques. Sushruta has been described as the first Indian cataract surgeon. Arab scientists are some of the earliest to have written about and drawn the anatomy of the eye—the earliest known diagram being in Hunain ibn Is-hâq's *Book of the Ten Treatises on the Eye*.

Ethnopediatrics

Ethnopediatrics is the study of parents and infants in our own and different cultures. It explores the way different care-taking styles affect the health, well-being and survival of infants. Ethnopediatrics has developed to help us understand what makes us bring up our children the way we do and to try to discover what is truly the best way to parent our babies.

All cultures are concerned with children: not only because children are vulnerable, but also because they are society's investment in the future. The human infant is perfectly designed: it knows when to sleep, when to eat and how to cry out to signal it's needs. Parenting, however, is not always straightforward. Conflict can arise in raising children not only between the baby and the caretaker, but also on the more basic level between biology and culture. Caretakers are "hard wired" to respond to a needy infant, but every adult carries personal and cultural "baggage" that determines how he or she will parent. In addition, every society has traditions that guide how adults "should" treat their offspring. The human child is slow to mature, giving parents years in which to make endless choices and decisions about how to bring up their children.

5

Use of Herbal Medicines and Alternative Medicine

In today's society, there have been many great advances in medical technology; however, with all the advancements, people are also suffering from many more chronic and terminal illnesses. One of these illnesses that have increased in today's population is cancer. Cancer is a diagnosis that evokes feelings of fear and helplessness within the individual. This disease is one that many people link with the diagnosis of certain death, but before death, there is much pain and suffering. One loses their quality of life to, not only the disease, but also to the cure itself. Usually the treatment for cancer itself is one that forces the patient to feel weak and even sicker than the illness itself.

Because of the side effects, many people choose to stop their cancer treatments of radiation or chemotherapy, though they are aware that their prognosis will be much worse without the treatments. There is very little that Western medicine can do to curb the side effects of cancer treatments.

The Western culture who are accustomed to a more natural way of healing, they tend to choose to stay with their old ways of treating illnesses, such as using herbs in Chinese medicine. Many immigrants will continue to follow their traditional ways of healing without informing their treating Western doctors for fear of ridicule or being looked down upon from their Western point of view. Therefore they may continue to use both Eastern and Western medicine together. However, if a professional who is knowledgeable of the effects does not monitor the mixing of both Eastern and Western medicine, there may be adverse reactions when the different drugs are used in conjunction. As with any patient who takes more than one medication, both the patient and the doctor need to know all of what is being used to avoid one medication affecting another, or to avoid the negative effects of mixing medications.

The ethnic backgrounds in our society, along with different traditions in healing, there needs to be an exchange of knowledge between the Western medical professionals and the traditional healing techniques of Eastern medicinal practices. There are benefits to both sides, and if combined correctly, tremendous benefits could be present for the patients. The benefits not only include the physical benefits in eliminating the cancer, but also the emotional wellbeing of the patient. In being able to explore some treatments that are familiar, the patient may feel more empowered to take the control away from the illness, and the helplessness that may come from taking a passive role in one's healing.

Complementary Medicine

The use of alternative or complementary medicine in the United States is steadily growing. People are drawn to the simplistic and holistic ideals of using more natural substances to cure the body. However, there is an unfound belief that because the herbs are all natural, they cannot harm, only heal the body. Unfortunately, this is not true. Just like medications produced in a lab, if herbal supplements are used incorrectly, they may cause more harm than good. Alternative or complementary medicine covers a wide range of options, from chiropractors, to herbs, to massage, acupuncture, acupressure, tai chi, qi gong, and may even include hypnosis and self-prayer.

The use of alternative medicine is steadily growing worldwide, estimating that 10 to 50% of the world's population is now utilizing alternative medicine on a daily basis. The use of herbal medicine has increased 380%. It is estimated that up to 50% of cancer patients utilize alternative medicine to treat their disease; however, very few inform their physicians of this use. Of this amount, 10% of patients choose to use alternative medicine in lieu of mainstream treatments. There are several reasons why people choose to use alternative medicine instead of conventional medicine, the main reason being that conventional modes of treatment may be painful or unpleasant, or tend to have a negative impact on a person's quality of life.

The use of herbs and alternative medicine, and the reluctance of patients to inform their doctors, there come risks and dangers of drug interactions. One example is there are herbs that may cause a patient to be overly sensitive to light, which increases the harm of radiation treatment. Other herbs also have anticoagulation effects on a person's blood, which poses danger to a patient during surgery. If a physician is unaware of the effects of the herbs, or of the patients' use of the herbs, it is difficult to set a beneficial treatment plan for the patient.

Physicians need to be made aware of their use of alternative medicines, therefore do not share this information. Some believe that their doctors are not familiar enough about complementary medicine, therefore there is no reason to inform them, and others do not tell their doctors because they are fearful that the doctors will discourage their continued use of alternative methods. Conventional medical treatment is the possibility of negative herb-drug interactions. This is even more of a problem if the physician prescribing the conventional treatment is unaware of the use of herbs, or the effects of specific herbs. If a physician is knowledgeable of the use of herbs and their effects, then there can be closer monitoring of specific characteristics of the patient. The doctor can make well-informed suggestions for tests and lab work to correctly monitor the patient's health. If the physician is aware of an herbs reaction with specific treatment, and it is shared with the patient, then this allows the patient the opportunity to make a well-informed decision on how to go about their own treatment of their illness. They can weigh the benefits and options of either continuing to pursue Complementary Alternative Medicine (CAM) with or without conventional treatment, or to forgo CAM and choose only conventional treatment.

Traditional Chinese Medicinal Practices

The lack of professionals within the medical setting that can broker between the modern Western practices and the traditional Chinese medicinal practices. With the possible benefits that traditional Chinese medicine has, and the large number of people who use Chinese medicine without a doctor's supervision, it will benefit the medical profession as well as the public to have trained professional social workers within oncology clinics to advocate for those who wish to choose alternative medicines along with Western medical treatments.

The purpose of this project is to create a social work position within a cancer treatment centre to assist patients in their treatment by helping bridge the gap between Western medicine and Traditional Chinese Medicine (TCM). The social worker will have training in the use and benefits of TCM, to be able to inform patients of their options. This will allow patients to make informed decisions about how to progress with their treatment. One of the responsibilities will be to advocate to the doctors for the patients' choice to use alternative medicine along with their Western methods of treatment.

Empowerment Perspective

The empowerment perspective states that an individual's feelings of powerlessness play a large role in an individual's experience, and how they interact and react to others. The term "empowerment" is described as the process of increasing the personal, interpersonal, and/or political power. By doing this, it allows the individual to take action in order to improve their life situation. This theoretical framework found its beginnings in community organization, adult education techniques, and feminist theory.

Eempowerment is the description of the development of the individual's feeling of increased power or control without any actual changes in structural arrangements. Through the process of empowering oneself, the person develops a sense of personal power. There are some psychological changes that appear to occur in individuals as they transition from a state of apathy and despair to action. One of these changes is described as increasing "self-efficacy" which is an individual's ability "to produce and to regulate events in one's life.". This is usually explained by examples of people who seem to display a sense of personal power or strength that seems to increase as they become more empowered. For many oncology patients, immediately after receiving a diagnosis of cancer, there are extreme feelings of fear and a feeling that they have lost control over their own lives, and their own bodies. This disease is controlling their physical bodies, mind and lives.

Some feelings that have been linked to self-blame are depression and feelings of being immobilized. By being able to reduce these feelings, and change patients' focus from feeling helpless, to feeling that they are able to change their situation increases feelings of control. Some cancer patients may begin to question what it is they may have done to bring on this diagnosis and suffering onto themselves. Some may blame the things they did to their physical bodies; did they eat the wrong things, should they have quit smoking or drinking earlier, should I have found a line of work that had better working conditions? Those that may be more spiritual may believe that they have done something sinful or wrong, and that the cancer diagnosis is punishment for their sinful deeds. By being able to move out of this mindset, patients begin to be able to see that perhaps the disease is not punishment and undeserved, this may assist them in being more open to suggestions and healing.

The empowerment perspective, there is an assumption of personal responsibility for change. By taking personal responsibility, patients may be more likely to take an active role, and put more effort into improving their lives and their health. This may cause patients to perform more research on their illness and which options are available to them. By taking action, and personal responsibility for their own health and well-being, they begin to take action against the disease and become active participants in their treatment plans.

Currently, in the medical field, the nurses and doctors are working from the paternalistic model where patients are expected to follow the directions of the doctor, who is seen as the knowledgeable and unquestionable one in the doctor-patient relationship. By changing the model to one of patient empowerment, there are benefits to this relationship, and may improve the patient's experience with one's doctor on five characteristics: acceptance, which is used to describe the doctors' need to accept the patient as they are. Affect, which describes how the patient and the doctor respond to each other as the partnership relationship evolves. Autonomy, which describes the patients' right to play as large or as small a role in the treatment as the patient wishes. Alliance is the description of the partnership, and the relationship building between doctor and patient that is supported by active participation by the patient. Patient empowerment is not only important in the eyes of the patient, but also from the healthcare professionals' opinion as well.

HISTORY OF HERBAL MEDICINE

Quite possibly the earliest form of herbal medicine was marshmallow root, which is a common grass chewed for settling an upset stomach, and has been eaten for (presumably) that reason by our closest evolutionary cousins, chimpanzees and bonobos. Likewise, hyacinth (a diuretic) causes the tissues to give up excess water, is rich in tannins and alkaloids, which have a bitter, or pungent taste.

As tribal human societies grew, a small body of knowledge over what plants were beneficial for what ailments grew, until the role of a tribal herb lore specialist became known; often times, in hunter-gatherer societies, this herbalist carries a lot of weight in the day to day running of the tribe.

As human societies shifted to an agronomical view of the world, the cultivation of plants for medicine was an important role in this; eventually, herbal lore and herbal remedies became codified, first with the Egyptians, then with the Greeks in the Western tradition, and the knowledge base was slowly accumulated upon by the Romans. It's from the Greeks in particular that the foundation of modern medicine-of not just prescribing a treatment, but recording what the treatment was, and what its impact was, got started.

In India, the herbalist tradition was Ayurvedic, focusing on the use of metals, herbs and parts of animals generally considered inedible, prepared in solution. These herbs and other compounds are used in varying proportions to remedy specific ills, and may be applied internally as pills or infusions, topically as ointments, inhaled as smoke, or pressed to the body as powders. In the Americas, without a written tradition to work from, most herbalism is carried by oral traditions from various tribes; this has proven invaluable when looking for herbal remedies in the rain forests and Andean uplands. Much of the American herbal tradition is tied to shamanism and spiritualism.

In China, herbalism and herbal remedies were used as an adjunct to acupuncture, and the medical morphology in use is of balancing qui or chi, the life force energies, which have yin and yang elements; in Chinese herbalism, the aim is to bring the systems of the body, treating it as an electrical system, back into balance, which is a tactic commonly expressed in modern, or syncretic herbalism.

Herbal Medicine Today

Modern herbal medicine takes a syncretic approach, trying to cross reference the benefits of various herbs and treatments from different traditions, and find the best combination of herbal remedies. It's estimated that upwards of three quarters of the people on the planet use herbal medicine as part of their primary health care regimen. Furthermore, it's estimated that nearly three quarters of all naturally derived medicines are used in ways conforming to their herbal component's or antecedents traditional use, and somewhere close to one third of all medical research begins with botanical research of samples collected from rain forests and other biomes.

Most traditional herbs are aromatics-the compounds we use to treat illness are an effect of plants conducting chemical warfare on each other and to fend off herbivores. The same compounds that make many herbs bitter or smell strongly are the ones used in herbal medicine and clinical trials. While there are countless claims that herbal remedies have "no side effect", this is not the case; it's more than the side effects cannot be attributed to one compound in the herbal repertoire, and sometimes this leads to dangers-for example, cochinea was used to treat gout (rheumatoid arthritis, and a number of related symptoms), but also has severe side effects on the function of the kidneys and liver, as it's a slow, cumulative toxin. The primary difference in side effects between herbal remedies and those listed in the Physician's Desk Reference is that the Physician's Desk Reference has double blind studies listing what dosages cause which side effects, while many herbal remedies lack this benchmark. That being said, most traditional therapeutic doses of herbal remedies are small enough to avoid the worst side effects. (Whether some herbs have their effect from the placebo effect is also open to dispute). While herbal remedies can be beneficial, do understand that they are not an either-or proposition with modern medicine, though there is a strong establishment precedent for treating them that way-up until the early part of this century, most of the remedies prescribed by doctors were herbal and natural remedies. Do consult with your health care provider about possible interactions between herbal remedies and prescription drugs.

HERBALISM: TRADITIONAL MEDICINE

Herbalism is a traditional medicinal or folk medicine practice based on the use of plants and plant extracts. Herbalism is also known as botanical medicine, medical herbalism, herbal medicine, herbology, and phytotherapy. The scope of herbal medicine is sometimes extended to include fungal and bee products, as well as minerals, shells and certain animal parts. Pharmacognosy is the study of medicines derived from natural sources.

Traditional use of medicines is recognized as a way to learn about potential future medicines. In 2001, researchers identified 122 compounds used in mainstream medicine which were derived from "ethnomedical" plant sources; 80% of these compounds were used in the same or related manner as the traditional ethnomedical use. Many plants synthesize substances that are useful to the maintenance of health in humans and other animals. These include aromatic substances, most of which are phenols or their oxygen-substituted derivatives such as tannins. Many are secondary metabolites, of which at least 12,000 have been isolated — a number estimated to be less than 10% of the total. In many cases, substances such as alkaloids serve as plant defense mechanisms against predation by microorganisms, insects, and herbivores. Many of the herbs and spices used by humans to season food yield useful medicinal compounds.

Similarly to prescription drugs, a number of herbs are thought to be likely to cause adverse effects. Furthermore, "adulteration, inappropriate formulation, or lack of understanding of plant and drug interactions have led to adverse reactions that are sometimes life threatening or lethal. Although such Adverse Drug Events are minuscule compared with the 20% of GP visitations said to be due to ADRs of conventional drugs. or the 6-7% of hospital admissions due to ADRs Well manufactured herbal products have far fewer ADRs and/or side effects generally than many drugs.

Anthropology of Herbalism

People on all continents have used hundreds to thousands of indigenous plants for treatment of ailments since prehistoric times. Medicinal herbs were found in the personal effects of *Ötzi the Iceman*, whose body was frozen in the Ötztal Alps for more than 5,300 years. These herbs appear to have been used to treat the parasites found in his intestines. Anthropologists theorize that animals evolved a tendency to seek out bitter plant parts in response to illness. Indigenous healers often claim to have learned by observing that sick animals change their food preferences to nibble at bitter herbs they would normally reject.

Field biologists have provided corroborating evidence based on observation of diverse species, such as chimpanzees, chickens, sheep and butterflies. Lowland gorillas take 90% of their diet from the fruits of *Aframomum melegueta*, a relative of the ginger plant, that is a potent antimicrobial and apparently keeps shigellosis and similar infections at bay. Current research focuses on the possibility that this plants also protects gorillas from fibrosing cardiomyopathy which has a devastating effect on captive animals.

Researchers from Ohio Wesleyan University found that some birds select nesting material rich in antimicrobial agents which protect their young from harmful bacteria. Sick animals tend to forage plants rich in secondary metabolites, such as tannins and alkaloids. Since these phytochemicals often have antiviral, antibacterial, antifungal and antihelminthic properties, a plausible case can be made for self-medication by animals in the wild.

Some animals have digestive systems especially adapted to cope with certain plant toxins. For example, the koala can live on the leaves and shoots of the eucalyptus, a plant that is dangerous to most animals. A plant that is harmless to a particular animal may not be safe for humans to ingest. A reasonable conjecture is that these discoveries were traditionally collected by the medicine people of indigenous tribes, who then passed on safety information and cautions.

The use of herbs and spices in cuisine developed in part as a response to the threat of food-borne pathogens. Studies show that in tropical climates where pathogens are the most abundant, recipes are the most highly spiced. Further, the spices with the most potent antimicrobial activity tend to be selected. In all cultures vegetables are spiced less than meat, presumably because they are more resistant to spoilage.

History

The use of plants as medicines predates written human history. A 60 000-year-old Neanderthal burial site, "SHANIDAR-4", in northern Iraq has yielded large amounts of pollen from 8 plant species, 7 of which are used now as herbal remedies. In the written record, the study of herbs dates back over 5,000 years to the Sumerians, who described well-established medicinal uses for such plants as laurel, caraway, and thyme. Ancient Egyptian medicine of 1000 B.C. are known to have used garlic, opium, castor oil, coriander, mint, indigo, and other herbs for medicine and the Old Testament also mentions herb use and cultivation, including mandrake, vetch, caraway, wheat, barley, and rye.

In Indian Ayurveda medicine has used many herbs such as turmeric possibly as early as 1900 B.C. Many other herbs and minerals used in Ayurveda were later described by ancient Indian herbalists such as Charaka and Sushruta during the 1st millennium BC. The Sushruta Samhita attributed to Sushruta in the 6th century BC describes 700 medicinal plants, 64 preparations from mineral sources, and 57 preparations based on animal sources.

The first Chinese herbal book, the Shennong Bencao Jing, compiled during the Han Dynasty but dating back to a much earlier date, possibly 2700 B.C., lists 365 medicinal plants and their uses-including ma-Huang, the shrub that introduced the drug ephedrine to modern medicine. Succeeding generations augmented on the Shennong Bencao Jing, as in the Yaoxing Lun (Treatise on the Nature of Medicinal Herbs), a 7th century Tang Dynasty treatise on herbal medicine. The ancient Greeks and Romans made medicinal use of plants. Greek and Roman medicinal practices, as preserved in the writings of Hippocrates and-especially-Galen, provided the pattern for later western medicine. Hippocrates advocated the use of a few simple herbal drugs-along with fresh air, rest, and proper diet. Galen, on the other hand, recommended large doses of drug mixtures-including plant, animal, and mineral ingredients. The Greek physician compiled the first European treatise on the properties and uses of medicinal plants, De Materia Medica. In the first century AD, Dioscorides wrote a compendium of more than 500 plants that remained an authoritative reference into the 17th century. Similarly important for herbalists and botanists of later centuries was the Greek book that founded the science of botany, Theophrastus' Historia Plantarum, written in the fourth century B.C.

Modern Era

The fifteenth, sixteenth, and seventeenth centuries were the great age of herbals, many of them available for the first time in English and other languages rather than Latin or Greek. The first herbal to be published in English was the anonymous *Grete Herball* of 1526. The two best-known herbals in English were *The Herball or General History of Plants* (1597) by John Gerard and *The English Physician Enlarged* (1653) by Nicholas Culpeper. Gerard's text was basically a pirated translation of a book by the Belgian herbalist Dodoens and his illustrations came from a German botanical work. The original edition contained many errors due to faulty matching of the two parts. Culpeper's blend of traditional medicine with astrology, magic, and folklore was ridiculed by the physicians of his day yet his book-like Gerard's and other herbals-enjoyed phenomenal popularity. The Age of Exploration and the Columbian Exchange introduced new medicinal plants to Europe. The *Badianus Manuscript* was an illustrated Aztec herbal translated into Latin in the 16th century.

The second millennium, however, also saw the beginning of a slow erosion of the pre-eminent position held by plants as sources of therapeutic effects. This began with the Black Death, which the then dominant Four Element medical system proved powerless to stop. A century later, Paracelsus introduced the use of active chemical drugs (like arsenic, copper sulfate, iron, mercury, and sulfur). These were accepted even though they had toxic effects because of the urgent need to treat Syphilis. The rapid development of chemistry and the other physical sciences, led increasingly to the dominance of chemotherapy-chemical medicine-as the orthodox system of the twentieth century.

Role in Modern Human Society

The use of herbs to treat disease is almost universal among non-industrialized societies. A number of traditions came to dominate the practice of herbal medicine at the end of the twentieth century:

- The "classical" herbal medicine system, based on Greek and Roman sources
- The Siddha and Ayurvedic medicine systems from various South Asian Countries
- Chinese herbal medicine (Chinese herbology)-No*f* (zhôngyào)
- Traditional African medicine
- Unani-Tibb medicine
- Shamanic herbalism: a catch-all phrase for information mostly supplied from South America and the Himalayas
- Native American medicine.

Many of the pharmaceuticals currently available to physicians have a long history of use as herbal remedies, including opium, aspirin, digitalis, and quinine. The World Health Organization (WHO) estimates that 80 percent of the world's population presently uses herbal medicine for some aspect of primary health care. Pharmaceuticals are prohibitively expensive for most of the world's population, half of which lives on less than $2 U.S. per day. In comparison, herbal medicines can be grown from seed or gathered from nature for little or no cost.

In addition to the use in the developing world, herbal medicine is used in industrialized nations by alternative medicine practitioners such as naturopaths. A 1998 survey of herbalists in the UK found that many of the herbs recommended by them were used traditionally but had not been evaluated in clinical trials. In Australia, a 2007 survey found that these Western herbalists tend to prescribe liquid herbal combinations of herbs rather than tablets of single herbs. The use of, and search for, drugs and dietary supplements derived from plants have accelerated in recent years. Pharmacologists, microbiologists, botanists, and natural-products chemists are combing the Earth for phytochemicals and leads that could be developed for treatment of various diseases. In fact, according to the World Health Organisation, approximately 25% of modern drugs used in the United States have been derived from plants.

- Among the 120 active compounds currently isolated from the higher plants and widely used in modern medicine today, 80 percent show a positive correlation between their modern therapeutic use and the traditional use of the plants from which they are derived.
- More than two thirds of the world's plant species-at least 35,000 of which are estimated to have medicinal value-come from the developing countries.
- At least 7,000 medical compounds in the modern pharmacopoeia are derived from plants.

Biological Background

All plants produce chemical compounds as part of their normal metabolic activities. These are divided into primary metabolites, such as sugars and fats, found in all plants, and secondary metabolites, compounds not essential for basic function found in a smaller range of plants, some useful ones found only in a particular genus or species. Pigments harvest light, protect the organism from radiation and display colors to attract pollinators. Many common weeds, such as nettle, dandelion and chickweed, have medicinal properties. The functions of secondary metabolites are varied. For example, some secondary metabolites are toxins used to deter predation, and others are pheromones used to attract insects for pollination. Phytoalexins protect against bacterial and fungal attacks. Allelochemicals inhibit rival plants that are competing for soil and light. Plants upregulate and downregulate their biochemical paths in response to the local mix of herbivores, pollinators and microorganisms. The chemical profile of a single plant may vary over time as it reacts to changing conditions. It is the secondary metabolites and pigments that can have therapeutic actions in humans and which can be refined to produce drugs.

Plants synthesize a bewildering variety of phytochemicals but most are derivatives of a few biochemical motifs.

- Alkaloids contain a ring with nitrogen. Many alkaloids have dramatic effects on the central nervous system. Caffeine is an alkaloid that provides a mild lift but the alkaloids in datura cause severe intoxication and even death.
- Polyphenol, also known as phenolics, contain phenol rings. The anthocyanins that give grapes their purple color, the isoflavones, the phytoestrogens from soy and the tannins that give tea its astringency are phenolics.
- Terpenoids are built up from terpene building blocks. Each terpene consists of two paired isoprenes. The names monoterpenes, sesquiterpenes, diterpenes and triterpenes are based on the number of isoprene units. The fragrance of rose and lavender is due to monoterpenes. The carotenoids produce the reds, yellows and oranges of pumpkin, corn and tomatoes.
- Glycosides consist of a glucose moiety attached to an aglycone. The aglycone is a molecule that is bioactive in its free form but inert until the glycoside bond is broken by water or enzymes. This mechanism allows the plant to defer the availability of the molecule to an appropriate time, similar to a safety lock on a gun. An example is the cyanoglycosides in cherry pits that release toxins only when bitten by a herbivore.

The word drug itself comes from the Dutch word "droog" (via the French word Drogue), which means 'dried plant'. Some examples are inulin from the roots of dahlias, quinine from the cinchona, morphine and codeine from the poppy, and digoxin from the foxglove. The active ingredient in willow bark, once prescribed by Hippocrates, is salicin, which is converted in the body into salicylic acid. The discovery of salicylic acid would eventually lead to the development of the acetylated form acetylsalicylic acid, also known as "aspirin", when it was isolated from a plant known as meadowsweet. The word *aspirin* comes from an abbreviation of meadowsweet's Latin genus *Spiraea*, with an additional "A" at the beginning to acknowledge acetylation, and "in" was added at the end for easier pronunciation. "Aspirin" was originally a brand name, and is still a protected trademark in some countries. This medication was patented by Bayer AG.

TYPES OF HERBAL MEDICINE SYSTEMS

Use of medicinal plants can be as informal as, for example, culinary use or consumption of an herbal tea or supplement, although the sale of some herbs considered dangerous is often restricted to the public. Sometimes such herbs are provided to professional herbalists by specialist companies. Many herbalists, both professional and amateur, often grow or "wildcraft" their own herbs.

Some researchers trained in both western and traditional Chinese medicine have attempted to deconstruct ancient medical texts in the light of modern science. One idea is that the yin-yang balance, at least with regard to herbs, corresponds to the pro-oxidant and anti-oxidant balance. This interpretation is supported by several investigations of the ORAC ratings of various yin and yang herbs.

In America, early settlers relied on plants imported from Europe, and also from local Indian knowledge. One particularly successful practitioner, Samuel Thomson developed a hugely popular system of medicine. This approach was subsequently broadened to include concepts introduced from modern physiology, a discipline called Physiomedicalism. Another group, the Eclectics, were a later offshoot from the orthodox medical profession, who were looking to avoid the then current medical treatments of mercury and bleeding, and introduced herbal medicine into their practices. Both groups were eventually overcome by the actions of the American Medical Association, which was formed for this purpose. Cherokee medicine tends to divide herbs into foods, medicines and toxins and to use seven plants in the treatment of disease, which is defined with both spiritual and physiological aspects, according to Cherokee herbalist David Winston.

In India, Ayurvedic medicine has quite complex formulas with 30 or more ingredients, including a sizable number of ingredients that have undergone "alchemical processing", chosen to balance "Vata", "Pitta" or "Kapha."

In Tamil Nadu, Tamils have their own medicinal system now popularly called the Siddha medicinal system. The Siddha system is entirely in the Tamil language. It contains roughly 300,000 verses covering diverse aspects of medicine such as anatomy, sex ("kokokam" is the sexual treatise of par excellence), herbal, mineral and metallic compositions to cure many diseases that are relevant even to-day. Ayurveda is in Sanskrit, but Sanskrit was not generally used as a mother tongue and hence its medines are mostly taken from Siddha and other local traditions. In addition there are more modern theories of herbal combination like William LeSassier's triune formula which combined Pythagorean imagery with Chinese medicine ideas and resulted in 9 herb formulas which supplemented, drained or neutrally nourished the main organ systems affected and three associated systems.

His system has been taught to thousands of influential American herbalists through his own apprenticeship programs during his lifetime, the William LeSassier Archive and the David Winston Centre for Herbal Studies. Different chemicals in herbs are more abundant than in a single drug. Some chemicals in herbs may work as growth hormones or antibiotics, nutrients, and toxin neutralizers. Many traditional African remedies have performed well in initial laboratory tests to ensure they are not toxic and in tests on animals. Gawo, a herb used in traditional treatments, has been tested in rats by researchers from Nigeria's University of Jos and the National Institute for Pharmaceutical Research and Development. According to research in the African Journal of Biotechnology, Gawo passed tests for toxicity and reduced induced fevers, diarrhoea and inflammation.

Routes of Administration

The exact composition of a herbal product is influenced by the method of extraction. A tisane will be rich in polar components because water is a polar solvent. Oil on the other hand is a non-polar solvent and it will absorb non-polar compounds. Alcohol lies somewhere in between. There are many forms in which herbs can be administered, these include:

- Tinctures-Alcoholic extracts of herbs such as Echinacea extract. Usually obtained by combining 100% pure ethanol (or a mixture of 100% ethanol with water) with the herb. A completed tincture has a ethanol percentage of at least 25% (sometimes up to 90%). The term tincture is sometimes applied to preparations using other solvents than ethanol.
- Herbal wine and elixirs-These are alcoholic extract of herbs; usually with an ethanol percentage of 12-38% Herbal wine is a maceration of herbs in wine, while an elixir is a maceration of herbs in spirits (e.g., vodka, grappa, etc.)

- Tisanes-Hot water extracts of herb, such as chamomile.
- Decoctions-Long-term boiled extract of usually roots or bark.
- Macerates-Cold infusion of plants with high mucilage-content as sage, thyme, etc. Plants are chopped and added to cold water. They are then left to stand for 7 to 12 hours (depending on herb used). For most macerates 10 hours is used.
- Vinegars-Prepared at the same way as tinctures, except using a solution of acetic acid as the solvent.
- Topicals:
    - o Essential oils-Application of essential oil extracts, usually diluted in a carrier oil (many essential oils can burn the skin or are simply too high dose used straight – diluting in olive oil or another food grade oil such as almond oil can allow these to be used safely as a topical).
    - o Salves, oils, balms, creams and lotions-Most topical applications are oil extractions of herbs. Taking a food grade oil and soaking herbs in it for anywhere from weeks to months allows certain phytochemicals to be extracted into the oil. This oil can then be made into salves, creams, lotions, or simply used as an oil for topical application. Any massage oils, antibacterial salves and wound healing compounds are made this way.
    - o Poultices and compresses-One can also make a poultice or compress using whole herb (or the appropriate part of the plant) usually crushed or dried and re-hydrated with a small amount of water and then applied directly in a bandage, cloth or just as is.
- Whole herb consumption-This can occur in either dried form (herbal powder), or fresh juice, (fresh leaves and other plant parts).
- Syrups-Extracts of herbs made with syrup or honey. Sixty five parts of sugar are mixed with 35 parts of water and herb. The whole is then boiled and macerated for three weeks.
- Extracts-Include liquid extracts, dry extracts and nebulisates. Liquid extracts are liquids with a lower ethanol percentage than tinctures. They can (and are usually) made by vacuum distilling tinctures. Dry extracts are extracts of plant material which are evaporated into a dry mass. They can then be further refined to a capsule or tablet. A nebulisate is a dry extract created by freeze-drying.
- Inhalation as in aromatherapy can be used as a mood changing treatment to fight a sinus infection or cough, or to cleanse the skin on a deeper level (steam rather than direct inhalation here).
- Apply fresh herb paste on skin.

- Ground herb and boil in water such as herbal tea.

Examples of Plants Used as Medicine

Few herbal remedies have conclusively demonstrated any positive effect on humans, possibly due to inadequate testing. Many of the studies cited refer to animal model investigations or in-vitro assays and therefore cannot provide more than weak supportive evidence.

- *Aloe vera* has traditionally been used for the healing of burns and wounds. A systematic review (from 1999) states that the efficacy of aloe vera in promoting wound healing is unclear, while a later review (from 2007) concludes that the cumulative evidence supports the use of aloe vera for the healing of first to second degree burns.
- Artichoke (*Cynara cardunculus*) may reduce production cholesterol levels according to *in vitro* studies and a small clinical study.
- Blackberry (*Rubus fruticosus*) leaf has drawn the attention of the cosmetology community because it interferes with the metalloproteinases that contribute to skin wrinkling.
- Black raspberry *(Rubus occidentalis)* may have a role in preventing oral cancer.
- Boophone (*Boophone disticha*) This highly toxic plant has been used in South African traditional medicine for treatment of mental illness. Research demonstrate *in vitro* and *in vivo* effect against depression.
- Butterbur *(Petasites hybridus)*
- Calendula *(Calendula officinalis)* has been used traditionally for abdominal cramps and constipation. In animal research an aqueous-ethanol extract of *Calendula officinalis* flowers was shown to have both spasmolytic and spasmogenic effects, thus providing a scientific rationale for this traditional use. There is "limited evidence" that calendula cream or ointment is effective in treating radiation dermatitis.
- Cannabis, see also medical cannabis.
- Cranberry *(Vaccinium oxycoccos)* may be effective in treating urinary tract infections in women with recurrent symptoms.
- Echinacea (*Echinacea angustifolia, Echinacea pallida, Echinacea purpurea*) extracts may limit the length and severity of rhinovirus colds; however, the appropriate dosage levels, which might be higher than is available over-the-counter, require further research.
- Elderberry (*Sambucus nigra*) may speed the recovery from type A and B influenza. However it is possibly risky in the case of avian influenza because the immunostimulatory effects may aggravate the cytokine cascade.

- Feverfew (*Chrysanthemum parthenium*) is sometimes used to treat migraine headaches. Although many reviews of Feverfew studies show no or unclear efficacy, a more recent RTC showed favourable results Feverfew is not recommended for pregnant women as it may be dangerous to the fetus.
- Gawo (*Faidherbia albida*), a traditional herbal medicine in West Africa, has shown promise in animal tests
- Garlic (*Allium sativum*) may lower total cholesterol levels.
- German Chamomile (*Matricaria chamomilla*) has demonstrated antispasmodic, anxiolytic, antiinflammatory and some antimutagenic and cholesterol-lowering effects in animal research. *In vitro* chamomile has demonstrated moderate antimicrobial and antioxidant properties and significant antiplatelet activity, as well as preliminary results against cancer. Essential oil of chamomile was shown to be a promising antiviral agent against herpes simplex virus type 2 (HSV-2) *in vitro*.
- Ginger (*Zingiber officinale*), administered in 250 mg capsules for four days, effectively decreased nausea and vomiting of pregnancy in a human clinical trial.
- Grapefruit (Naringenin) components may prevent obesity.
- Green tea (*Camelia sinensis*) components may inhibit growth of breast cancer cells and may heal scars faster.
- Purified extracts of the seeds of *Hibiscus sabdariffa* may have some antihypertensive, antifungal and antibacterial effect. Toxicity tested low except for an isolated case of damage to the testes of a rat after prolonged and excessive consumption.
- Honey may reduce cholesterol. May be useful in wound healing.
- Lemon grass (*Cymbopogon citratus*), administered daily as an aqueous extract of the fresh leaf, has lowered total cholesterol and fasting plasma glucose levels in rats, as well as increasing HDL cholesterol levels. Lemon grass administration had no effect on triglyceride levels.
- Magnolia
- Meadowsweet (*Filipendula ulmaria, Spiraea ulmaria*) can be used for a variety of anti-inflammatory and antimicrobial purposes due to presence of salicylic acid. Effective for fevers and inflammations, pain relief, ulcers and bacteriostatic. Listed as therapeutical in 1652 by Nicholas Culpeper. In 1838, salicylic acid was isolated from the plant. The word Aspirin is derived from spirin, based on Meadowsweet's synonym name Spiraea ulmaria.
- Milk thistle (*Silybum marianum*) extracts have been recognized for many centuries as "liver tonics.". Research suggests that milk thistle extracts

both prevent and repair damage to the liver from toxic chemicals and medications.

- Morinda citrifolia (noni) is used in the Pacific and Caribbean islands for the treatment of inflammation and pain. Human studies indicate potential cancer preventive effects.
- Nigella sativa (Black cumin) has demonstrated analgesic properties in mice. The mechanism for this effect, however, is unclear. In vitro studies support antibacterial, antifungal, anticancer, anti-inflammatory and immune modulating effects. However few randomized double blind studies have been published.
- Ocimum gratissimum and tea tree oil can be used to treat acne.
- Oregano (*Origanum vulgare*) may be effective against multi-drug resistant bacteria.
- Pawpaw can be used as insecticide (killing lice, worms).,
- Peppermint oil may have benefits for individuals with irritable bowel syndrome.
- Phytolacca or Pokeweed can be applied topically or taken internally. Topical treatments have been used for acne and other ailments. It is used as a treatment for tonsilitis, swollen glands and weight loss.
- Pomegranate contains the highest percentage of ellagitannins of any commonly consumed juice. Punicalagin, an ellagitannin unique to pomegranate, is the highest molecular weight polyphenol known. Ellagitannins are metabolized into urolithins by gut flora, and have been shown to inhibit cancer cell growth in mice.
- Rauvolfia Serpentina, high risk of toxicity if improperly used, used extensively in India for sleeplessness, anxiety, and high blood pressure.
- Rooibos (*Aspalathus linearis*) contains a number of phenolic compounds, including flavanols, flavones, flavanones, flavonols, and dihydrochalcones. Rooibos has traditionally been used for skin ailments, allergies, asthma and colic in infants. In an animal study with diabetic mice, aspalathin, a rooibos constituent improved glucose homeostasis by stimulating insulin secretion in pancreatic beta cells and glucose uptake in muscle tissue.
- Rose hips – Small scale studies indicate that hips from *Rosa canina* may provide benefits in the treatment of osteoarthritis. Rose hips show anti COX activity.
- Salvia lavandulaefolia may improve memory
- Saw Palmetto can be used for BPH. Supported in some studies, failed to confirm in others.
- Shiitake mushrooms (*Lentinus edodes*) are edible mushrooms that have been reported to have health benefits, including cancer-preventing

properties. In laboratory research a shiitake extract has inhibited the growth of tumor cells through induction of apoptosis. Both a water extract and fresh juice of shiitake have demonstrated antimicrobial activity against pathogenic bacteria and fungi in vitro.

- Soy and other plants that contain phytoestrogens (plant molecules with estrogen activity) (black cohosh probably has serotonin activity) have some benefits for treatment of symptoms resulting from menopause.
- St. John's wort, has yielded positive results, proving more effective than a placebo for the treatment of mild to moderate depression in some clinical trials A subsequent, large, controlled trial, however, found St. John's wort to be no better than a placebo in treating depression However, more recent trials have shown positive results or positive trends that failed significance. A 2004 meta-analysis concluded that the positive results can be explained by publication bias but later analyses have been more favourable. The Cochrane Database cautions that the data on St. John's wort for depression are conflicting and ambiguous.
- Stinging nettle In some clinical studies effective for benign prostatic hyperplasia and the pain associated with osteoarthritis. In-vitro tests show antiinflammatory action. In a rodent model, stinging nettle reduced LDL cholesterol and total cholesterol. In another rodent study it reduced platelet aggregation.
- Umckaloabo (*Pelargonium sidoides*): an extract of this plant showed efficacy in the treatment of acute bronchitis in a controlled trial and is approved for this use in Germany.
- Valerian root can be used to treat insomnia. Clinical studies show mixed results and researchers note that many trials are of poor quality.
- Vanilla
- Willow bark (*Salix alba*) can be used for a variety of anti-inflammatory and antimicrobial purposes due to presence of salicylic acid and tannins. Has been in use for aprox. 6000yrs and was described in the 1st century AD by Dioscorides.

Name Confusion

The common names of herbs (folk taxonomy) may not reflect differences in scientific taxonomy, and the same (or a very similar) common name might group together different plant species with different effects.

For example, in 1993 in Belgium, medical doctors created a formula including some Traditional Chinese medicine (TCM) herbs for weight loss. One herb (*Stephania tetrandra*) was swapped for another (*Aristolochia fangchi*) whose name in Chinese was extremely similar but which contained higher levels of a renal toxin, aristolochic acid; this mistake resulted in 105 cases of kidney damage.

Note that neither herb used in a TCM context would be used for weight loss or given for long periods of time. In Chinese medicine these herbs are used for certain forms of acute arthritis and edema.

For this reason, Western herbalists use binomial nomenclature in their terminology within the profession.

Effectiveness

The highest standard for pharmaceutical testing is repeated, small-scale, randomized, double-blind tests. In 2002 the U.S. National Centre for Complementary and Alternative Medicine of the National Institutes of Health began funding clinical trials into the effectiveness of herbal medicine. In a 2010 survey of 1000 plants, 356 had clinical trials published evaluating their "pharmacological activities and therapeutic applications" while 12% of the plants, although available in the Western market, had "no substantial studies" of their properties.

Many herbs have shown positive results in-vitro, animal model or small-scale clinical tests but many studies on herbal treatments have also found negative results. The quality of the trials on herbal remedies is highly variable and many trials of herbal treatments have been found to be of poor quality, with many trials lacking an intention to treat analysis or a comment on whether blinding was successful. The few randomized, double-blind tests that receive attention in medical publications are often questioned on methodological grounds or interpretation. Likewise, studies published in peer-reviewed medical journals such as Journal of the American Medical Association receive more consideration than those published in specialized herbal journals.

One study found that non-impact factor alternative medicine journals published more studies with positive results than negative results and that trials finding positive results were of lower quality than trials finding negative results. High impact factor mainstream medical journals, on the other hand, published equal numbers of trials with positive and negative results. In high impact journals, trials finding positive results were also found to have lower quality scores than trials finding negative results. Another study reported that some clinical studies of herbal medicines were not inferior to similar medical studies. However, this study used a matched pair design and excluded all herbal trials that were not controlled, did not use a placebo or did not use random or quasi random assignment.

Herbalists criticize mainstream studies on the grounds that they make insufficient use of historical usage, which has been shown useful in drug discovery and development in the past and present They maintain that tradition can guide the selection of factors such as optimal dose, species, time of harvesting and target population.

Dosage is in general an outstanding issue for herbal treatments: while most medicines are heavily tested to determine the most effective and safest dosages (especially in relation to things like body weight, drug interactions, etc.), there are fewer varieties of dosages for various herbal treatments on the market. Furthermore, from a conventional pharmacological perspective, herbal medicines taken in whole form cannot generally guarantee a consistent dosage or drug quality, since certain samples may contain more or less of a given active ingredient.

Several methods of standardization may be applied to herbs. One is the ratio of raw materials to solvent. However different specimens of even the same plant species may vary in chemical content. For this reason, thin layer chromatography is sometimes used by growers to assess the content of their products before use. Another method is standardization on a signal chemical.

Standards and Quality Control

The issue of regulation is an area of continuing controversy in the EU and USA. At one end of the spectrum, some herbalists maintain that traditional remedies have a long history of use, and do not require the level of safety testing as xenobiotics or single ingredients in an artificially concentrated form. On the other hand, others are in favour of legally enforced quality standards, safety testing and prescription by a qualified practitioner. Some professional herbalist organizations have made statements calling for a category of regulation for herbal products. Yet others agree with the need for more quality testing but believe it can be managed through reputation without government intervention. The legal status of herbal ingredients varies by country. In the EU, herbal medicines are now regulated under the European Directive on Traditional Herbal Medicinal Products.

In the United States, most herbal remedies are regulated as dietary supplements by the Food and Drug Administration. Manufacturers of products falling into this category are not required to prove the safety or efficacy of their product, though the FDA may withdraw a product from sale should it prove harmful.

The National Nutritional Foods Association, the industry's largest trade association, has run a program since 2002, examining the products and factory conditions of member companies, giving them the right to display the GMP (Good Manufacturing Practices) seal of approval on their products. In the UK, herbal remedies that are bought over the counter are regulated as supplements, as in the US. However, herbal remedies prescribed and dispensed by a qualified "Medical Herbalist", after a personal consultation, are regulated as medicines. A Medical Herbalist can prescribe some herbs which are not available over the counter, covered by Schedule III of the Medicines Act. Forthcoming changes to laws regulating herbal products in the UK, are intended to ensure the quality of herbal products used. Some herbs, such as Cannabis, are outright banned in most countries. Since 2004, the sales of ephedra as an dietary supplement is prohibited in the United States by the Food and Drug Administration., and subject to Schedule III restrictions in the United Kingdom.

HISTORY OF USE OF TRADITIONAL HERBAL MEDICINES

Through definition, 'traditional' use of herbal medicines implies substantial historical use, and this is certainly true for many products that are available as 'traditional herbal medicines'. In many developing countries, a large proportion of the population relies on traditional practitioners and their armamentarium of medicinal plants in order to meet health care needs. Although modern medicine may exist side-by-side with such traditional practice, herbal medicines have often maintained their popularity for historical and cultural reasons. Such products have become more widely available commercially, especially in developed countries. In this modern setting, ingredients are sometimes marketed for uses that were never contemplated in the traditional healing systems from which they emerged. An example is the use of ephedra (= Ma huang) for weight loss or athletic performance enhancement. While in some countries, herbal medicines are subject to rigorous manufacturing standards, this is not so everywhere. In Germany, for example, where herbal products are sold as 'phytomedicines', they are subject to the same criteria for efficacy, safety and quality as are other drug products. In the USA, by contrast, most herbal products in the marketplace are marketed and regulated as dietary supplements, a product category that does not require pre-approval of products on the basis of any of these criteria.

HERBALISM

Herbal medicine (or "herbalism") is the study and use of medicinal properties of plants.

Plants have the ability to synthesize a wide variety of chemical compounds that are used to perform important biological functions, and to defend against attack from predators such as insects, fungi and herbivorous mammals. Many of these phytochemicals have beneficial effects on long-term health when consumed by humans, and can be used to effectively treat human diseases. At least 12,000 such compounds have been isolated so far; a number estimated to be less than 10% of the total. Chemical compounds in plants mediate their effects on the human body through processes identical to those already well understood for the chemical compounds in conventional drugs; thus herbal medicines do not differ greatly from conventional drugs in terms of how they work. This enables herbal medicines to be as effective as conventional medicines, but also gives them the same potential to cause harmful side effects.

The use of plants as medicines predates written human history. Ethnobotany (the study of traditional human uses of plants) is recognized as an effective way to discover future medicines. In 2001, researchers identified 122 compounds used in modern medicine which were derived from "ethnomedical" plant sources; 80% of these have had an ethnomedical use identical or related to the current use of the active elements of the plant.Many of the pharmaceuticals currently available to physicians have a long history of use as herbal remedies, including aspirin, digitalis, quinine, andopium.

The use of herbs to treat disease is almost universal among non-industrialized societies, and is often more affordable than purchasing expensive modern pharmaceuticals. The World Health Organization (WHO) estimates that 80 percent of the population of some Asian and African countries presently use herbal medicine for some aspect of primary health care. Studies in the United States and Europe have shown that their use is less common in clinical settings, but has become increasingly more in recent years as scientific evidence about the effectiveness of herbal medicine has become more widely available.

History

The use of plants as medicines predates written human history. Many of the herbs and spices used by humans to season food also yield useful medicinal compounds. The use of herbs and spices in cuisine developed in part as a response to the threat of food-borne pathogens. Studies show that in tropical climates where pathogens are the most abundant, recipes are the most highly spiced. Further, the spices with the most potent antimicrobial activity tend to be selected. In all cultures vegetables are spiced less than meat, presumably because they are more resistant to spoilage. Many of the common weeds that populate human settlements, such as nettle, dandelion and chickweed, also have medicinal properties.

A large amount of archaeological evidence exists which indicates that humans were using medicinal plants during the Paleolithic, approximately 60,000 years ago.

Ancient Times

In the written record, the study of herbs dates back over 5,000 years to the Sumerians, who created clay tablets with lists of hundreds of medicinal plants (such as myrrh and opium). In 1500 B.C., the Ancient Egyptians wrote the Ebers Papyrus, which contains information on over 850 plant medicines, including garlic,juniper, cannabis, castor bean, aloe, and mandrake.

In India, Ayurveda medicine has used many herbs such as turmeric possibly as early as 1900 BC.Sanskrit writings from around 1500 B.C., such as the *Rig Veda*, are some of the earliest available documents detailing the medical knowledge that formed the basis of the Ayurveda system.

Many other herbs and minerals used in Ayurveda were later described by ancient Indian herbalists such as Charaka and Sushrutaduring the 1st millennium BC. The *Sushruta Samhita* attributed to Sushruta in the 6th century BC describes 700 medicinal plants, 64 preparations from mineral sources, and 57 preparations based on animal sources.

The Chinese emperor Shen Nung (of the Han Dynasty) is said to have written the first Chinese herbal, the *Pen Tsao*. The *Pen Tsao* lists 365 medicinal plants and their uses - including Ephedra (the shrub that introduced the drug ephedrine to modern medicine), hemp, and chaulmoogra (one of the first effective treatments for leprosy). Succeeding generations augmented on the *Shennong Bencao Jing*, as in the *Yaoxing Lun* (*Treatise on the Nature of Medicinal Herbs*), a 7th century Tang Dynasty treatise on herbal medicine.

The earliest known Greek herbals were those of Diocles of Carystus, written during the 3rd century B.C, and one by Krateuas from the 1st century B.C. Only a few fragments of these works have survived intact, but from what remains scholars have noted that there is a large amount of overlap with the Egyptian herbals. Greek and Roman medicinal practices, as preserved in the writings of Hippocrates (e.g. *De herbis et curis*) and - especially - Galen (e.g. *Therapeutics*), provided the pattern for later western medicine. Sometime between 50 and 68 A.D., a compendium of more than 600 plants, 35 animal products, and ninety minerals. *De Materia Medica* remained the authoritative reference of herbalism into the 17th century. Similarly important for herbalists and botanists of later centuries was Theophrastus' *Historia Plantarum*, written in the fourth century BC, which was the first systematization of the botanical world.

Middle Ages

Benedictine monasteries were the primary source of medical knowledge in Europe and England during the Early Middle Ages. However, most of these monastic scholars' efforts were focused on translating and copying ancient Greco-Roman and Arabic works, rather than creating substantial new information and practices. Many Greek and Roman writings on medicine, as on other subjects, were preserved by hand copying of manuscripts in monasteries. The monasteries thus tended to become local centers of medical knowledge, and their herb gardens provided the raw materials for simple treatment of common disorders. At the same time, folk medicine in the home and village continued uninterrupted, supporting numerous wandering and settled herbalists. Among these were the "wise-women", who prescribed herbal remedies often along with spells and enchantments. It was not until thelate Middle Ages that women who were knowledgeable in herb lore became the targets of the witch hysteria. One of the most famous women in the herbal tradition was Hildegard of Bingen. A twelfth century Benedictine nun, she wrote a medical text called *Causes and Cures*.

Medical schools known as Bimaristan began to appear from the 9th century in the medieval Islamic world among Persians and Arabs, which was generally more advanced than medieval Europe at the time. The Arabs venerated Greco-Roman culture and learning, and translated tens of thousands of texts into Arabic for further study. As a trading culture, the Arab travellers had access to plant material from distant places such as China and India. Herbals, medical texts and translations of the classics of antiquity filtered in from east and west. Muslim botanists and Muslim physicians significantly expanded on the earlier knowledge of materia medica. For example, al-Dinawari described more than 637 plant drugs in the 9th century, and Ibn al-Baitar described more than 1,400 different plants, foods and drugs, over 300 of which were his own original discoveries, in the 13th century. The experimental scientific method was introduced into the field of materia medica in the 13th century by the Andalusian-Arab botanist Abu al-Abbas al-Nabati, the teacher of Ibn al-Baitar. Al-Nabati introduced empirical techniques in the testing, description and identification of numerous materia medica, and he separated unverified reports from those supported by actual tests and observations. This allowed the study of materia medica to evolve into the science of pharmacology.

Baghdad was an important centre for Arab herbalism, as was Al-Andalus between 800 and 1400. Abulcasis (936-1013) ofCordoba authored *The Book of Simples*, an important source for later European herbals, while Ibn al-Baitar (1197–1248) of Malaga authored the *Corpus of Simples*, the most complete Arab herbal which introduced 200 new healing herbs, including tamarind, *Aconitum*, and nux vomica. Avicenna's *The Canon of Medicine* (1025) lists 800 tested drugs, plants and minerals. Book Two is devoted to a discussion of the healing properties of herbs, including nutmeg, senna, sandalwood, rhubarb, myrrh, cinammon, and rosewater. The *Canon of Medicine* remained a medical authority, used at many European and Arab medical schools, until the early 19th century. Other pharmacopoeia books include that written by Abu-Rayhan Biruni in the 11th century and Ibn Zuhr (Avenzoar) in the 12th century (and printed in 1491), Peter of Spain's *Commentary on Isaac*, and John of St Amand's *Commentary on the*

Antedotary of Nicholas. In particular, the *Canon* introduced clinical trials,randomized controlled trials, and efficacy tests.

Modern Herbal Medicine

The use of herbs to treat disease is almost universal among non-industrialized societies.

Many of the pharmaceuticals currently available to physicians have a long history of use as herbal remedies, including opium, aspirin, digitalis, andquinine. The World Health Organization (WHO) estimates that 80 percent of the population of some Asian and African countries presently use herbal medicine for some aspect of primary health care. Pharmaceuticals are prohibitively expensive for most of the world's population, half of which lives on less than $2 U.S. per day. In comparison, herbal medicines can be grown from seed or gathered from nature for little or no cost.

The use of, and search for, drugs and dietary supplements derived from plants have accelerated in recent years. Pharmacologists, microbiologists, botanists, and natural-products chemists are combing the Earth for phytochemicals and leads that could be developed for treatment of various diseases. In fact, according to the World Health Organisation, approximately 25% of modern drugs used in the United States have been derived from plants.

Among the 120 active compounds currently isolated from the higher plants and widely used in modern medicine today, 80 percent show a positive correlation between their modern therapeutic use and the traditional use of the plants from which they are derived. More than two thirds of the world's plant species - at least 35,000 of which are estimated to have medicinal value - come from the developing countries. At least 7,000 medical compounds in the modern pharmacopoeia are derived from plants In many medicinal and aromatic plants (MAPs) significant variations of plants characteristics have been ascertained with varying soil traits, and the selective recovery and subsequent release in food of certain elements have been demonstrated. Great attention must be paid to choose soil and cropping strategies, to obtain satisfactory yields of high quality and best-priced products, respecting their safety and nutritional value.

Biological Background

All plants produce chemical compounds as part of their normal metabolic activities. These phytochemicals are divided into (1) primary metabolites such as sugars and fats, which are found in all plants; and (2) secondary metabolites—compounds which are found in a smaller range of plants, serving a more specific function. For example, some secondary metabolites are toxins used to deter predation and others are pheromones used to attract insects for pollination. It is these secondary metabolites and pigments that can have therapeutic actions in humans and which can be refined to produce drugs—examples are inulin from the roots of dahlias, quinine from the cinchona, morphine and codeine from the poppy, and digoxin from thefoxglove.

Plants synthesize a bewildering variety of phytochemicals but most are derivatives of a few biochemical motifs:

- Alkaloids are a class of chemical compounds containing a nitrogen ring. Alkaloids are produced by a large variety of organisms, including bacteria, fungi, plants, and animals, and are part of the group of natural products (also called secondary metabolites). Many alkaloids can be purified from crude extracts by acid-base extraction. Many alkaloids are toxic to other organisms. They often have pharmacological effects and are used as medications, as recreational drugs, or in entheogenic rituals. Examples are the local anesthetic and stimulant cocaine; the psychedelic psilocin; the stimulant caffeine; nicotine; the analgesic morphine; the antibacterial berberine; the anticancer compound vincristine; the antihypertension agent reserpine; the cholinomimeric galatamine; the spasmolysis agent atropine; the vasodilator vincamine; the anti-arhythmia compound quinidine; the anti-asthma therapeutic ephedrine; and the antimalarial drug quinine. Although alkaloids act on a diversity of metabolic systems in humans and other animals, they almost uniformly invoke a bitter taste.
- Polyphenols (also known as phenolics or polyphenols) are compounds contain phenol rings. The anthocyanins that give grapes their purple color, the isoflavones, the phytoestrogens from soyand the tannins that give tea its astringency are phenolics.
- Glycosides is a molecule in which a sugar is bound to a non-carbohydrate moiety, usually a small organic molecule. Glycosides play numerous important roles in living organisms. Many plants store chemicals in the form of inactive glycosides. These can be activated by enzyme hydrolysis, which causes the sugar part to be broken off, making the chemical available for use. Many such plant glycosides are used as medications. In animals and humans, poisons are often bound to sugar molecules as part of their elimination from the body. An example is the cyanoglycosides in cherry pits that release toxins only when bitten by a herbivore.
- Terpenes are a large and diverse class of organic compounds, produced by a variety of plants, particularly conifers, which are often strong smelling and thus may have had a protective function. They are the major components of resin, and of turpentine produced from resin. (The

name "terpene" is derived from the word "turpentine"). Terpenes are major biosynthetic building blocks within nearly every living creature. Steroids, for example, are derivatives of the triterpene squalene. When terpenes are modified chemically, such as by oxidation or rearrangement of the carbon skeleton, the resulting compounds are generally referred to as *terpenoids*. Terpenes and terpenoids are the primary constituents of the essential oils of many types of plants and flowers. Essential oils are used widely as natural flavor additives for food, as fragrances in perfumery, and in traditional and alternative medicines such as aromatherapy. Synthetic variations and derivatives of natural terpenes and terpenoids also greatly expand the variety of aromas used in perfumery and flavors used in food additives. Vitamin A is an example of a terpene. The fragrance of rose and lavender is due to monoterpenes. The carotenoids produce the reds, yellows and oranges of pumpkin, corn and tomatoes.

A consortium of plant molecular researchers at Washington State University, the Donald Danforth Plant Science Centre, the National Centre for Genome Resources, and the University of Illinois at Chicago began an NIH-sponsored study of over thirty medicinal plant species late 2009. The initial work, to develop a sequence reference for the transcriptome of each, has led to the development of the Medicinal Plant Transcriptomics Database.

Clinical Tests

Many herbs have shown positive results in-vitro, animal model or small-scale clinical tests, while studies on some herbal treatments have found negative results. In 2002, the U.S. National Centre for Complementary and Alternative Medicine of the National Institutes of Health began funding clinical trials into the effectiveness of herbal medicine. In a 2010 survey of 1000 plants, 356 had clinical trials published evaluating their "pharmacological activities and therapeutic applications" while 12% of the plants, although available in the Western market, had "no substantial studies" of their properties.

Herbalists criticize the manner in which many scientific studies make insufficient use of historical knowledge, which has been shown useful in drug discovery and development in the past and present. They maintain that this traditional knowledge can guide the selection of factors such as optimal dose, species, time of harvesting and target population.

Prevalence of Use

A survey released in May 2004 by the National Centre for Complementary and Alternative Medicine focused on who used complementary and alternative medicines (CAM), what was used, and why it was used. The survey was limited to adults, aged 18 years and over during 2002, living in the United States. According to this survey, herbal therapy, or use of natural products other than vitamins and minerals, was the most commonly used CAM therapy (18.9%) when all use of prayer was excluded.

Herbal remedies are very common in Europe. In Germany, herbal medications are dispensed by apothecaries (e.g., Apotheke). Prescription drugs are sold alongside essential oils, herbal extracts, or tisanes. Herbal remedies are seen by some as a treatment to be preferred to pure medical compounds which have been industrially produced.

In India, the herbal remedy is so popular that the Government of India has created a separate department - AYUSH - under the Ministry of Health & Family Welfare. The National Medicinal Plants Board was also established in 2000 by the Govt. of India in order to deal with the herbal medical system.

Avid public interest in herbalism in the UK has been recently confirmed by the popularity of the topic in mainstream media, such as the prime-time hit TV series BBC's Grow Your Own Drugs, which demonstrated how to grow and prepare herbal remedies at home.

Herbal Preparations

There are many forms in which herbs can be administered, the most common of which is in the form of a liquid that is drunk by the patient—either a tisane or a (possibly diluted) plant extract. Whole herb consumption is also practiced either fresh, in dried form or as fresh juice.

Several methods of standardization may be determining the amount of herbs used. One is the ratio of raw materials to solvent. However different specimens of even the same plant species may vary in chemical content. For this reason, thin layer chromatography is sometimes used by growers to assess the content of their products before use. Another method is standardization on a signal chemical.

Tisanes, or "herbal teas", are the resultant liquid of extracting herbs into water, though they are made in a few different ways. Infusions are hot water extracts of herbs, such as chamomile or mint, through steeping. Decoctions are the long-term boiled extracts, usually of harder substances like roots or bark. Maceration is the old infusion of plants with high mucilage-content, such as sage, thyme, etc. To make macerates, plants are chopped and added to cold water. They are then left to stand for 7 to 12 hours (depending on herb used). For most macerates 10 hours is used.

Tinctures are alcoholic extracts of herbs, which are generally stronger than tisanes. Usually obtained by combining 100% pure ethanol (or a mixture of 100% ethanol with water) with the herb. A completed tincture has an ethanol percentage of at least 25% (sometimes up to 90%). Herbal wine andelixirs are alcoholic extract of herbs; usually with an ethanol percentage of 12-38% Herbal wine is a maceration of herbs in wine, while an elixir is a maceration of herbs in spirits (e.g., vodka, grappa, etc.) Extracts include liquid extracts, dry extracts and nebulisates. Liquid extracts are liquids with a lower ethanol percentage than tinctures. They can (and are usually) made by vacuum distilling tinctures. Dry extracts are extracts of plant material which are evaporated into a dry mass. They can then be further refined to a capsule or tablet. A nebulisate is a dry extract created by freeze-drying. Vinegars are prepared at the same way as tinctures, except using a solution of acetic acid as the solvent. Syrups are extracts of herbs made with syrup or honey. Sixty five parts of sugar are mixed with 35 parts of water and herb. The whole is then boiled and macerated for three weeks.

The exact composition of a herbal product is influenced by the method of extraction. A tea will be rich in polar components because water is a polar solvent. Oil on the other hand is a non-polar solvent and it will absorb non-polar compounds. Alcohol lies somewhere in between.

Many herbs are applied topically to the skin in a variety of forms. Essential oil extracts can be applied to the skin, usually diluted in a carrier oil (many essential oils can burn the skin or are simply too high dose used straight – diluting in olive oil or another food grade oil such as almond oil can allow these to be used safely as a topical). Salves, oils, balms, creams and lotions are other forms of topical delivery mechanisms.Most topical applications are oil extractions of herbs. Taking a food grade oil and soaking herbs in it for anywhere from weeks to months allows certain phytochemicals to be extracted into the oil. This oil can then be made into salves, creams, lotions, or simply used as an oil for topical application. Any massage oils, antibacterial salves and wound healing compounds are made this way. One can also make a poultice or compress using whole herb (or the appropriate part of the plant) usually crushed or dried and re-hydrated with a small amount of water and then applied directly in a bandage, cloth or just as is.

Inhalation as in aromatherapy can be used as a mood changing treatment to fight a sinus infection or cough, or to cleanse the skin on a deeper level (steam rather than direct inhalation here)

Safety

A number of herbs are thought to be likely to cause adverse effects. Furthermore, "adulteration, inappropriate formulation, or lack of understanding of plant and drug interactions have led to adverse reactions that are sometimes life threatening or lethal." Proper double-blind clinical trials are needed to determine the safety and efficacy of each plant before they can be recommended for medical use. Although many consumers believe that herbal medicines are safe because they are "natural", herbal medicines and synthetic drugs may interact, causing toxicity to the patient. Herbal remedies can also be dangerously contaminated, and herbal medicines without established efficacy, may unknowingly be used to replace medicines that do have corroborated efficacy.

Standardization of purity and dosage is not mandated in the United States, but even products made to the same specification may differ as a result of biochemical variations within a species of plant. Plants have chemical defense mechanisms against predators that can have adverse or lethal effects on humans. Examples of highly toxic herbs include poison hemlock and nightshade. They are not marketed to the public as herbs, because the risks are well known, partly due to a long and colourful history in Europe, associated with "sorcery", "magic" and intrigue.

Although not frequent, adverse reactions have been reported for herbs in widespread use. On occasion serious untoward outcomes have been linked to herb consumption. A case of major potassium depletion has been attributed to chronic licorice ingestion., and consequently professional herbalists avoid the use of licorice where they recognise that this may be a risk. Black cohosh has been implicated in a case of liver failure.

Few studies are available on the safety of herbs for pregnant women, and one study found that use of complementary and alternative medicines are associated with a 30% lower ongoing pregnancy and live birth rate during fertility treatment. Examples of herbal treatments with likely cause-effect relationships with adverse events include aconite, which is often a legally restricted herb, ayurvedic remedies, broom, chaparral, Chinese herb mixtures, comfrey, herbs containing certain flavonoids, germander, guar gum, liquorice root, and pennyroyal. Examples of herbs where a high degree of confidence of a risk long term adverse effects can be asserted include ginseng, which is unpopular among herbalists for this reason, the endangered herb goldenseal, milk thistle, senna, against which herbalists generally advise and rarely use, aloe vera juice, buckthorn bark and berry, cascara sagrada bark, saw palmetto, valerian, kava, which is banned in the European Union, St. John's wort, Khat, Betel nut, the restricted herb Ephedra, and Guarana.

There is also concern with respect to the numerous well-established interactions of herbs and drugs. In consultation with a physician, usage of herbal remedies should be clarified, as some herbal remedies have the potential to cause adverse drug interactions when used in combination with various prescription and over-the-counterpharmaceuticals, just as a patient should inform a herbalist of their consumption of orthodox prescription and other medication.

For example, dangerously low blood pressure may result from the combination of an herbal remedy that lowers blood pressure together with prescription medicine that has the same effect. Some herbs may amplify the effects of anticoagulants. Certain herbs as well as common fruit interfere with cytochrome P450, an enzyme critical to much drug metabolism.

Practitioners

A herbalist is:

1. A person whose life is dedicated to the economic or medicinal uses of plants.
2. One skilled in the harvesting and collection of medicinal plants (see wildcrafter).
3. Traditional Chinese herbalist: one who is trained or skilled in the dispensing of herbal prescriptions; traditional Chinese herb doctor. Similarly, Traditional Ayurvedic herbalist: one who is trained or skilled in the dispensing of herbal prescriptions in the Ayurvedic tradition.
4. One trained or skilled in the therapeutic use of medicinal plants.

Herbalists must learn many skills, including the wildcrafting or cultivation of herbs, diagnosis and treatment of conditions or dispensing herbal medication, and preparations of herbal medications. Education of herbalists varies considerably in different areas of the world. Lay herbalists and traditional indigenous medicine people generally rely upon apprenticeship and recognition from their communities in lieu of formal schooling.

In some countries formalised training and minimum education standards exist, although these are not necessarily uniform within or between countries. For example, in Australia the currently self-regulated status of the profession (as of April 2008) results in different associations setting different educational standards, and subsequently recognising an educational institution or course of training. The National Herbalists Association of Australia is generally recognised as having the most rigorous professional standard within Australia. In the United Kingdom, the training of medical herbalists is done by state funded Universities. For example, Bachelor of Science degrees in herbal medicine are offered at Universities such as University of East London, Middlesex University, University of Central Lancashire, University of Westminster, University of Lincoln and Napier University in Edinburgh at the present.

Government Regulations

In the EU, herbal medicines are now regulated under the European Directive on Traditional Herbal Medicinal Products.

In the United States, most herbal remedies are regulated as dietary supplements by the Food and Drug Administration. Manufacturers of products falling into this category are not required to prove the safety or efficacy of their product, though the FDA may withdraw a product from sale should it prove harmful.

The National Nutritional Foods Association, the industry's largest trade association, has run a program since 2002, examining the products and factory conditions of member companies, giving them the right to display the GMP (Good Manufacturing Practices) seal of approval on their products.

Some herbs, such as cannabis and coca, are outright banned in most countries. Since 2004, the sales of ephedra as a dietary supplement is prohibited in the United States by the Food and Drug Administration., and subject to Schedule III restrictions in the United Kingdom.

Traditional Herbal Medicine Systems

Native Americans medicinally used about 2,500 of the approximately 20,000 plant species that are native to North America. With great accuracy, the plants they chose to use for medicine were in those families of plants that modern phytochemical studies show contain the most bioactive compounds.

Some researchers trained in both western and traditional Chinese medicine have attempted to deconstruct ancient medical texts in the light of modern science. One idea is that the yin-yang balance, at least with regard to herbs, corresponds to the pro-oxidant and anti-oxidant balance. This interpretation is supported by several investigations of the ORAC ratings of various yin and yang herbs.

In India, Ayurvedic medicine has quite complex formulas with 30 or more ingredients, including a sizable number of ingredients that have undergone "alchemical processing", chosen to balance "Vata", "Pitta" or "Kapha. ".

In Ladakh, Lahul-Spiti and Tibet, the Tibetan Medical System is prevalent, which is also called as 'Amichi Medical System'. Over 337 species ofmedicinal plants has been documented by C.P. Kala those are used by Amchis - the practitioners of this medical system.

In Tamil Nadu, Tamils have their own medicinal system now popularly called the Siddha medicinal system. The Siddha system is entirely in the Tamil language. It contains roughly 300,000 verses covering diverse aspects of medicine such as anatomy, sex ("kokokam" is the sexual treatise of par excellence), herbal, mineral and metallic compositions to cure many diseases that are relevant even to-day. Ayurveda is in Sanskrit, but Sanskrit was not generally used as a mother tongue and hence its medines are mostly taken from Siddha and other local traditions.

Herbal Philosophy and Spiritual Practices

As Eisenburg states in his book, Encounters with Qi: "The Chinese and Western medical models are like two frames of reference in which identical phenomena are studied. Neither frame of reference provides an unobstructed view of health and illness. Each is incomplete and in need of refinement." Specifically, the traditional Chinese medical model could effect change on the recognized, and expected, phenomena of detachment to patients as people and estrangement unique to the clinical and impersonal relationships between patient and physician of the Western school of medicine.

Four approaches to the use of plants as medicine include:

1. The magical/shamanic—Almost all non-modern societies recognize this kind of use. The practitioner is regarded as endowed with gifts or powers that allow him/her to use herbs in a way that is hidden from the average person, and the herbs are said to affect the spirit or soul of the person.
2. The energetic—This approach includes the major systems of Traditional Chinese Medicine, Ayurveda, and Unani. Herbs are regarded as having actions in terms of their energies and affecting the energies of the body. The practitioner may have extensive training, and ideally be sensitive to energy, but need not have supernatural powers.
3. The functional dynamic—This approach was used by early physiomedical practitioners, whose doctrine forms the basis of contemporary practice in the UK. Herbs have a functional action, which is not necessarily linked to a physical compound, although often to a physiological function, but there is no explicit recourse to concepts involving energy.
4. The chemical—Modern practitioners - called Phytotherapists - attempt to explain herb actions in terms of their chemical constituents. It is generally assumed that the specific combination of secondary metabolites in the plant are responsible for the activity claimed or demonstrated, a concept called synergy.

Herbalists tend to use extracts from parts of plants, such as the roots or leaves but not isolate particular phytochemicals. Pharmaceutical medicine prefers single ingredients on the grounds that dosage can be more easily quantified. It is also possible to patent single compounds, and therefore generate income. Herbalists often reject the notion of a single active ingredient, arguing that the different phytochemicals present in many herbs will interact to enhance the therapeutic effects of the herb and dilute toxicity. Furthermore, they argue that a single ingredient may contribute to multiple effects. Herbalists deny that herbal synergism can be duplicated with synthetic chemicals. They argue that phytochemical interactions and trace components may alter the drug response in ways that cannot currently be replicated with a combination of a few putative active ingredients. Pharmaceutical researchers recognize the concept of drug synergism but note that clinical trials may be used to investigate the efficacy of a particular herbal preparation, provided the formulation of that herb is consistent.

In specific cases the claims of synergy and multifunctionality have been supported by science. The open question is how widely both can be generalized. Herbalists would argue that cases of synergy can be widely generalized, on the basis of their interpretation of evolutionary history, not necessarily shared by the pharmaceutical community. Plants are subject to similar selection pressures as humans and therefore they must develop resistance to threats such as radiation, reactive oxygen species and microbial attack in order to survive. Optimal chemical defenses have been selected for and have thus developed over millions of years. Human diseases are multifactorial and may be treated by consuming the chemical defences that they believe to be present in herbs. Bacteria, inflammation, nutrition and ROS (reactive oxygen species) may all play a role in arterial disease. Herbalists claim a single herb may simultaneously address several of these factors. Likewise a factor such as ROS may underlie more than one condition. In short herbalists view their field as the study of a web of relationships rather than a quest for single cause and a single cure for a single condition.

In selecting herbal treatments herbalists may use forms of information that are not applicable to pharmacists. Because herbs can moonlight as vegetables, teas or spices they have a huge consumer base and large-scale epidemiological studies become feasible. Ethnobotanical studies are another source of information. For example, when indigenous peoples from geographically dispersed areas use closely related herbs for the same purpose that is taken as supporting evidence for its efficacy. Herbalists contend that historical medical records and herbals are underutilized resources. They favour the use of convergent information in assessing the medical value of plants. An example would be when in-vitro activity is consistent with traditional use.

Uses of Herbal Medicines by Animals

Indigenous healers often claim to have learned by observing that sick animals change their food preferences to nibble at bitter herbs they would normally reject. Field biologists have provided corroborating evidence based on observation of diverse species, such as chickens, sheep, butterflies, and chimpanzee. The habit has been shown to be a physical means of purging intestinal parasites,. Lowland gorillas take 90% of their diet from the fruits of *Aframomum melegueta,* a relative of the ginger plant, that is a potent antimicrobial and apparently keeps shigellosis and similar infections at bay. Current research focuses on the possibility that this plants also protects gorillas from fibrosing cardiomyopathy which has a devastating effect on captive animals.

Researchers from Ohio Wesleyan University found that some birds select nesting material rich in antimicrobial agents which protect their young from harmful bacteria.

Sick animals tend to forage plants rich in secondary metabolites, such as tannins and alkaloids. Since these phytochemicals often have antiviral, antibacterial, antifungal and antihelminthicproperties, a plausible case can be made for self-medication by animals in the wild.

Some animals have digestive systems especially adapted to cope with certain plant toxins. For example, the koala can live on the leaves and shoots of the eucalyptus, a plant that is dangerous to most animals. A plant that is harmless to a particular animal may not be safe for humans to ingest. A reasonable conjecture is that these discoveries were traditionally collected by the medicine men of indigenous tribes, who then passed on safety information and cautions.

Extinction of Medicinal Plant Species

Because "over 50% of prescription drugs are derived from chemicals first identified in plants," a 2008 report from the Botanic Gardens Conservation International (representing botanic gardensin 120 countries) warned that "cures for things such as cancer and HIV may become 'extinct before they are ever found'." They identified 400 medicinal plants at risk of extinction from over-collection and deforestation, threatening the discovery of future cures for disease. These included Yew trees (the bark is used for the cancer drug paclitaxel); Hoodia (from Namibia, a potential source of weight loss drugs); half of Magnolias (used as Chinese medicine for 5,000 years to fight cancer, dementia and heart disease); and Autumn crocus (for gout). Their report said that "five billion people still rely on traditional plant-based medicine as their primary form of health care."

TYPES OF HERBAL MEDICINES

Medicinal plants can be used by anyone, for example as part of a salad, an herbal tea or supplement, although some herbs considered dangerous are restricted from sale to the public. Sometimes such herbs are provided to professional herbalists by specialist companies. Many herbalists, both professional and amateur, often grow or wildcraft their own herbs. Many common weeds have medicinal properties (*e.g.* dandelion).

In the herbal "Healing Wise" by Susun S Weed, the three traditions of healing include" the Wise Woman Tradition, the Heroic Tradition, and the

Scientific Tradition. The Scientific tradition relies on use of herbal medicines in the form of isolating the active ingredients in herbs, many modern pharmaceuticals are derived from isolating active ingredients from herbs. The Heroic Tradition relies on the belief that the body is dirty and must be cleansed, it promoted the use of purifying herbs and diuretics.

The Wise Woman Tradition uses herbs to nourish and tonify the body, herbs are used in the most natural forms possible, and they are used to support the body in healing itself. Learn more about the Wise Woman Tradition of healing with Herbal Medicine from this article, which includes the Six Steps of Healing by Susun Weed Medicinal herbs can be used in various forms:

Herbal Teas

There are two methods of making herbal teas, infusion and decoction. Infusion is steeping lighter parts of the plant (leaves, flowers, light stems) in boiled water for four to eight hours. Decoction is boiling tougher parts, such as roots or bark for a longer period of time. Herbal teas are often used as a home remedy, and as an alternative to tea and coffee.

Some popular herbal teas include borage, chamomile, dandelion, elderflower, hibiscus, nettle, and various species of mint. Each herb has unique medicinal properties, and a range of secondary effects; and this is linked to its use as a casual drink. For instance, Borage can be used medicinally (amongst other things) as an aid against depression; and it may be drunk more casually to lift the spirits. It was traditionally served as a pep drink for weary travellers. Secondary effects include use as an anti-inflammatory or balsam; and hormonal and metabolic regulation. Other herbs may have similar side-effects, but in different proportions and are used in different ways.

Mixing Herbs: To counteract the various complications and side-effects of an ailment, or to produce a more rounded taste, a number of herbs may be mixed. A well-known mixture used against a cold includes eucalyptus leaf, mint leaf (which contains Menthol) and juniper berry. Another is the age-old favourite "dandelion and burdock", from which the popular fizzy drink was derived.

Fresh or Dried? Many flower and leaf herbs lose volatile compounds within a few hours, as the juices and oils evaporate, the scent leaks away, and the chemicals change their form. Drying concentrates other compounds as water is removed. Most herbal traditions use dried material and the reported effects for each herb tend to be based upon dried herbs unless otherwise specified.

If you are using fresh herbs, you will need more of them, and the tea will have a somewhat different effect. Finely chop the leaf immediately before using it. Generic Western Tea is usually the leaf of one specific plant, Camelia Sinensis, which grows mainly in India and China. It can be seen as just one of many herbal teas. It is a stimulant, and its main property is to increase alertness, along with a slightly sedative or calming effect. But unlike a fresh herbal tea, it may include artificial additives to enhance the taste and to preserve it in the shops. More expensive recipes include Darjeeling (from Darjeeling in India) and Earl Grey (which has bergamot added).

Making a Nourishing Herbal Infusion

Typically, one ounce by weight (about a cup by volume) of dried herb is placed in a quart jar which is then filled to the top with boiling water, tightly lidded and allowed to steep for 4-10 hours. After straining, a cup or more is consumed, and the remainder chilled to slow spoilage. Drinking 2-4 cups a day is usual. Since the minerals and other phytochemicals in nourishing herbs are made more accessible by drying, dried herbs are considered best for infusions.

Stinging nettle (Urtica dioica) builds energy, strengthens the adrenals, and is said to restore youthful flexibility to blood vessels. A cup of nettle infusion contains 500 milligrams of calcium plus generous amounts of bone-building magnesium, potassium, silicon, boron, and zinc. It is also an excellent source of vitamins A, D, E, and K. For flexible bones, a healthy heart, thick hair, beautiful skin, and lots of energy, make friends with sister stinging nettle. It may make you feel so good you'll jump up and exercise.

Oatstraw (Avena sativa) reduces high cholesterol, increases libido, and strengthens the nerves. A cup of oatstraw infusion contains more than 300 milligrams of calcium plus generous amounts of many other minerals. Its steroidal saponins nourish the pancreas and liver, improving digestion and stabilizing moods. Oatstraw is best known however for its ability to enhance libido and mellow the mood. Do be careful whom you share it with, or you may find yourself sowing some wild oats. In Auryuvedic medicine, oatstraw is considered the finest of all longevity tonics.

Red clover (Trifolium pratense) is better in every way than its cousin soy. It contains four phytoestrogens; soy has only one (isoflavone). Red clover infusion has ten times more phytoestrogens than soy "milk," fewer calories, more calcium, and no added sugars. Red clover is the world's leading anti-cancer herb; soy isoflavone encourages the growth of breast cancer cells in the lab. Red clover improves the memory; Japanese men who ate tofu twice a week doubled their risk of Alzheimer's disease. Soy beverage can contain up to 1000 times more aluminum than milk, according to Sally Fallon, lipid researcher and fat specialist. She believes that "the highly processed soy foods of today are perpetuating... nutrient deficiencies...."

Comfrey (Symphytum) leaf is free of the compounds (PAs) found in the root that can damage the liver. I have used comfrey leaf infusion regularly for decades with no liver problems, ditto for the group of people at the Henry Doubleday Research Foundation who have eaten cooked comfrey leaves as a vegetable for four generations. Comfrey is also known as "knitbone," and no better ally for the woman with thin bones can be found. And, don't forget, comfrey contains special proteins used in the formation of short-term memory cells. Its soothing mucilage adds flexibility to joints, eyes, vagina, and lungs.

HERBAL MEDICINE FOR CANCER PATIENTS

In Traditional Chinese Medicine (TCM), herbal prescriptions are given to patients as complex formulations containing multiple herbs. Notably, this approach amounts to the administration of several chemical entities at once.

The underlying theory is, that interaction among the chemicals present within a single plant, as an entity, and also the different herbs in a formula exert synergistic pharmaco-dynamic actions not present when administered in form of an isolated active ingredient. Synergy of many different chemical components within the plant is responsible for these effects and involves a number of different processes. Whilst the exact mechanisms behind plant synergy and the allelopathic properties of the plant are still not fully understood, a great deal of research has been done in this field. Today's understanding of basic molecular cell biochemistry and the consequent possibility of elucidating the actual mechanism of action of chemical components at the cellular level, or even gene level, have resulted in a rational explanation of the action of medicinal plants.

Molecular Cancer Therapeutics

Multi-drug resistance (MDR) is an important biological behaviour of tumour cells in chemotherapy and it is also one of the major causes of clinical chemotherapy failure. There is increasing interest into the exact mechanism of tumour cells' MDR and its reversion by Chinese herbs. Organ preservation protocols in head and neck squamous cell carcinoma (HNSCC) are limited by tumours that fail to respond. We observed that larynx preservation and response to chemotherapy is significantly associated with p53 over-expression, and that most HNSCC cell lines with mutant p53 are more sensitive to cisplatin than those with wild-type p53. To investigate cisplatin resistance, we studied two HNSCC cell lines, UM-SCC-5 and UM-SCC-10B, and two resistant sublines developed by cultivation in gradually increasing concentrations of cisplatin. The cisplatin-selected cell lines, UM-SCC-5PT and UM-SCC-10BPT, are 8 and 1.5 times more resistant to cisplatin than the respective parental cell lines, respectively. The parental lines over-express p53 and contain *p53* mutations but the cisplatin-resistant cell lines do not, indicating that cells containing mutant *p53* were eliminated during selection. Bcl-x_L expression increased in the cisplatin-resistant lines relative to the parental lines, whereas Bcl-2 expression was high in the parental lines and decreased in the cisplatin-resistant lines. Thus, cisplatin selected for wild-type p53 and high Bcl-x_L expression in these cells. We tested a small-molecule BH3 mimetic, (–)-gossypol, which binds to the BH3 domain of Bcl-2 and Bcl-x_L, for activity against the parental and cisplatin-resistant cell lines. At physiologically attainable levels, (–)-gossypol induces apoptosis in 70% to 80% of the cisplatin-resistant cells but only in 25% to 40% of the parental cells. Thus, cisplatin-resistant cells seem to depend on wild-type p53 and Bcl-x_L for survival and BH3 mimetic agents, such as (–)-gossypol, may be useful adjuncts to overcome cisplatin resistance in HNSCC.

Growth and Metastasis of Solid Tumours

Triptolide (TPL), a diterpenoid triepoxide purified from the Chinese herb Tripterygium wilfordii (Lei Gong Teng) was tested for its anti-tumour properties in several model systems. *In vitro*, TPL inhibited the proliferation and colony formation of tumour cells at extremely low concentrations (2–10 ng/ml) and was more potent than Taxol. Likewise, *in vivo*, treatment of mice with TPL for 2–3 weeks inhibited the growth of xenografts formed by four different tumour cell lines (B16 melanoma, MDA-435 breast cancer, TSU bladder cancer, and MGC80-3 gastric carcinoma), indicating that TPL has a broad spectrum of activity against tumours that contain both wild-type and mutant forms of p53.

In addition, TPL inhibited experimental metastasis of B16F10 cells to the lungs and spleens of mice. The anti-tumour effect of TPL was comparable or superior with that of conventional anti-tumour drugs, such as Adriamycin, mitomycin, and cisplatin.

Importantly, tumour cells that were resistant to Taxol attributable to the over-expression of the multi-drug resistant gene 1 were still sensitive to the effects of TPL. Studies on cultured tumour cells revealed that TPL induced apoptosis and reduced the expression of several molecules that regulate the cell cycle. Taken together, these results suggest that TPL has several attractive features as a new anti-tumour agent.

Independent Apoptosis induced by Evodiamine

Evodiamine is one of the major bioactive compounds that have been isolated and purified from the fruit of Evodiae fructus (Wu Zhu Yu).Evodiamine exhibits anti-tumour activities against the human tumor cells, including multi-drug-resistant tumour cells. However, the molecular mechanism involved in cell death induced by evodiamine treatment remains poorly understood. In the present study, we showed that evodiamine activated the caspase-dependent apoptotic pathway.

This apoptosis was only partially inhibited by a pancaspase inhibitor benzyloxycarbonyl-Val-Ala-Asp-fluoromethyl ketone, which suggested that evodiamine-induced apoptosis in leukemic U937 cells is partially caspase independent.

We observed the nuclear translocation of apoptosis-inducing factor in evodiamine-induced apoptosis of U937 cells, which may be responsible for the caspase-independent apoptotic execution.

We next showed that evodiamine induced the substantial amount of apoptosis both in Bcl-2- and Akt-overexpressing U937 cells but not in human peripheral blood mononuclear cells. Although benzyloxycarbonyl-Val-Ala-Asp-fluoromethyl ketone inhibited caspase activity in Bcl-2-overexpressing U937 cells, it completely prevented neither the induction of apoptosis or the nuclear translocation of apoptosis-inducing factor, which suggests that evodiamine is, at least in part, able to bypass the resistance of leukemia cells via caspase-independent apoptotic pathways. Thus, therapeutic strategy using evodiamine may warrant further evaluation.

Mediated Pathways in Myeloid Leukaemia Cells

The Chinese herb Ru Xiang (Boswellia carterii) is investigated for its antineoplastic properties in this article. The mechanism of the cytotoxic effect of boswellic acid acetate, a 1:1 mixture of -boswellic acid acetate and ß-boswellic acid acetate, isolated from *Boswellia carterri* Birdw on myeloid leukaemia cells was investigated in six human myeloid leukaemia cell lines (NB4, SKNO-1, K562, U937, ML-1, and HL-60 cells).

Morphologic and DNA fragmentation assays indicated that the cytotoxic effect of boswellic acid acetate was mediated by induction of apoptosis. More than 50% of the cells underwent apoptosis after treatment with 20 μg/mL boswellic acid for 24 hours.

This apoptotic process was *p53* independent. The levels of apoptosis-related proteins Bcl-2, Bax, and Bcl-X_L were not modulated by boswellic acid acetate. Boswellic acid acetate induced Bid cleavage and decreased mitochondrial membrane potential without production of hydrogen peroxide. A general caspase inhibitor (Z-VAD-FMK) and a specific caspase-8 inhibitor II (Z-IETD-FMK) blocked boswellic acid acetate–induced apoptosis. The mRNAs of death receptors 4 and 5 (DR4 and DR5) were induced in leukaemia cells undergoing apoptosis after boswellic acid acetate treatment. These data taken together suggest that boswellic acid acetate induces myeloid leukaemia cell apoptosis through activation of caspase-8 by induced expression of DR4 and DR5, and that the activated caspase-8 either directly activates caspase-3 by cleavage or indirectly by cleaving Bid, which in turn decreases mitochondria membrane potential.

Ginseng Enhances Anti-cancer Effect

Panax notoginseng is a commonly used Chinese herb. Although a few studies have found that notoginseng shows anti-tumor effects, the effect of this herb on colorectal cancer cells has not been investigated.

5-Fluorouracil (5-FU) is a chemotherapeutic agent for the treatment of colorectal cancer that interferes with the growth of cancer cells. CONCLUSIONS: This study demonstrates that the herb can enhance the anti-proliferation effect of 5-FU on HCT-116 human colorectal cancer cells and may decrease the dosage of 5-FU needed for colorectal cancer treatment.

Sensitizes Resistant Malignant Cells

We show here that wogonin, derived from the popular Chinese herb Huang-Qin, attenuates NF-kappaB activity by shifting TNFalpha-induced free radical.O(2)(-) to a more reduced nonradical product, H(2)O(2), and thereby sensitizes TNFalpha-resistant leukemia cells to TNFalpha-induced apoptosis. Importantly, wogonin does not affect the viability of normal peripheral blood T cells.

Wogonin also sensitizes TRAIL-induced apoptosis. Our data suggest a potential use of wogonin as a TNFalpha or TRAIL adjuvant for cancer treatment. Our data also demonstrate how a herbal compound enhances killing of tumor cells with reduced side effects compared with other treatments.

Potent Inhibition of Lewis Lung Cancer Growth by Heyneanol

Vitis amurensis Rupr. (Shan Pu Tao) has long been used for the treatment of cancer to this end, we isolated from its root heyneanol A (HA), which is a tetramer of resveratrol (RES), and established the in vivo anti-tumour activity of HA using the Lewis lung carcinoma (LLC) model. Remarkably, HA was fairly stable in cell culture medium and did not undergo intracellular conversion to RES. Therefore, HA is an active anti-cancer compound that induces caspase-mediated cancer cell apoptosis and inhibits angiogenesis rivaling the potency of RES and merits further evaluation for cancer chemoprevention.

THE ROLE OF HERBAL MEDICINES IN TRADITIONAL HEALING

The pharmacological treatment of disease began long ago with the use of herbs. Methods of folk healing throughout the world commonly used herbs as part of their tradition.

Traditional Chinese Medicine

Traditional Chinese medicine has been used by Chinese people from ancient times. Although animal and mineral materials have been used, the primary source of remedies is botanical. Of the more than 12 000 items used by traditional healers, about 500 are in common use (Li, 2000). Botanical products are used only after some kind of processing, which may include, for example, stir-frying or soaking in vinegar or wine. In clinical practice, traditional diagnosis may be followed by the prescription of a complex and often individualized remedy. Traditional Chinese medicine is still in common use in China. More than half the population regularly uses traditional remedies, with the highest prevalence of use in rural areas. About 5000 traditional remedies are available in China; they account for approximately one fifth of the entire Chinese pharmaceutical market.

Japanese Traditional Medicine

Many herbal remedies found their way from China into the Japanese systems of traditional healing. Herbs native to Japan were classified in the first pharmacopoeia of Japanese traditional medicine in the ninth century.

Indian Traditional Medicine

Ayurveda is a medical system primarily practised in India that has been known for nearly 5000 years. It includes diet and herbal remedies, while emphasizing the body, mind and spirit in disease prevention and treatment.

If traditional herbal medicines into Europe, the USA and other developed countries. The desire to capture the wisdom of traditional healing systems has led to a resurgence of interest in herbal medicines, particularly in Europe and North America, where herbal products have been incorporated into so-called 'alternative', 'complementary', 'holistic' or 'integrative' medical systems.

During the latter part of the twentieth century, increasing interest in self-care resulted in an enormous growth in popularity of traditional healing modalities, including the use of herbal remedies; this has been particularly true in the USA. Consumers have reported positive attitudes towards these products, in large part because they believe them to be of 'natural' rather than 'synthetic' origin, they believe that such products are more likely to be safe than are drugs, they are considered part of a healthy lifestyle, and they can help to avoid unnecessary contact with conventional 'western' medicine.

While centuries of use in traditional settings can be used as testimony that a particular herbal ingredient is effective or safe, several problems must be addressed as these ingredients are incorporated into modern practice.

One problem is that ingredients once used for symptomatic management in traditional healing are now used in developed countries as part of health promotion or disease prevention strategies; thus, acute treatment has been replaced by chronic exposure (*e.g.*, herbal products used for weight loss, Allison et al., 2001). This means that a statement about 'thousands of years of evidence that a product is safe' may not be valid for the way the product is now being used. This does not expressly mean that an ingredient is unsafe; it does mean that safety in the modern context cannot be assumed. A second problem is that efficacy and effectiveness have rarely been demonstrated using modern scientific investigations. An evidence-based approach to this issue has only recently been implemented, and the results reveal that for most herbal products, considerable gaps in knowledge need to be remedied before one can be convinced about their efficacy.

One of the most difficult issues to contend with in translating traditional herbal practices into conventional 'western' medicine is the individualization of prescriptions containing multiple herbal and other ingredients. There is little incentive for standardization of products for a mass market, when the intention has been to provide an individual prescription. To the small grower or the traditionally trained herbalist, standardization means understanding the growth conditions, the time of harvesting, the manner of extraction or other preparation of material so that a reliable (albeit small amount of) active ingredient can be offered to people. To the manufacturer or distributor of large quantities that will be sold in a supermarket or a health food store, standardization refers to industrial production under defined conditions, using so-called Good Manufacturing Practices (GMP) (Food & Drug Administration, 2002) akin to those used for drug production.

In the USA, there is both small-scale and large-scale production of herbal products and there can be wide variation in their content and quality in the marketplace. Regulations in the USA do not yet require that dietary supplement manufacturers adhere to standard manufacturing practices, and so quality is not guaranteed. The public becomes discouraged by reports that products taken from store shelves do not consistently contain the ingredients — or in the amounts — that are claimed on the label. For herbal products in common use, evidence of efficacy may be based upon traditional use, testimonials, clinical studies, both controlled and uncontrolled, and randomized, double-blind, placebo-controlled trials. For the most part, however, there is a lack of systematic clinical studies to support claims.

Safety of some herbal ingredients has been recently called into question, in part because of the identification of adverse events associated with their use and, increasingly, because of the demonstration of clinically relevant interactions between herbs and prescription drugs.

Adverse events (stroke, heart attacks, heart-rate irregularities, liver toxicity, seizures, psychoses and death) associated with use of ephedra for weight loss, body-building effects and increased energy or kava-kava (also known as kawa), widely used in Europe and increasingly in Canada to treat anxiety, nervousness, insomnia, pain and muscle tension, for example, have caused some countries to issue regulations restricting or banning these products. Only a few herbs in common use have been suspected of causing cancer.

TRADITIONAL HERBAL MEDICINES IN DEVELOPED COUNTRIES

Plants and their secondary metabolite constituents have a long history of use in modern 'western' medicine and in certain systems of traditional medicine, and are the sources of important drugs such as atropine, codeine, digoxin, morphine, quinine and vincristine. Use of herbal medicines in developed countries has expanded sharply in the latter half of the twentieth century. Monographs on selected herbs are available from a number of sources, including the European Scientific Cooperative on Phytotherapy, German Commission E and the World Health Organization.

The WHO monographs, for example, describe the herb itself by a number of criteria (including synonyms and vernacular names) and the herb part commonly used, its geographical distribution, tests used to identify and characterize the herb (including macroscopic and microscopic examination and purity testing), the active principles (when known), dosage forms and dosing, medicinal uses, pharmacology, contra-indications and adverse reactions. Other resources that provide detailed information about herbal products in current use include the Natural Medicines Comprehensive Database and NAPRALERT (NAtural PRoducts ALERT) (2001). Information about other available databases has been published by Bhat (1995).

Beneficial effects and active components

In some cases, the active principles of plant-derived products have been isolated and characterized, and their mechanisms of action are understood (*e.g.*, ephedrine alkaloids in some species of Ephedra). For many, however, including virtually all of the most common products in the marketplace, such information is incomplete or unavailable. This is in large part due to the complexity of herbal and botanical preparations; they are not pure compounds. It is also a function of the traditionally-held belief that the synergistic combination of several active principles in some herbal preparations is responsible for their beneficial effects.

HERBAL MEDICINES FOR INJECTION

In history, Chinese have made 5 major inventions to the world civilization. 1) Chinese herbal medicine for effective treatment of variety of chronic diseases and tumors, 2) Gun powders for the development of rockets and space science, 3) Navigator for sailing on ships and airplanes, 4) Manufacture of papers, and

5) Printing technology. Herbal cancer therapy comprises a number of alternative treatments in the fight against cancer. As early as more than 3,000 years ago, Chinese doctors had used herbs in treatment of cancer patients. Chinese medicine has been used widely in Japan, Korea, India, and South East Asia countries since long time ago.

According to the reliability of therapeutic effects, Chinese medicinal herbs divide into 3 main categories. The first is the Classical Medicinal Herbs, including approximate 265 kinds of medicinal herbs and plants and a few of medicinal minerals that have been identified by scientific works and proven by clinic studies. The second is the folk herbs (folk experienced recipe herbs) that have approximately 600 sorts of herbs. The third is the hi-tech made herbal medicines, the concentrated herbal extract, which is 5 to 10-fold more effective than their raw materials. From the modality of administration of herbal medication, anti-cancer herbal medicines are herein classified into 3 groups, including take by mouth, topical use and injectable preparations (not available at our HCC and HMC).

Since 1990, a research group of hi-tech herbal medicine directed by Dr. David Liu has conducted many studies on herbal treatments in chronic diseases and tumors. We have screened all of 66 sorts of anti-cancer medicinal herbs using our unique techniques, including identify and analysis of ester-soluble active ingredients, ethanol-soluble active ingredients and hydrate-soluble active ingredients in each potential anti-cancer medicinal herb or plant.

We have demonstrated that LDL-110 anti-cancer herbal active ingredient is 6-fold powerful than chemotherapy drug mitomycin in killing 14 types of human cancer cell lines in tissue culture, including 3 types of breast cancer and cancer of prostate, 4 types of lymphoma, 2 types of leukemia and melanoma, and 2 types of colorectal carcinoma. Furthermore, clinic studies have shown LPY-80 herbal capsule is a high potent broad-spectrum anti-leukemia and lymphoma herbal remedy. More importantly, both LDL-110 anti-cancer herbal capsules and LPY-80 anti-leukemia-lymphoma herbal capsules are convenient and safe to patients, they are available in capsules which are taken by mouth and are free of side-effects if clients follow the service directions.

Commonly used Chinese Anti-cancer Herbs

The commonly used Chinese anti-cancer herbs that have been investigated, identified, tested, and clinically proven in over hundred thousand patients every year in China. These herbs are allowed to be used as herbal supplements in the USA. One should understand that a single herb or a single herbal extract may only give little anti-cancer therapeutic effect when it is used alone. However, when several herbs or herbal extracts scientifically formulated together will result in highly effective anti-cancer recipe and the side-effects of the formulated herbs would be attenuated, minimized or neutralized. For example, when Glossy Privet fruit is used alone, it may give about 20 to 30% anti-cancer efficacy in some patients with leukemia or lymphoma and it may cause some adverse effects as well. However, our experience indicated that Glossy Privet fruit combines with Milkvetch root herb and others that may attain 90% anti-cancer efficacy and brings about 10% side-effects. Therefore, a correct herbal therapy regimen is not a simple accumulation picking several kinds of anti-cancer herbs together. Self-prescription of herbs by clients is not advised that may be harmful or even fatal.

For cancer patient, this chapter is a good self-education booklet and reference from which patients will understand what anti-cancer herbal treatment is. For cancer patient, you need always consulting your primary care physician or herbal specialist before you use any anti-cancer herb or herbal product. Particular attention should be paid to whom the below herbs are not for use in children under 18 of age. Safety during pregnancy and in lactating mothers has not yet been established. The HCC and HMC will not take any legal responsibility to one who has used raw herbal materials or herbal remedies from the outside resources of our facilities.

The FDA Regulations: Although these anti-cancer herbs, herbal supplements or herbal remedies are clinically proven high potent for patients with malignant tumor, cancer, leukemia and lymphoma in China and other countries, according to the USA-FDA regulations of herbal supplements, each of the below described herbs or herbal remedies is labeled as "This statement has not been evaluated by the FDA. This product is not intended to diagnosis, treat, cure or prevent disease".

Camptotheca Acuminata

Camptotheca acuminata is one of the Nyssaceae family members and it is native only to China and Tibet, where it is known as Xi Shu ("happy tree"). Its primary anti-cancer ingredient is a quinoline alkaloid called camptothecin, which in turn has been modified to create a group of new anti-cancer drugs, including irinotecan, topotecan, 9-aminocamptothecin, and CPT-11. Camptothecin and these analogs are being investigated to treat a variety of cancers, but the compounds are quite toxic, and only topotecan (Hycamtin®) and irinotecan HCl (Camptosar®) have met with the FDA approval; Hycamtin® has been approved for ovarian cancer therapy, and Camptosar® is approved for metastatic colorectal cancer.

Western researchers (Dr. Monroe E. Wall and Jonathon Hartwell of the National Cancer Institute) first discovered anticancer properties of Camptotheca in 1958. In 1966 camptothecin was isolated. A camptothecin analog (camptothecin sodium) was tested on gastrointestinal cancer patients in the early 70's, but the clinical trials were discontinued because the patients had severe side effects. In China, camptothecin has been used in the treatment of leukemia and cancers of the stomach and liver.

Injectable preparations of Camptotheca and camptothecin are using in China but they are not available at the Herbal Cancer Centre and Herbal Medical Centre in Boston.

Catharanthus Roseus

Traditionally, Catharanthus roseus has been used in folk medicine to treat diabetes and high blood pressure. Catharanthus roseus has function of diureses. During the 1950s, however, Catharanthus roseus was discovered to contain a number of chemicals in the alkaloid class.

Alkaloids are bitter-tasting plant compounds that contain nitrogen. Many of them have pain-relieving or anticancer properties. At least two of the alkaloids in Catharanthus roseus (vinblastine and vincristine) have been isolated and developed into prescription anti-cancer drugs.

These injectable drugs and their derivatives (such as vinorelbine) interfere with the division of cancer cells. These drugs should only be used by licensed medical professionals in the USA. Using vinblastine and vincristine in combination chemotherapy has resulted in 80% remission in Hodgkin's disease, 99% remission in acute lymphocitic leukemia, 80% remission in Wilm's tumor, 70% remission in gestational chorioarcinoma, and 50% remission in Burkitt's lymphoma.

Synthetic vincristine, used to treat leukemia, is only 20% as effective as the natural product derived from Catharanthus roseus. Further research is needed especially on bioactive compounds, means of preparation, and effectiveness of plants and herbal remedies.

Catharanthus roseus extract and vinblastine and vincristine are injectable herbal preparations that are not available at the Herbal Cancer Centre and Herbal Medical Centre in Boston. For more information consult your primary care physicians.

Taxus Cuspidata

Taxus cuspidata grows in China (NS~FIg), Japan, Korea and Manchuria, where it grows to 50 feet tall. In North America, it is usually grown as a compact, spreading shrub. Studies have shown that Taxus cuspidata contains the substance 'taxol' in their shoots and bark. Taxol is a broad-spectrum anti-cancer chemotherapy drug in Western medicine for treatment of cancer of breast, uterus, ovary, kidney and lung. This drug is toxic; even it is surface used or topical used. It therefore should be only used under the supervision of a licensed medical professional. For more information consult your primary care physicians. Taxus cuspidata and Taxol are injectable medicines that are not available at the Herbal Cancer Centre and Herbal Medical Centre in Boston.

SALIENT FEATURES OF ALTERNATIVE MEDICINES

Efficacy: Advocates of alternative medicine hold that the various alternative treatment methods are effective in treating a wide range of major and minor medical conditions, and contend that recently published research proves the effectiveness of specific alternative treatments. They assert that a PubMed search revealed over 370,000 research papers classified as alternative medicine published in Medline-recognized journals since 1966 in the National Library of Medicine database.

Advocates of alternative medicine hold that alternative medicine may provide health benefits through patient empowerment, by offering more choices to the public, including treatments that are simply not available in conventional medicine:

"Most Americans who consult alternative providers would probably jump at the chance to consult a physician who is well trained in scientifically based medicine and who is also open-minded and knowledgeable about the body's innate mechanisms of healing, the role of lifestyle factors in influencing health, and the appropriate uses of dietary supplements, herbs, and other forms of treatment, from osteopathic manipulation to Chinese and Ayurvedic medicine. In other words, they want competent help in navigating the confusing maze of therapeutic options that are available today, especially in those cases in which conventional approaches are relatively ineffective or harmful."

It must be added though that most practitioners do not hold a degree in official medicine or even have a solid understanding of scientific principles, as can be deduced from many of their publications. And providing more choice has no bearing as to the efficacy of the proposed treatment. Although advocates of alternative medicine acknowledge that the placebo effect may play a role in the benefits that some receive from alternative therapies, they point out that this does not diminish their validity. Researchers who judge treatments using the scientific method are concerned by this viewpoint, since, according to standard controlled studies, it is an acknowledgement of the inefficacy of alternative treatments.

Danger Reduced when Used as a Complement to Conventional Medicine

A major objection to alternative medicine is that it may be done in place of conventional medical treatments. As long as alternative treatments are used alongside standard conventional medical treatments, most medical doctors find most forms of complementary medicine acceptable. Consistent with previous studies, the CDC recently reported that the majority of individuals in the United States (*i.e.*, 54.9%) used CAM in conjunction with conventional medicine.

It would be ideal for patients to inform their medical doctor when they are using alternative medicine. Some alternative treatments may interact with orthodox medical treatments, and such potential conflicts should be explored in the interest of the patient. However, many conventional practitioners are biased or uninformed about alternatives, and the exhortations to disclose alternative treatments to one's doctor do not address the complexities involved. Patients are often reluctant to share this information with their medical doctors since they fear it will hurt their patient-doctor relationship.

The issue of alternative medicine interfering with conventional medical practices is minimized when it is only turned to after the conventional medicine path has been exhausted. Many patients believe alternative medicine can help in coping with chronic illnesses for which conventional medicine offers no cure and only management. It is becoming more common for a patient's own MD to suggest alternatives when they cannot offer a treatment.

There are also the patients who have made it a habit to turn to alternatives for non-threatening disorders that may only need medical intervention in rare recalcitrant cases. They typically utilize mainstream medicine for diagnosis and basic information, while turning to alternatives for what are believed to be health-enhancing measures.

Criticism of Alternative Medicine

Due to the wide range of therapies that are considered to be "alternative medicine" few criticisms apply across the board, except possibly that of not being scientifically supported or even testable. Criticisms directed at specific branches of alternative medicine range from the fairly minor (conventional treatment is believed to be more effective in a particular area) to incompatibility with the known laws of physics (for example, in homeopathy). Critics argue that alternative medicine practitioners may not have an accredited medical degree or be licensed physicians or general practitioners and make sweeping claims without demonstrated expertise. This cannot always be considered a serious criticism, because unless a new system of medicine becomes established, it does not receive accreditation of any kind, except by its own professional organizations. This is the route homeopathy, ayurveda, siddha, unani, and naturopathy had to follow in those countries where it is now offered by accredited institutions. Proponents of the various forms of alternative medicine reject criticism as being founded in prejudice, financial self-interest, or ignorance. Refutations of criticism sometimes take the form of an appeal to nature.

Efficacy

Lack of proper testing: Evidence-based medicine (EBM) applies the scientific method to medical practice, and aims for the ideal that healthcare professionals should make "conscientious, explicit, and judicious use of current best evidence" in their everyday practice. Prof. Edzard Ernst is a notable proponent of applying EBM to CAM.

Although proponents of alternative medicine often cite the large number of studies which have been performed, critics point out the fact that there are no statistics on exactly how many of these studies were controlled, double-blind peer-reviewed experiments or how many produced results supporting alternative medicine or parts thereof.

They contend that many forms of alternative medicine are rejected by conventional medicine because the efficacy of the treatments has not been demonstrated through double-blind randomized controlled trials; this is not a moot point, since all conventional drugs reach the market only after such trials have proved their efficacy. One is led to wonder why whole categories of drugs or treatments should be excused from these routine tests. Also, some skeptics of alternative practices point out that a person may attribute symptomatic relief to an otherwise ineffective therapy due to the natural recovery from or the cyclical nature of an illness (the regression fallacy), the placebo effect, or the possibility that the person never originally had a true illness.

Problems with known tests and studies: Critics contend that observer bias and poor study design invalidate the results of many studies carried out by alternative medicine promoters.

A review of the effectiveness of certain alternative medicine techniques for cancer treatment, while finding that most of these treatments are not merely "unproven" but are proven not to work, notes that several studies have found evidence that the psychosocial treatment of patients by psychologists is linked to survival advantages (although it comments that these results are not consistently replicated). The same review, while specifically noting that "complementary therapies for cancer-related symptoms were not part of this review", cites studies indicating that several complementary therapies can provide benefits by, for example, reducing pain and improving the mood of patients.

Some argue that less research is carried out on alternative medicine because many alternative medicine techniques cannot be patented, and hence there is little financial incentive to study them. Drug research, by contrast, can be very lucrative, which has resulted in funding of trials by pharmaceutical companies. Many people, including conventional and alternative medical practitioners, contend that this funding has led to corruption of the scientific process for approval of drug usage, and that ghostwritten work has appeared in major peer-reviewed medical journals.

Increasing the funding for research of alternative medicine techniques was the purpose of the National Centre for Complementary and Alternative Medicine. NCCAM and its predecessor, the Office of Alternative Medicine, have spent more than $200 million on such research since 1991. The German Federal Institute for Drugs and Medical Devices Commission E has studied many herbal remedies for efficacy.

Safety

Critics contend that some people have been hurt or killed directly from the various practices or indirectly by failed diagnoses or the subsequent avoidance of conventional medicine which they believe is truly efficacious.

Alternative medicine critics agree with its proponents that people should be free to choose whatever method of healthcare they want, but stipulate that people must be informed as to the safety and efficacy of whatever method they choose. People who choose alternative medicine may think they are choosing a safe, effective medicine, while they may only be getting quack remedies. Grapefruit seed extract is an example of quackery when multiple studies demonstrate its universal antimicrobial effect is due to synthetic antimicrobial contamination.

COMMERCIAL TRADE IN MEDICINAL PLANTS

The large and growing demand for plant-based medicines and changing population patterns have prompted a growing domestic and international trade in medicinal plants. The following information from Lange (1997, 1998) gives an indication of the scale of the trade.

According to Customs data, approximately 440 000 t of medicinal and aromatic plants were traded internationally in 1996, with a reported value of USD1.3 billion. Hong Kong, Japan and Germany were the largest importers during 1994 and 1995, the United States being the third largest importer overall during the period 1992 to 1996. Approximately 60% of imports into Germany in 1996 originated from non-European countries, with exports from Asia dominating the trade, followed by exports from Africa. China was also by far the largest exporter of medicinal and aromatic plants to world markets during the mid-1990s, with average exports topping 140 000 t from 1992 to 1996. The second largest exporter was India, with export volumes averaging approximately 36 000 t during this period.

A wide diversity of medicinal plant species are used and traded for medicinal purposes. A recent TRAFFIC 1 study of the European medicinal plant trade (Lange, 1998) estimates that over 2000 medicinal and aromatic plant species are used commercially in Europe, of which 1200 to 1300 are native. Approximately 90% of the European species are collected from the wild, with eastern Europe and the Mediterranean regions being the main suppliers (Lange, 1998). In India it has been estimated that approximately 7500 species are used for medicinal and veterinary purposes. Over 10,000 species are used medicinally in China, with 1,000 species commonly used in medicinal preparations, of which 80% are wild-collected.

Harvest of medicinal plants to supply domestic and foreign markets provides an important source of cash income in many countries. In Nepal, for example, Olsen has estimated that 470 000 households are engaged in commercial collection of medicinal plants. Several publications in the FAO Non-Wood Forest Product Series have drawn attention to the current and potential role of medicinal plants in economic development.

Declines in Medicinal Plant Populations

There is growing evidence that the populations of many medicinal plant species are declining in the wild. These declines are the result of several factors, key among them being habitat degradation and expanding harvests. TRAFFIC's study of the European medicinal plant trade identified approximately 150 European species reported to be threatened in at least one European country; a TRAFFIC study in East/Southern Africa identified approximately 100 species of conservation concern in one or more countries (Marshall, 1998). Reviews of the status of medicinal plant species according to the 'Red List' (threat) criteria of IUCN-The World Conservation Union in three regions of India identified approximately 70 species considered at risk.

Fourteen species have been included in the Appendices of the Convention on International Trade in Endangered Species of Wild Fauna and Flora (CITES) owing to concern that they might be threatened unless international trade is subject to specific controls.

USE AND DIVERSITY IN MEDICINAL PLANTS

In India, of the 17,000 species of higher plants, 7500 are known for medicinal uses. This proportion of medicinal plants is the highest proportion of plants known for their medical purposes in any country of the world for the existing flora of that respective country. Ayurveda, the oldest medical system in Indian sub-continent, has alone reported approximately 2000 medicinal plant species, followed by Siddha and Unani. The Charak Samhita, an age-old written document on herbal therapy, reports on the production of 340 herbal drugs and their indigenous uses. Currently, approximately 25% of drugs are derived from plants, and many others are synthetic analogues built on prototype compounds isolated from plant species in modern pharmacopoeia.

The northern part of India harbours a great diversity of medicinal plants because of the majestic Himalayan range. So far about 8000 species of angiosperms, 44 species of gymnosperms and 600 species of pteridophytes have been reported in the Indian Himalaya, of these 1748 species are known as medicinal plants. The maximum medicinal plants (1717 species) have been reported around the 1800 m elevation range. On the regional scale, the maximum species of medicinal plants have been reported from Uttaranchal, followed by Sikkim and North Bengal. The trans-Himalaya sustains about 337 species of medicinal plants, which is low compared to other areas of the Himalaya due to the distinct geography and ecological marginal conditions.

Several plant species are endemic to the Himalayan region. Out of total known number of higher plants from India, approximately 46% are endemic to the Himalaya. Of the total medicinal plant species, sixty-two species of medicinal plants are endemic to the Himalaya and 208 extend their distribution to the adjacent areas, and are therefore classified as near endemic.

Over 200 species of Himalayan medicinal plants are consumed raw, roasted, boiled, fried, cooked, or they are used in the form of oil, spices, jams or pickles.

The indigenous communities use some medicinal plant species as a source of food, fodder, timber as well as various other ethnobotanical purposes. For example, apart from the use of Myrica esculenta and Terminalia bellirica as medicines, the fruits of these species are edible, the leaves are used for fodder and the wood is used for fuel. Approximately 81 species of Himalayan medicinal plants are known to be used for the extraction of oil. Of the total 675 species of Himalayan wild edibles, 171 are used for the treatment of diseases. The crop plants diversity is also a source of traditional medicine.

Apart from the human use, animal husbandry uses many plant species as its primary source of healthcare in northern India. The reliance on medicinal plants is also due to cultural preferences. Medicinal plants have strong acceptance in religious activities of north Indian native communities, who worship the plants in the form of various gods, goddesses and minor deities.

Origanum vulgare, Saussurea obvallata, Ocimum sanctum, Cedrus deodara, Cynodon dactylon, Aegle marmelos, Juniperus communis, Musa paradissica, Nardostachys grandiflora, Zanthoxylum armatum, Ficus benghalensis, and Ficus religiosa are examples of the medicinal plants highly used for medicinal as well as a religious purposes by the Hindus in northern India.

The Buddhist community in northern India regards Terminalia chebula as an important medicine as well as sacred fruit. It has been stated long ago that the therapeutic potency of medicinal plants is more effective and better suited to a person of a particular region or culture in which the plant is naturally growing. This idea has given a way to the development of a new drug for heart patients of specific ethnic groups in African countries.

Challenges in Medicinal Plants Sector

The continuous increase in human population is one of the causes for concern in meeting the daily requirements of food and medicine as the economy and livelihoods of human societies living in developing countries primarily depend on forest products. This phenomenon is leading to continuous erosion of forest and the forest products, thus making challenge to meet the requirements as well as to conserve useful bio-resources.

More and more species are being gradually added in the Materia Medica; however, the standards of their purity and correct identification do not keep pace with the process of expansion. The market prices for medicinal plants and derived materials provide only a limited insight into the workings of the market, and not on the precise information of profits, supply and demand. We have identified the following major features and challenges on the basis of examining the existing knowledge on the medicinal plants sector.

Rising Demand

The World Health Organization (WHO) has estimated the present demand for medicinal plants is approximately US $14 billion per year. The demand for medicinal plant-based raw materials is growing at the rate of 15 to 25% annually, and according to an estimate of WHO, the demand for medicinal plants is likely to increase more than US $5 trillion in 2050. In India, the medicinal plant-related trade is estimated to be approximately US $1 billion per year.

The projected escalating demand of medicinal plants has led to the over-harvesting of many plants from wild, which subsequently results in the loss of their existing populations. For example, the large quantity of Himalayan yew (Taxus baccata) has been gathered from the wild since its extract, taxol, was established as a use in the treatment of ovarian cancer. Aconitum heterophyllum, Nardostachys grandiflora, Dactylorhiza hatagirea, Polygonatum verticillatum, Gloriosa superba, Arnebia benthamii and Megacarpoea polyandra are other examples of north Indian medicinal plant species which have been overexploited for therapeutic uses and have subsequently been placed today in rare and endangered categories.

Many medicinal plant species are used in curing more than one disease, and as a result, these species are under pressure due to over collection from wild. For example, Hemidesmus indicus is used to cure 34 types of diseases; Aegle marmelos 31, Phyllanthus emblica 29, and Gloriosa superba 28. Overexploitation and continuous depletion of medicinal plants have not only affected their supply and loss of genetic diversity, but have seriously affected the livelihoods of indigenous people living in the forest margins.

More than 95% of the 400 plant species used in preparing medicine by various industries are harvested from wild populations in India. Harvesting medicinal plants for commercial use, coupled with the destructive harvest of underground parts of slow reproducing, slow growing and habitat-specific species, are the crucial factors in meeting the goal of sustainability. Harvesting shoots and leaves of medicinal plants may decline their photosynthetic capacity, and as well as the potential for survival and effective propagation. Medicinal plants tolerance to harvest varies with climatic conditions as the temperate herbs become highly vulnerable to harvest of individuals. Furthermore, rising demand with shrinking habitats may lead to the local extinction of many medicinal plant species.

Increasing Rarity

The continuous exploitation of several medicinal plant species from the wild and substantial loss of their habitats during past 15 years have resulted in population decline of many high value medicinal plant species over the years. The primary threats to medicinal plants are those that affect any kind of biodiversity used by humans. The weakening of customary laws, which have regulated the use of natural resources, are among the causes of threatening the medicinal plant species.

These customary laws have often proved to be easily diluted by modern socio-economic forces. There are many other potential causes of rarity in medicinal plant species, such as habitat specificity, narrow range of distribution, land use disturbances, introduction of non-natives, habitat alteration, climatic changes, heavy livestock grazing, explosion of human population, fragmentation and degradation of population, population bottleneck, and genetic drift. Additionally, natural enemies (*i.e.*, pathogens, herbivores, and seed predators) could substantially limit the abundance of rare medicinal plant species in any given area.

In addition to the consumption of medicinal plants by animals, there are physical ailments in humans, which are cured by different species of the same genera. For example, the malarial fever is treated by many species of Swertia (*e.g.* Swertia chiraiyta, S. angustifolia, and S. cordata). Similarly, different species of Berberis (*e.g.* Berberis aristata, B. asiatica, B. lycium, B. chitria and B. jaeschkeana) are used as a source of berberidine to cure certain eye diseases. Furthermore, different species of the same genera contain different proportions of chemical quantity, and there is a preference over their demand; however, the degree of threat for their exploitation is relatively lower than those species, which do not have alternatives. An estimated 4,000 to 10,000 species of medicinal plants face potential local, national, regional or global extinction, with subsequent serious consequences for livelihoods, economies and health care systems. Although, a few studies exist on the rare and endangered medicinal plant species of the northern India, none of these studies have complete data set for even a single species. In 2003, 71 rare and endangered medicinal plant species have been assessed for the northwest Himalaya during the Conservation Assessment and Management Plan workshop, according to the guidelines of the World Conservation Union. In northern India, Aconitum is the rarest genus with 5 species, followed by Rheum with 4 rare species. Out of the 71 rare medicinal plants, 92% are in active trade; 74% are traded nationally and 35% are traded internationally.

The meager availability of data on the population and quantum of rare species in nature, however, has restricted their categorization to a few species on the basis of herbarium collection and by consultation by a few experts. The present assessments are also questioned for their validity on the assignment of threat categories to the species, including the number of taxa in danger for specific area.

The problems in assessing the species is increased in the mountainous region, especially high altitude areas because of tough and inaccessibility of the terrain, inhospitable climatic conditions, and short life cycle of plants. Most of the available data have been collected from the easily accessible areas in these mountains.

Indigenous communities and commercial herb gatherers also raid these same areas for collection of medicinal plants. Therefore, the estimated population density of categorized rare medicinal plants is not precise because it differs the areas that never and hardly undergone any collection of such rare medicinal plant species.

6

Ethnomedicine and Health Care

The Sonowal Kacharis is an endogamous group of Kachari tribe and a popular plain scheduled tribe population of Assam. Various types of locally available herbs and leaves of wild plants are used by them as medicine. Like many other communities of the region, there are few herbal specialists among the Sonowal Kachari. These specialists or medicine-men have considerable knowledge about the herbs and its medicinal use. Normally they learn about these medicinal plants and its uses from their ancestor. These medicine-men are referred by different term according to the cultural norms. Among the Sonowal Kachari's they are called as Bez. Of course in rural Assam, they are mainly known by this term. It has been observed in the villages that use of herbal medicine for curing certain diseases are quite known to the people and besides medicine-men, many elderly persons known about the use of herbal medicines. Some of the diseases and their indigenous methods of treatment are given below:

(1) Fever: Lime (Citrus auran tifolia) juice mixed with sugar is applied on the forehead of the patient to get relief from fever.

(2) Diarrhoea: Dry goose berry (Emblica officinalis) powder and black salt mixed with cold water is taken. Bark of Long Pepper (Pipoli tree) mixed with Misiri water is also used to cure the disease.

(3) Dysentery: Lime (Citrus auran tifolia) juicewith hot water and little salt is used in dysentery. The juice of black Tulsi leaves (Ocimum sanctum) and Sirata (Swertiachirata) is also used for the purpose. The juice of tender leaves (three numbers) of mango (Mangifera indica), black berry (S.cuminii) and goose berry (Emblica officinalis) (equal proportions) together with honey are mixed with goat milk and is taken to cure blood dysentery. Honey together with the juice of Dubari grass (Family-Gramineae) can cure blood dysentery and need to be taken for three/ four days. They also use a kind of wild herb, locally called Manimuni (Centila asiatica). The juice of this herb mixed with sugar or honey

should be taken continuously for a month to cure the disease. They also use limewater (chun pani) mixed with juice of turmeric (Purcuma domestica) leave to get relief from blood dysentery and mucous.

(4) Blood Vomiting: A table spoon of carrot (Dancus carota) juice mixed with honey can cure blood vomiting.

(5) Liver Disease: Two to three raw or ripe Papayas (Carica papaya) daily can cure liver disease. A curry prepared from the bud of banana (Musa paradisiaca) and the meat of pigeon is also used as a medicine for the purpose.

(6) Jaundice: The medicine is prepared by pounding five or six number of Silikha (Myroballum) mixing with jaggery and it can cure jaundice. A glass of sugarcane (Saccharum officinarum) juice twice daily prescribed for the purpose. Boiled raw papaya (Carica papaya) is said to be good for curing the disease. Kardoi (Averrhoa carambola), Goose Berry (Emblica officinalis), Sugar cane (Saccharun officinarum), Neem leave (Azadirachta indica), a wild herb known as Duran ban (Lecas aspera), Brahmi sak (Herpestis monnieria), Purakol (Musa sapientum) are prescribed edibles for the patient.

(7) Nose Bleeding: Flower of Pomegranate (Punica granatum Linn) is crushed and 3-4 drops of juice is poured inside the nose to give immediate relief.

(8) Tonsilities: Juice is prepared by mixing one Amara seed (Sponolias mangifera), one Silikha seed (Mysoballum) and a piece of Turmeric (Purcuma domestica) and advice the patient gargles for a week regularly.

(9) Worms: Paste of five lemon seeds (Citrus aurantifolia) mixed with water and is prescribed to eat in empty stomach for a few days. The twigs of Chirata (Swertia chirata) are soaked in the water overnight and the water is prescribed to drink in empty stomach in the morning for one week regularly.

(10) Scabies: Lemon juice (Citrus aurantifolia) mixed with coconut oil is massaged for curing scabies. To remove scabies they take bath with hot water in which leaves of Neem (Azadirachta officinarum) were boiled. Twigs of Chirata (Swertia chirata) arecrushed into paste with water to be used as an ointment and applied on the skin. Chirata water is prescribed to drink in the morning in empty stomach.

(11) Pain in the Ear: Juice of Tulsi (Ocimum sanctum) is boiled and put it in the ears to heal earache.

The patient is treated with available herbs, flora and minerals. Some of these are home remedies and some are specially prescribed by herbalist or folk medicine man available in the community.

The practice of ethno-medicine is a complex multi-disciplinary system constituting the use of plants, spirituality and the natural environment and has been the source of healing for people for millennia.

The spiritual aspects of health and sickness have been an integral component of the ethno-medicinal practice for centuries.

Present Position of Tribes

The tribal health care practices and system of treating diseases are based on their deep observation and belief in nature.

But with the development of education and their awareness towards importance of health and health care and also with the advent of modern health care facilities, Government health measures these people are becoming more interested in taking modern medicine instead of traditional herbal medicine.

Saving the Plant is Saving the Life

According to the text of Vishnu Samhita, causing any harm to the plants/animals is a sin. Even purloining of parts/products of any of these living beings is a crime. The sinner/criminals are liable to chastisement in this life and also after death. The punishments are of diverse nature:-pecuniary, corporal, expiatory and donation of specific articles to Brahmins.

ZINC NUTRITION AND TRIBAL HEALTH IN INDIA

Zinc is an essential trace element that contributes immensely to human health and development. It is an important structural component of most proteins and contributes to the function of more than 200 enzymes in humans. Zinc also plays a central role in cellular growth and differentiation because of its critical role in RNA and DNA synthesis and it is important for brain function. Body functions affected by zinc nutriture include growth, immune system development and function, normal integrity of intestinal mucosa, pregnancy outcome and neuro-behavioural development.

Zinc deficiency therefore results in adverse consequences on the body, the magnitude of which depends on whether the ensuing deficit is marginal or severe. Marginal zinc deficiency is the most common and, although asymptomatic, it is associated with impaired immune function, anorexia, dysfunction of smell and taste, irritability, depression, anger, sleepiness, reduced sperm production in men and decreased mental ability. Severe zinc deficiency, which rarely occurs, is characterized by severely impaired immune function, dermatitis, growth impairment, alopecia, lethargy and recurrent infections such as diarrhoea.

Marginal zinc deficiency appears to be an important public health problem in many developing countries. Data derived from FAO National Food Balance

Sheets suggests, for example, that about half of the world's population is at risk of inadequate zinc intake. Furthermore, a third of pre-school children (34.0 %) worldwide have stunted physical growth.

The recognition of childhood stunting as an indirect indicator of a population's risk of zinc deficiency supports the proposition that inadequate zinc nutriture is a widespread public health problem. Stunting is recognized as an indirect indicator of zinc status in some populations because zinc nutrition has been shown to have a significant impact on growth of young children. A meta-analysis of 25 studies of the effect of zinc supplementation on growth in children less than 13 years of age showed that zinc supplementation has a highly statistically significant effect on linear growth and weight gain. About 70 % of the world's stunted children under five years of age live in Asia and each year, zinc deficiency is estimated to contribute to more than a million deaths worldwide with a significant proportion of the zinc related morbidity and mortality occurring in South Asia. However little is known about the zinc status of the Indian population due to a lack of nationally representative data on this micronutrient and the absence of an appropriate indicator for assessing zinc status of individuals. Nevertheless, some studies from different parts of India have suggested that marginal zinc deficiency is common, though these studies used plasma zinc, a measure of zinc status that is affected by the acute phase response, and indirect indicators like stunting. The national prevalence of childhood stunting stands at 42.6% among preschool children (NFHS-2, 1998) and the International Zinc Nutrition Consultative Group estimates that over 25 % of the total population in India is at risk of inadequate zinc intake.

In a vast and multiethnic country like India, the extent of zinc deficiency is likely to vary from state to state and even within each state, from one area to another, depending upon several factors such as socioeconomic status, food habits, level of literacy, climate, religion and cultural practices. Various tribal populations are among the most underprivileged people since they occupy the lowest part of the socioeconomic strata in Indian society and therefore have the highest likelihood of any form of malnutrition including zinc deficiency. How ever the scarcity of data on the zinc status of the Indian tribal populations makes it difficult to draw any conclusive evidence on the extent of the deficiency and the need for programmatic inter-ventions to address this problem. This paper attempts to provide reasons for studying zinc nutriture among tribes, why this is an issue that needs addressing in this indigenous population and possible programmatic approaches to meaningfully address this condition.

Dietary Sources and Zinc Bioavailability

Individual zinc status is influenced by intake of zinc from the diet, its absorption (or bioavailability) and the loss of it from the body. Pertaining to zinc intake, the richest dietary sources of zinc are the organs and flesh of mammals, fowls, fish and crustaceans, and zinc-fortified foods. Organ and flesh meat and poultry do not contain any known specific anti-nutritional factors that hinder zinc absorption. Eggs and dairy products are also rich in zinc and free of phytates, but they have slightly lower zinc content than can be found in organ and flesh foods. Absorption of zinc takes place in the small intestine and the extent of uptake of this nutrient is determined largely by the presence of specific dietary factors that either inhibit or enhance its absorption. Among the several factors that interfere with digestion and absorption of dietary zinc, the phytate content of the diet is most important. The higher order phytates, like inositol hexaphosphate and pentaphosphates found in most cereal and legumes, are known to bind to zinc and form poorly soluble complexes that lead to reduced absorption from the intestinal lumen.

Although most cereals and legumes have relati-vely high amounts of zinc, they contain high concentrations of phytates, which reduce the amount of absorbable zinc from these foods, and therefore they are relatively poor sources of zinc. Starchy roots and tubers have much lower zinc content than legumes and cereals. In general, fruits and vegetables are not considered rich sources of zinc, although some green leafy vegetables like spinach have moderate amounts of zinc but with uncertain bioavailability.

It is clear from the above discussion that a cereal or legume based diet without an adequate inclusion of animal source foods or an external source of zinc often will not allow individuals to meet their daily zinc requirements. The diet of an average Indian is mainly cereal based and is said to be low in zinc and rich in zinc inhibitors that reduce zinc absorption. A study by Chakravarty and Sinha (2002) in rural areas of five Indian states (Assam, Bihar, Orissa, Tripura and West Bengal) found the average consumption of zinc among various age groups to be much lower than their recommended daily allowance (RDA).

A large proportion of the families in this study (about 84.0%) had deficient zinc intakes with more than 50.0 % of the families in all the surveyed areas having moderate to severe deficiency in dietary zinc intake.

In general, poor Indian families are often vulnerable to zinc deficiency since majority of Indians are vegetarians and vegetarian diets are often lower in zinc content and contain factors that hinder zinc absorption in contrast to meat-based diets.

Hence vegetarian families unable to meet their zinc intake through adequate inclusion of non-meat sources of bioavailable zinc in the diet (e.g. eggs and diary products), zinc fortified foods or zinc supplements are at higher risk of zinc deficiency. Such is the case in most tribal communities in India.

Tribal Populations and Zinc Deficiency

Tribal groups constitute about 8.2 % of the total population in India (Indian Government Census, 2001). According to government statistics, tribes can be found in approximately 461 communities (Ajumder, 2001) with almost 92 % of them residing in rural areas, mostly in remote underserved forest regions with little or no basic civic amenities like transport, roads, markets, health care, safe drinking water or sanitation (Indian Government Census, 2001).

Tribal communities therefore lag behind other commu-nities with respect to attainment of income, education, health and other requisites for good community nutrition (Srinivasan and Mohanty, 2004). A study by Mishra (2005) using the National Family Health Survey (NFHS-2) found that in almost all the states of India, tribal households had a higher incidence of childhood stunting (52.3%) than non-tribal households (42.8%).

Using the same dataset, Nagda (2004) reported an anemia prevalence of more than 80% among tribal children. Several studies have also reported deficient intake of calories and protein among tribal populations relative to the Indian RDA, which may be an explanation for the high rates of stunting among this group.

Iron deficiency is recognized as the major cause of anemia in tribal communities and several studies have reported that deficiencies of micronutrients such as iron and zinc often occur together.Hence the high rates of anemia among tribal populations provide additional evidence of the possibility of marginal zinc deficiency in tribal areas.

This is further supported by the high prevalence of stunting and the highly deficient dietary energy intakes in the tribal populations since intake of both zinc and iron are known to be highly correlated with dietary energy intake (Willett, 1998). At least one study has shown that zinc intake of populations in tribal regions was significantly lower than that of any of the other regions studied.

Tribal populations still largely depend on agriculture and forest products for their livelihood and they follow a relatively homogenous lifestyle with their food habits, dietary practices and general pattern of living. Most tribes still rely on their indigenous foods, which usually consist of wild unconventional forest products although some cultivate grains and other farm products for subsistence. The most frequently used cereals are maize, millet or rice and these form part of a major meal at least once daily. Since the tribal diet is usually plant based with significant amounts of anti-nutritional factors, which limit the absorption, and/or bioavailability of zinc and because very limited amounts of animal source foods are consumed, these populations are at high risk for zinc deficiency.

Kapil et al. (2003) assessed the serum zinc levels of tribal adults in Jharkhand and found that 53% of the study subjects were zinc deficient (serum zinc < 70 μg/dl), with deficiency occurring more frequently among women (61.3%) than men (38.7%). The authors recommended the need to assess the zinc status of tribals in other parts of the country in order to establish the magnitude of the problem. Despite the fact that most tribals are vegetarians as is much of the Indian population as a whole, the non-vegetarian tribals still find it difficult to afford frequent consumption of animal products.

The nutritional value of most of the wild plants used in tribal diets has been evaluated in recent years but a review of the literature reveals that, although most of these plants contain significant amounts of micronutrients, they also contain large amounts of anti-nutritional components that inhibit absorption of such minerals from the diet. Sundriyal and Sundriyal (2004) analysed the nutritional content of 27 of the most frequently used wild edible plants among tribal groups in Sikkim and found that the zinc content of some of these plants ranged from as high as 1490 μg/g to as low as 212 μg/g; however, the fibre contents of these plants ranged from 5.1% to as high as 39.9%.

Apart from low supply and poor bioavailability of dietary zinc, increased urinary and fecal excretion and high needs of zinc under certain physiologic conditions such as infection also contribute to zinc deficiency.

Earlier studies indicated that, comparatively, the overall health of the tribal population is inferior to that of people elsewhere in India and that poor environmental sanitation and unhygienic personal practices predispose tribal populations to high risk of infection.

Findings from a recent national survey showed that 82.4% of tribal households did not have latrines and 78.1% did not have drainage facilities in their homes (NFHS-2, 1998), a situation that predis-poses children to diarrhoeal disease. The survey also found that the prevalence of diarrhoea and acute respiratory infection (ARI) was higher among tribal children than children of non-tribal mothers. Similarly, the study by Nagda (2004) suggested that childhood diarrhoea, ARI, anemia and fever were major causes of infant mortality in tribal areas.

Diarrhoea for instance leads to reduced intake of dietary zinc as a result of anorexia and increased loss of body zinc as a result of malabsorption or rapid gut transit time, since the main route by which zinc is lost from the body is through the gastrointestinal tract. Another highly prevalent infection that may negatively affect zinc status in tribal areas is intestinal helminthes.

Zinc is also lost from the body through urine, menstrual flow, semen and sloughed skin, nails, and hair, but the quantity lost through these routes are small and may not significantly contribute to zinc deficiency.

THE TRIBAL HEALTH INITIATIVE MODEL

The THI healthcare delivery model is based on a 3-tiered framework of healthcare staff (doctors, health workers and health auxiliaries) with a base hospital as its nodal point. The base hospital functions as the centre and administrator of the health system, which was our primary reason for choosing the hospital as the setting of our study.

The first phase of the base hospital, the outpatient facility, was a mud and thatched hut erected in 1993. By the end of 1996, the hospital had expanded to a 10-bedded facility with an operation theatre, labour room, neonatal care facility, emergency room and a laboratory. Currently, the hospital has 20 beds. Tubal ligations and intrauterine devices are provided on a voluntary basis to tribal women who desire to end or limit their reproductive capabilities. While on-site doctors oversee up to the secondary level of curative treatment in the hospital setting, the roles of the health worker and health auxiliary involve a limited combination of clinical and preventive services, both in the hospital and in the 21 tribal villages to which the THI provides health services. The hospital has a multimedia centre that organizes weekly screening of health education videos for inpatients. The THI, however, does not provide immunizations to its target population.

The THI health workers are tribal women who have studied up to the eighth standard of school, and received one-and-a-half years of hospital-based residential training in primary and secondary care. After successful completion of their training, they are deployed at the base hospital to function as nurses. They also participate in the technical aspects of peripheral health activities that take place in the field.

Health auxiliaries are illiterate tribal women, past childbearing age, who function as the THI's first point of contact for patients in each of the 21 villages. They receive a total of 25 days of training at the base hospital. Health auxiliaries register births, deaths, marriages and pregnancies in their respective villages, register and periodically weigh children under 5 years of age, collect pregnant mothers for village antenatal clinics, and refer complicated diseases and deliveries to the base hospital. Health auxiliaries are also trained to provide services for the prevention, detection and treatment of malnutrition, as well as for the early detection and treatment of respiratory infections.

Six medicines are provided by the THI's base hospital to the health auxiliaries to aid in managing minor medical conditions of patients with common ailments. Graphical methods, including colour coding, are used to familiarize health auxiliaries with the medicines provided to them (e.g. 'the red medicine [paracetamol] is for mild fever'), and descriptive methods are used to teach health auxiliaries to make a symptomatic diagnosis of common morbidities such as a cold, fever and respiratory infections. Children are weighed with the aid of Teaching Aids at Low Cost™ (TALC) weighing scales that allow the documenter to make graphical notations on pre-formatted weight charts to track the growth status of children. These qualitative methods have obviated the need for literate village-based health staff. To examine an allopathic healthcare model for tribal populations, however, it is important to realize that the alternative medicinal systems including Ayurveda and Siddha are often rooted in tribal assumptions of healthcare delivery. Not surprisingly, the health status and health-seeking behaviour in the area of study before the THI intervention, as documented by Karunakaran, is highly skewed towards alternative medicine. Implementation of an allopathic healthcare delivery system in tribal areas requires considerable time to surmount the cultural and social barriers associated with these medical interventions.

Methods

We chose the year 2000 as the starting point for this study based on our observation of general tribal confidence in the allopathic inpatient services provided by the THI. Specifically, door-to-door interviews of tribals in selected villages during 1999 revealed that a majority (77.9%) of the individuals had confidence in the efficacy of the allopathic health services provided by the base hospital. This was in contrast to the Karunakaran study of 1987, which showed that tribal confidence in allopathic medicines varied dramatically as a function of the disease.

While a multidisease surveillance system to monitor the incidence of morbidities in the village setting was not available at the time, we used the base hospital of the THI to observe the incidence and treatment of severe and predominant gastrointestinal diseases, mental health-related disorders, typhoid and anaemia in the in-patient setting.

We know that the use of a hospitalized population as a denominator for calculating the incidence of specific conditions may not be an accurate indicator of the health status of the population as a whole. The data may be reflective of the sector of the population that is willing to receive allopathic services from the THI system.

To that end, we specifically denote these epidemiological observations as 'inpatient incidence' in contrast to incidence data that could be calculated from an active and comprehensive surveillance methodology. The gastrointestinal disorders under observation were acid peptic disease, acute gastritis, acute gastroenteritis (diarrhoea), cholecystitis, colitis and duodenal ulcers. Given that THI's implementation of the Revised National Tuberculosis Control Programme (RNTCP) began in early 2000, we felt it appropriate to begin monitoring tuberculosis disease management and incidence both among inpatients and out-patients. Mortality patterns, however, were delineated through a combination of inpatient and field data collected by the base hospital via THI's health auxiliaries deployed in the villages. The health auxiliaries also reported deaths occurring in the 21 villages, as well as the symptoms associated with the deaths.

Diagnosis of patients in the inpatient, outpatient and field setting of the THI with the morbidities under examination took place using the diagnostic rubric outlined with the exception of tuberculosis, which was diagnosed and treated using the RNTCP protocol.

Statistics

Selection of sample size and method of allocation. The statistical universe for monitoring of the incidence of severe gastrointestinal disorders, mental health-related ailments, typhoid and anaemia included only those patients who were admitted as inpatients to the THI in 2000 (558 patients), 2001 (644 patients), 2002 (733 patients), and 2003 (850 patients). All outpatients, therefore, were excluded from the study sample, as their illnesses were minor. From the inpatient sample, those diagnosed with the observed morbidities were analysed by gender.

Mental health-related cases were further categorized according to both gender and age groups at 5-year intervals of age. Incidence monitoring of tuberculosis, however, included both inpatients and outpatients in 2000 (12 947 patients), 2001 (12 796 patients), 2002 (14 124 patients) and 2003 (17 033 patients). Individual cases were categorized according to gender, sputum positivity/negativity and extrapulmonary diagnosis, and RNTCP treatment regimens.

The statistical universe for the analysis of mortality patterns included inpatients, outpatients and village populations within THI's geographical scope of health services. The subjects were divided into 5 representative age groups beginning with the infant group (0–1 year), the child group (2–5 years), the youth age group (6–15 years), the 'age of productivity' group (16–50 years) and the geriatric age group (51+ years). To illustrate tribal social factors that may detract from THI's allopathic interventions, infant mortality was separated into deaths occurring from medical morbidities, and those occurring from male or female infanticide. The presence of infanticide was determined through direct questioning of the parent(s), who often clearly stated their involvement in the death, and observations of induced asphyxiation or the presence of poisoning-related symptoms.

Finally, mortality patterns as functions of predominant morbidities in the area were examined through diagnosis and allocation of deaths occurring from neonatal causes (neonatal death), suicide (mental health), pneumonia (lower respiratory tract infection), meningitis (neurological disease), acute gastroenteritis and dysentery (gastrointestinal disorders).

Statistical analysis: We calculated the incidence rate of gastrointestinal disorders, mental-health related ailments, anaemia and typhoid in the inpatient setting by considering the population at risk to be the total number of inpatients in a given year. The incidence rate of tuberculosis, however, was calculated by considering the population at risk to be a combination of inpatients and outpatients for that given year. While these incidence rates do not provide a comprehensive measure of population health with respect to the morbidities under observation that would be attainable through a multidisease surveillance system, our goal was to examine an allopathic healthcare model from a clinical and epidemiological perspective.

Taking into consideration the ability of an allopathic healthcare delivery system to single-handedly provide health services to a relatively small tribal population with confidence in allopathic health services, we believe that calculating incidence rates using inpatient and outpatient admissions provides a relatively accurate description of the healthcare model's influence on the target population. As previously mentioned, however, a bias does arise when using hospital-based data to reflect the health status of the population in general, given that persons who avail of hospital services are (i) those individuals who are sick, and (ii) those who are confident in allopathic interventions.

Gender-dependent susceptibility of examined morbidities required the use of previously described gender categorizations to assign a percentage of a given disease's incidence to the appropriate gender in the inpatient and/or outpatient setting.

Determination of age-and selected disease-specific mortality involved standard percentage calculations based on the number of deaths associated with previously categorized age groups and selected morbidities, respectively.

Infant mortality rates were calculated through standard formulas, where the number of births and deaths corresponded to those occurring both at the base hospital and in THI's geographic area from information furnished by THI's health auxiliaries. For infant mortality rates, 95% confidence intervals were calculated, while the relatively small number of events and sample size used in calculating disease incidence rates (limited to inpatients and outpatients) did not necessitate the calculation of invariably wide confidence intervals.

MISSIONARIES AND THEIR MEDICINE: A CHRISTIAN MODERNITY FOR TRIBAL INDIA

In a novel written in 1958, the Bengali literary critic Pramathanath Bishi suggested that there was a meeting of the medieval and modern ages in late eighteenth-century Bengal in the persons of the British Baptist missionary William Carey and his Bengali *munshi*, Ramram Basu. In Bishi's view, Carey belonged to the Christian medieval age, seeking all explanations in religion, while Basu belonged to the modern age, determined to replace God with knowledge.

Bishi's tongue-in-cheek reversal of the usual narratives of colonial modernity (and of the role played by Christian missions in it) has not proved popular with scholars of South Asia. Christian missions therefore remain secure as pilots of modernity, especially in its imperial form, and implicated in all its coercive and contradictory aspects.

With or without the analytical framework of 'Christian modernity' that Hardiman deploys, this rich and meticulously connected historical study of a Church Missionary Society (CMS) medical mission to the Bhil 'tribes' of western India, which stretches over a period of about 80 years (1880–*c.* 1960), would have been an important contribution to Indian history. To begin with, although education and medical service have historically been the two principal 'specializations' of Christian public works in India, only the former has received significant attention from historians, and in recent times mostly in order to reveal the allegedly hegemonic political functions of such education. Hardiman does propose a similar project of transformation and legitimation for medical missions, but by presenting a complex story involving a variety of agents over a sustained period of time, he achieves something quite different.

What we have is a story of how this particular CMS mission came to be established among a distinctive group of 'subaltern' people deemed primitive in official as well as higher-status Indian views. Hardiman shows how the strategies of the mission were shaped in response to ongoing social changes within that selected constituency, as well as the power dynamics of the region. In addition, the medical 'specialization' of the mission arose out of theological developments in Britain but also outstanding local events, such as a tremendous famine in the region in 1899–1900 when the mission became the most important relief supplier to the afflicted.

Certainly this, or any other, medical mission was not just about treating bodily diseases. But is this a story of the encounter of two belief systems—European scientific modernity (hitched to a miracle-free Christianity) and Bhil cosmology, the former underpinning claims to civilisational superiority and exclusive right to rule?

In Hardiman's article-length work on the same theme in an earlier edited volume of essays on medical missions in Asia and Africa, this appeared to be his argument. In the present volume, Hardiman makes the argument more complex and more satisfying by referring to the structures of authority that authorise 'belief': not only Bhil belief, but also Christian and scientific belief.

This allows him to open up the practically effaced history of racial hierarchy and conflict within missions and churches in colonial India, and subsequently describe the tortuous process of a parallel 'decolonization', during which time the argument of expertise continued to justify white missionary domination in 'specialist' areas such as the medical mission even after the churches themselves had been handed over to Indian Christian authority. Parallel to this institutional transformation is the story of a cultural transformation, such that by the 1940s, respect for Gandhian nationalism, as well as deference for Bhil beliefs and customs, came to be perceived by the Christian authorities, including the remaining European missionaries, as less of a threat to Christian faith and medical science alike.

One leaves the book with the impression of a scattering rather than a resounding resistance by a subaltern community, which does appear to have been Hardiman's own intention. While a few years ago a reviewer might have inevitably suggested the alternative of 'hybridity', my only complaint is that the book gave no more than tantalizing glimpses of several leading characters in this complex historical drama.

We learn only in passing for instance that one of the principal missionaries, Arthur Birkett, had his faith in the efficacy of European Christian civilisation undermined together with his attachment to that outstanding sartorial investiture of racial distinction: the *sola topi*. Perhaps the greatest value of this book by an eminent historian of India is to contribute, by the practice of his trade, to the superannuation of tools that have served him and others better in the past.

INDIA: TRIBAL AREA MEDICAL PROGRAM TRADITIONAL & MODERN-GENDER

Gadchiroli (Women's Feature Service)-Deep in the forests of Gadchiroli, a tribal area of eastern Maharashtra, live the Gond 'adivasis' (tribals), some of the poorest and most neglected people of the state. The region is considered dangerous because large parts of it have come under the sway of Maoist rebels, also known as Naxalites, who have taken up the challenge of organising the Gonds to fight for a society they claim is based on justice and equality. The ensu[illegible]nflict between the rebels and the state has turned the region into a "p[illegible]e", where anti-insurgency security forces are constantly on the vigil, [illegible]laoist hide-outs and eliminating suspects. The word 'encounter'-a eup[illegible]mism for such extra-judicial killings-has become a part of local vocabulary.

The forest is usually not a place where one would expect to find qualified doctors, especially ones who have studied at the world renowned Johns

Hopkins University in the US. But then Dr Rani Bang and her husband, Dr. Abhay Bang, who are both in their fifties, founders of the Society for Education, Action and Research in Community Health (SEARCH), are not "usual". They were determined to take the road less travelled.

Rani Bang (nee Chari), daughter of a doctor and the granddaughter of a prominent Congress Party Member of Parliament (MP) from Chandrapur, met Abhay, the son of the famous Gandhian, Thakurdas Bang of Wardha, at Nagpur's Government Medical College. Abhay was involved in the Sampoorna Kranti (Complete Revolution) movement initiated by political leader Jayaprakash Narayan. On returning from Johns Hopkins, where the couple had gone to pursue higher studies after their marriage, Rani and Abhay resolved to put their powers of healing, as gynaecologist and physician respectively, in the service of government Primary Health Centres (PHCs) for the benefit of ordinary people.

In 1985, the couple set up SEARCH, a multifarious village within a village. Located in Shodhgram, about 15 kilometres from the district headquarters of Gadchiroli on the Dhanora road, SEARCH is a hospital, a de-addiction centre, a voluntary organisation that runs various projects on tribal welfare, health, adolescent sex education and so on. It is also a research institute that has brought out many publications. Reminiscent of a tribal village, it is equipped with all the modern amenities necessary to meet its objectives.

Mud houses amidst trees built around a common courtyard, hutments for in-house patients to live in with their families, a temple dedicated to Danteswari Devi, worshipped by the Gonds, and other symbols of tribal culture, are around to make patients feel at home. "We asked the people what kind of a hospital they would like and then designed this facility," says Dr. Rani Bang. Of course, the funds to do all the good work come from various government schemes and donors like the Ford Foundation.

The greatest achievements of the SEARCH project have been to bring about a fall in the maternal mortality rate (MMR) of the area through improved neo-natal childcare. This has been done by introducing modern medicine and practices of hygiene into the tribal lifestyle, through camps, visits to villages, training of birth attendants and health workers from among the community and by encouraging city-trained doctors to work in the area.

According to Sunanda, Women's Health Coordinator, SEARCH, maternal mortality has been high in this region because childbirth is carried out at home in the most primitive way. "Women arrive at the hospital only in cases of an emergency, due to factors such as lack of transport, finances and, initially, a lack of faith in modern medicine. But this is gradually changing." This positive behavioural change-including a growing preference for institutional deliveries-is largely because workers of SEARCH take the pains to explain the danger signs to pregnant women so that they understand when they must go to a hospital. "We explain about the anatomy, nutritious food and convince the mothers-in-law to feed the pregnant women well," elaborates Sunanda, who has been with the project for 15 years. Sunanda is originally from Nagpur and has done her MA in Sociology. She and her husband are both social workers employed by SEARCH.

Local customs are the reason for infant deaths, too. Traditionally, Gond mothers starve themselves for an easier birth, don't nurse for three days after their babies are born, and don't clothe the newborn for five weeks.

As a result, pneumonia kills a large number of infants. In an attempt to address this concern, SEARCH has been encouraging mothers to check the weight of their newborns, among other measures. SEARCH has also trained birth attendants (TBAs), who can be any committed person who has attended to around four child births in the village.

Another SEARCH intervention has been in improving the hygiene of the traditional Gond 'korma'-the rather dark and dirty hut in which women are isolated during menstruation. While it has been difficult to convince the community to do away with this practice of isolation, SEARCH health workers have managed to at least improve the 'korma', turning it into a clean, comfortable place, with perhaps a bed and a tiled roof. The 'korma' has, in fact, been transformed into a 'women's room', where women meet during their difficult days, rest and share experiences.

Elucidating the SEARCH approach to improving the well-being of the Gonds, Sunanda speaks of the need to understand the essentials of Gond culture and build on their tribal heritage. "We don't laugh at the tribals, their beliefs or superstitions," she says. "Their medicine is mainly herbal medicine and black magic practised by traditional healers. We tell the people that they should also take our modern medicine. We encourage them to bring their healer along and try to train him in modern medicine. Now the traditional healers trained by us carry malaria slides and give tablets."

At the other end of the spectrum, Rani Bang has been working on the Gond tribal medicine, conducting scientific experiments to ascertain their veracity. She feels that the use of asafoetida (hing) to treat fungal infections of the skin; garlic for vaginal infections; and boiled guava leaves for anal fissures probably have a sound scientific basis. Her book 'Goin', a Gondi word for 'friend', has a study of the flora of the area as seen through the eyes of Gond women and traditional healers. Her research has introduced her to a wealth of tribal knowledge and anecdotes. Yet, despite her wide exposure to tribal customs, there are times when she is left startled. Once she was taken aback when a woman casually pointed to a plant which she claimed was useful to "kill a husband"!

But how can people work so selflessly in an area of conflict? Don't Rani Bang and her colleagues sometimes feel intimidated by their difficult circumstances? Says Rani, the recipient of the National Award for Women's Development Through Application of Science and Technology, 2008, as well as many national and international awards, "What is there to fear? After all, everybody has to die some day?"

TRIBAL MEDICINE IN THE 21ST CENTURY

"Medicine is medicine, there's no other name for it," Janu Bhai Thakrey responds as we watch him chop a piece of wood into two-centimetre-thick slices. He turns to his 'patient' from Surat and tells her, "Grind these, boil them in water for half an hour. Then filter the water and drink it twice a day. Your cancer will become better." The patient notes down the prescription on a yellow chit as others wait impatiently for their turn. Thakrey is just one of the *bhagats* (tribal healers) that The Dangs, Gujarat boasts off. Sitting in his own 'clinic' (a shabby corner storage room at the back of a run-down *chai* joint in Ahwa) he doles out ancient tribal remedies – fruits, shoots and roots – to the throng of patients from all over Gujarat and even beyond.

Nature Cure in its Purest Form

The Dangs is Gujarat's densest forest that extends into Maharashtra and Madhya Pradesh. Besides Valsadi teak, the forest produces an array of medicinal trees such as:

1. *Solanum indicum*: Roots are diaphoretic, diuretic, expectorant, stimulant. The root is used against bronchitis, itch and for body aches, for asthma and to cure wounds while the seeds are used to treat toothache.
2. *Embelia ribes*: The dried fruits are anti-bacterial, anti-inflammatory, anti-diuretic and anti-astringent.
3. *Tylophora indica*: The leaves and roots have emetic, cathartic, laxative, expectorant, diaphoretic and purgative properties. It has also been used for the treatment of allergies, cold, dysentery, hay fever and arthritis. It has reputation as an alterative and as a blood purifier, often used in rheumatism. Root or leaf powder is used in diarrhoea, dysentery and intermittent fever.
4. *Nordostachys jatamansi*: The roots or rhizomes are used for medicinal purpose. *Jatamamsi* can be used both, internally as well as externally. The paste prepared in cold water is beneficial to reduce the burning sensation. It also imparts fair complexion to the skin and alleviates the pain and swelling. It also effectively relieves the symptoms like vertigo, seizures, etc.

5. *Coleus forskohlii*: It is found to be effective in skin conditions as eczema and psoriasis. It can aid in weight loss due to its ability to breakdown stored fat as well as inhibit the synthesis of adipose tissue, additionally, it increases thyroid hormone production and release thereby increasing metabolism. Ophthalmic preparation of the chief alkaloid forskolin to the eyes lowers eye pressure thus reducing the risk of glaucoma.

Wave Theory and Black Magic

While naturopathy is the most important healing technique in all of The Dangs, the *bhagats* also use black magic to heal those who can't be cured by the herbs.

During the annual food festival called *Kurmari*, thousands of tribal healers assemble during the full moon night to demonstrate their knowledge and skills. As tribal men sway to the beats of drums and pipes and chain dance around a pole, the *bhagats* compete with each other and exchange their knowledge of herbs and black magic. Tribals from all over The Dangs come to witness the competitions. Those looking for cures to serious ailments often come with goats, chickens and calves for sacrifice to the Food God, Dangar Devta.

"The tribals believe in the Wave Theory. When you come in contact with another person there is an exchange of waves. This exchange could be positive or negative. When someone abuses you, the impact is different from when someone speaks to you with love and affection. Healing processes here too have two different roles. On one side, they can help make you feel better. On the other hand, they can weaken your immune system and make you ill," says Anil Patel, a filmmaker who has been documenting the lives of the tribals in The Dangs.

"Rather die than go to a hospital" : "The tribals are humanists and find all their cures in nature. In the whole district, there's only one civil hospital in Ahwa. Most people here are familiar with basic natural remedies. They know what to do in case of cuts, bruises and a mild case of fever. For more complex diseases such as malaria and typhoid they go to the bhagat.

Only in very, very serious cases do they think of leaving the forest to go to the hospital. In many cases they'd rather die than get treated in a 'closed' hospital," says Patel.

Urban diseases such as diabetes, coronary artery disease and cancer are rare among the tribal population. The average life expectancy is around 80 (in Mumbai it is 56.8) and the most common diseases are malaria (only during the monsoon) and skin disorders such as acne and eczema.

Prevention may be cure in urban India, but here the cure is nature and the faith that tribals have in its power to tackle all human problems.

ALCOHOL: ITS HEALTH AND SOCIAL IMPACT IN INDIA

Alcohol and tobacco are important products of the global addictive demand and have experienced a rapid increase in per capita consumption.

The fastest growth has been in developing countries in the Asian subcontinent where the per capita pure alcohol consumption has increased by over 50% between 1980 and 2000.1 Alcoholic beverages, and the problems they engender, have been familiar in human societies since the beginning of recorded history. Accompanying the near ubiquity of alcoholic beverages in human history has been an appreciation of the social and health problems caused by drinking.

Whether in Greece, Palestine or China, ancient texts speak eloquently of such problems. Scientific attention to problems of alcohol consumption has increased during the past 30 years. Every major world religion has at least some strands that counsel abstinence from alcoholic beverages.

Alcohol is no longer viewed as a threat to all, but rather to a small subclass of 'alcoholics' or, in today's technical terms, people who are 'alcohol dependent'. Alcohol is causally related to more than 60 medical conditions. Overall, 3.5% of the global burden of disease is attributable to alcohol, which accounts for as much death and disability as tobacco and hypertension.

ALCOHOL AND GLOBAL BURDEN

Taking into account both recorded and unrecorded consumption, the highest amount of alcohol consumed per adult resident is in Europe, especially in Russia and its surrounding countries, and in the established market economies of western Europe and North America.

The least amount of alcohol consumed per resident is in the mostly Islamic regions of the Eastern Mediterranean and in the lesser developed region of Southeast Asia, dominated by India. Between the subregion with the highest estimated consumption level (Europe C) and the subregion with the lowest (Eastern Mediterranean D) the difference in consumption is more than 20-fold.

Indian Scenario

Although the recorded alcohol consumption per capita has fallen since 1980 in most developed countries, it has risen steadily in developing countries, alarmingly so in India. The per capita consumption of alcohol by adults 15 years in India increased by 106.7% between 1970–72 and 1994–96!5 The pattern of drinking in India has changed from occasional and ritualistic use to social use. Today, the common purpose of consuming alcohol is to get drunk. These developments have raised concerns about the health and the social consequences of excessive drinking.

SOURCES OF DATA

Measuring alcohol use and alcoholic liver disease in an individual or a country has several limitations. Most studies rely on interviews with patients and their families to estimate the amount, frequency and duration of alcohol consumption. However, patients may not accurately report the quantity of alcohol they consume and the definition of a 'standard drink' varies from country to country. Studies of the incidence and prevalence of alcoholic liver disease, rather than decompensated cirrhosis alone, in the general population are difficult to conduct because patients with compensated liver disease usually do not seek medical attention.

Financial constraints among patients suffering from excessive alcohol use may hamper the ability to obtain routine healthcare and further delay the diagnosis of alcoholic liver disease. Because of this, alcohol-related problems are usually not detected until hepatic decompensation occurs.

The adult per capita data are available from the Global Status Report on Alcohol11 and the WHO Global Alcohol Database created by the Marin Institute for the Prevention of Alcohol and Other Drug Problems, and presently maintained by the Swiss Institute for the Prevention of Alcohol Problems.

There are three principal sources of data for per capita estimates: national government data, data from international organizations and alcohol industry data. In most cases the best and most reliable source is national government data, which are usually based on sales figures, tax revenues, and/or production data. Generally, sales data are considered the most accurate, provided that sales of alcoholic beverages are separated from sales of any other items sold at the location, and that sales data are beverage-specific.

Indian Sources

Large or nationally representative epidemiological studies on alcohol consumption have not been conducted in India due to resource constraints. The following agencies collect some data, usually incomplete, regarding alcohol:

Ministry of Chemicals, Government of India; Ministry of Welfare, Government of India; Department of Excise, Ministry of Finance, Government of India; Indian Distillery Association, New Delhi; and the All-India Prohibition Council, New Delhi. In addition, the corresponding Ministries at the state level also collect information for their state.

The Indian beer industry currently produces 4.32 million hectolitres of beer per year, and is growing at a annual rate of 17%. The spirits industry in India is divided into three segments: 'India-made foreign liquor' (IMFL: whisky, gin, rum, brandy, liqueurs, vodka); 'India-made country liquor' (licensed distilled spirits, made locally); and the illicit liquor sectors.

1. Daru, a drink distilled from the flowers of the mahwa tree, has an alcohol content ranging from 20% to 40%.
2. Spirit produced from solvents, which varies greatly in alcohol content and, at the time of the study, was drunk only by 'untouchables' and members of other lower castes.
3. 'English alcohol,' a distilled liquor—usually whisky or gin—associated with the British rule.

The consumption of alcoholic beverages in India predates colonization by the British. However, in contrast to other countries, alcohol consumption was not considered central to normal social life or daily meals in pre-colonial India.

Nevertheless, in certain tribal groups throughout the country, alcoholic beverages still are considered 'a gift to humankind and, in turn, were reverently offered to the nature gods and other sacred powers'.

One reason for the specific drinking patterns in India may be the strong advocacy of abstinence by Indian religious groups. For example, among the Hindus, alcoholic beverages are forbidden for Brahmins and other upper caste groups who are strict vegetarians. Drinking is acceptable for members of all other caste groups who are meat-eaters (the warrior, farmer and scavenger-untouchable castes). Muslims are also not supposed to drink, although some Muslim men consume alcohol. Finally, Buddhists and Jains, who are strict vegetarians, are forbidden to drink. In addition, political prohibition policies in certain states may contribute to the drinking patterns seen in India.

India is a diverse nation with cultural variations among ethnic, religious and linguistic groups, and there are major differences between the urban and rural areas. One cannot accurately characterize the drinking patterns of all Indian ethnic and cultural groups based on the findings from just one of these groups. Indian attitudes to drinking include both permissive and abstinent features, especially when different population groups are considered.

Epidemiology

Alcohol abuse can be found among all age groups, predominantly in men. Notable ethnic differences observed were in the prevalence of alcohol-related liver disease and associated mortality. Overall consumption or the average volume of alcohol consumption has been the usual measure of exposure linking alcohol to disease in recent decades.

The average volume of consumption works as a risk factor mainly through biological and biochemical effects, including dependence, to produce long term health consequences. Although research shows that the average volume of alcohol consumption is correlated with measures of acute consequences such as injury and injury-related death, several studies indicate that the ability to predict these injury measures is improved by taking patterns of drinking into account. There is an exponential relationship between the amount of alcohol consumed and criminal behaviour, including drunken driving and legal arrests.

The Food and Agriculture Organization (FAO) of the United Nations observed that with increasing marginalization and alienation, excessive alcohol consumption has become widespread among tribal men in Madhya Pradesh and Bihar. Not only do the men's incomes decline but they also forcibly use up even the women's earnings. Resistance invites domestic violence and abuse. Household food security becomes a major casualty. Social functioning is also affected by the amount of alcohol consumed per day. Gupta et al. noted that, among the study subjects, the number of people consuming alcohol was lower than, for example, in developed countries; but the amount of alcohol consumed by drinkers was high, which suggests the risk of serious public health problems.The volume of consumption as well as the patterns of drinking, especially irregular heavy drinking, have been shown to determine the burden of disease. In other words, the impact of the average volume of consumption on mortality or morbidity is partly moderated by the way alcohol is consumed by the individual, which in turn is influenced by the cultural context. Patterns of drinking have been linked not only to acute health outcomes such as injuries, but also to chronic diseases such as coronary heart disease (CHD) and sudden cardiac death.

There is general agreement that excessive alcohol consumption is associated with an increased risk of cirrhosis. However, there is no consensus on the exact dose or a specific dose–response relationship for cirrhosis.

Evidence suggests that there is an increased risk with ingestion >60–80 g/day of alcohol in men and >20 g/day in women. However, 6%–41% of those drinking these amounts will develop cirrhosis. Bellentani *et al.* showed that even in patients with an extremely high daily alcohol intake (>120 g/day), only 13.5% developed alcohol-induced liver damage. It is believed that other factors such as genetic susceptibility and dietary intolerance may be co-factors in alcohol-induced liver damage.

Breast Cancer

Meta-analyses have shown a linear increase in the risk of breast cancer with increasing average volumes of consumption of alcohol.

Coronary Heart Disease

A meta-analysis on the average volume of alcohol consumption and CHD yielded a J-shaped curve. Compared with not drinking, low-to-moderate consumption of alcohol is associated with lower CHD incidence and mortality. For higher average volumes of alcohol consumption, the risk reverses. Several the seventh place in the world for its area. The tribal population is 8 percentage of the total population of the country. The rural population is about 70 percent of the total population. The proverbial statement notwithstanding, agriculture is probably the oldest profession and it is still the occupation of a majority of people in rural areas. It continues to be the principal source of our national income.

Our rural people continue to be in perpetual poverty due to various reasons. In rural areas agriculture holds the key to the economic development of the community. Our rural communities lack the basic infrastructure facilities to sustain their life. Their small land holdings provide them with minimal yield to support their existence. The opportunities to a better standard of living in rural areas of our country are minimal. The health facilities are remote and expensive to the rural poor communities. In rural areas marriage at young age is a reason for more children in a family and the health of women is deteriorating at motherhood due to more deliveries and prolonged period of pregnancies. The family size is also increasing which needs to be supported from the minimal yield of the fields. This leads to recurring effects on children's health and ill effects in their growth and development. The sickness and morbidity are more in rural and tribal areas due to the poor sanitary conditions and degrading environment around.

HIV/AIDS

Regarding HIV/AIDS one of the most important lessons that has emerged over the years is that a safe and supportive environment is a crucial element in effective HIV prevention. Countless intervention studies and grassroots initiatives have demonstrated one telling fact. Even when individuals are well aware of the dangers of AIDS, know full well how to avoid HIV infection, and are motivated to avoid HIV infection) several factors in the immediate and wider environment play an important role in determining whether or not individuals can protect themselves from AIDS.

Some of these factors are restrictive laws and policies, economic constraints, social and cultural pressures, lack of availability and accessibility to health services in both in rural and tribal areas. This means that along with carefully tailored actions directed at the level of the individual a complementary set of actions is also required at the level of the environment. For instance, providing individuals with the information they need, motivating them to take the necessary steps to protect themselves, and strengthening their abilities to deal with challenges in every day situations through "life-skills" training to overcome the environmental factors that hinder one's 'abilities' to protect oneself.

Safeguarding Sexual Health

The importance of community action (Rural & Tribal) in promoting and safeguarding sexual health cannot be overestimated. One of the positive outcomes of the growing interest in environmental factors that influence HIV/STD transmission is the focus on the contribution of community action in this area. Communities everywhere have responded in one way or another to the threat posed by HIV/AIDS to their health and wellbeing. As Elizabeth Reid, Development Worker and AIDS activist, pointed out some years ago: "wherever the virus has spread, communities have responded, to provide care and support, to stop further infection, to assure the rights of the affected, to minister to spiritual, emotional and physical need".

These inspiring community responses have emerged not only from people living in specific localities, but also from groups of individuals unified by common interests and concerns.

The involvement of communities in their own health care is neither a new concept nor a new practice. Twenty years ago, the Declaration of Alma Ata called for international commitment to involving the communities in the design, choice and delivery of their own health care. Today, the concept of community involvement is receiving even greater interest and support than before. In developed and developing countries alike, families and communities every where are realizing that they must assume greater responsibility for their own health and welfare, and that every thing possible must be done to develop and strengthen their capacity.

Stalwarts of Ancient Medicine

a) Aswin Twins. In the Rig Veda, the Aswini twins were described as divine physicians who used herbs and medicinal plants against diseases, could even ward off death. In the legendary account of their marvels, it is said that they could restore youth to the old. They rejuvenated the debilitated body of the sage Chyavana and invigorated the aged kal. Legend has it that Sage Rebha, who was stabbed and hidden under the waters for ten days and nights, was pulled out of waters and revived.

b) Dhanvantri. Believed to have established his school in the 6th century B. C.

c) Charaka. Believed to be most famous in ayurvedic medicine. According to Charaka Samhita, treatment of dertratoses consists of purification, systematic therapy and local medication. In case of leucoderma Charaka Samhita recommends exposure to sunlight after oil massage. There are Muslim practitioners on herbal medicine like Hakim Muhammad Sharif Khan, Iban-Al-Baitar, Iban Rusad.

d) Nagarjuna. Author of Rasaratnakara deals with the use of metallic compounds and recipes in which vegetable or animal products are used to transform other metals into compounds.

e) Sushruta. Authored of a book on garlic and other therapeutic substances.

Even in ancient times India had visitors, guests and scientists from other countries. In medieval period the influence of Muslim dynasties enriched the herbal drug therapy.

Modern Times & Stress

Due to various demands on mankind, increasing mental and emotional stress producing negative effects in different organs of the body, resulting to premature death. Abnormal physical and psychological activity greatly alters the degree of functioning of nerve's stimulation. Skeletal muscular activity leads to progressive body fatigue, inability to make decisions and loss of concentration. These conditions force mankind to depend on drugs and medicines to prop up the system instead of rebuilding. The extracts from herbs and medicinal plants work in harmony with the body and revitalize energy. It is the best alternative medicine economically available to rural and tribal people.

Role of Plants

Medicinal plants and herbs have been used for healing purposes and maintaining good health. Herbal healing has been sustained over a long period since ancient times. From a botanical point of view, a herb is a plant with a non woody stem which withers and dies down after flowering. In common use all plants whose leaves, stems, roots, barks, flowers, fruits or seeds are used to heal or to provide vital energy to a patient.

The practice of herbal medicine dates back to the ancient period known to human history. There are numerous evidences that herbs and plants have been used in the treatment of diseases and for revitalizing body systems in all ancient civilizations like Indian, Egyptian, Chinese, Greek and Roman.

In India, the records highlight herb's curative properties in Rig-Veda and Atharva-Veda (3500-1800 BC) Information about herbs has been recorded in Charaka Samhita and Shusruta Samhita – the most important books on Ayurvedic system of medicine. Well over 1500 plants were used in indigenous medicine in India. The Chinese also have a compilation of 1000 herbs. Pen Ts'ao Ching as an important ancient Chinese work dating back to 2800 BC, describes various plant medicaments and instructions on their use.

Bibliography

Akerele, O.: *Medicinal Plants: Policies and Priorities*, Cambridge, UK; Cambridge University Press, 1991.

Bankoti T. S. : *Encyclopaedic Ethnography of the Himalayan Tribes*, Global Vision, Delhi, 2004.

Bhasin M. K. : *Genetics of Castes and Tribes of India*, Kamla-Raj Enterprises, Delhi, 2001.

Chakraborty, P.: *The Inner-Line Regulation of the NorthEast*, Linkman Publication, India, 1995.

Chandrasekar B: *Blood sugar lowering potentiality of selected Cucurbitaceae plants of Indian origin*. Ind J Med Res. 1989.

Chattopadhyay RR: *A Comparative Evaluation of Some Blood Sugar Lowering agents of Plant Origin*. J Ethnopharmacology. 1999.

Dasgupta Samira : *Ethno Ecology of Indian Tribes : Diversity in Cultural Adaptation*, Rawat, Delhi, 2000.

De Silva T.: *A Manual on the Essential Oil Industry*, Vienna, Austria; United Nations Industrial Development Organisation, 1996.

Donellan, C.: *Endangered Species*. Independence, Cambridge, 1995.

Donellan, C.: *Endangered species*. Independence, Cambridge, 1995.

Bergman M, Felig C.: *The Endocrine Pancreas: Diabetes mellitus*, New York: MacGraw-Hill; 1995.

Morton H. : *The Notion of Tribe*, Menlo Park: Cummings Publishing Co, 1975.

Fuller, D.: *Medicine from the Wild*. Washington, DC; Traffic USA, 1991.

Goldsmith, F.B.: *Monitoring for conservation and ecology*. Chapman and Hall, London, 1991.

Bakshi, A S : *A Lexicon of Medicinal Plants in India*, Naya Prokash, Delhi, 2001.

Synge, H.: *Conservation of medicinal plants*. Cambridge Univ. Press, Cambridge, UK, 1991.

Hutchinson, R. H. S.: *Chittagong Hill Tracts*, Vivek Publishing House, Delhi, 1978.

Khan, Borhan Uddin: *CHT Governance Study: An Institutional Review*, CARE-Bangladesh, Dhaka, 2004.

Lewington, A.: *Medicinal Plant and Plant Extracts*, Cambridge, UK; Traffic International, 1993.

Mankin, Albert: *The Rights of Adivasis on Land and Forests: Bangladesh Government's Perspectives*, Centre for Indigenous Peoples Research and development (CIPRAD), Dhaka, 2004.

Lal Bahadur Shastri

Lal Bahadur Shastri

Dr. C.P. Raj
Dr. Ved Prakash

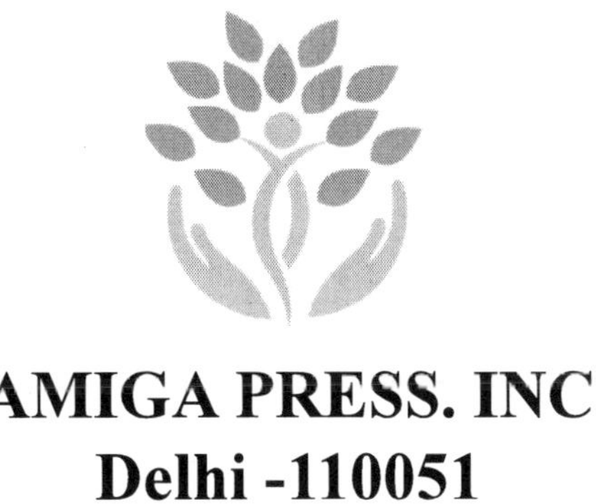

AMIGA PRESS. INC
Delhi -110051

AMIGA PRESS. INC
H.O :- 28-A, Indra Park, Chander Nagar
Delhi :- 110051 (India)
Tel :- 011-22504028, +91-98736-57000
Email :- amigapress@gmail.com
amigaeditorial@gmail.com
Website :- www.amigapress@co.in

This edition is published by Amiga Press.Inc

ISBN : 978-93-84533-30-4

First Published 2018

PRINTED : Replika Press Pvt. Ltd.

Preface

Shri Lal Bahadur Shastri was born on October 2, 1901 at Mughalsarai, a small railway town seven miles from Varanasi in Uttar Pradesh. His father was a school teacher who died when Lal Bahadur Shastri was only a year and half old. His mother, still in her twenties, took her three children to her father's house and settled down there.

As he grew up, Lal Bahadur Shastri became more and more interested in the country's struggle for freedom from foreign yoke. He was greatly impressed by Mahatma Gandhi's denunciation of Indian Princes for their support of British rule in India. Lal Bahadur Sashtri was only eleven at the time, but the process that was end day to catapult him to the national stage had already begun in his mind.

Lal Bahadur Shastri joined the Kashi Vidya Peeth in Varanasi, one of the many national institutions set up in defiance of the British rule. There, he came under the influence of the greatest intellectuals, and nationalists of the country. 'Shastri' was the bachelor's degree awarded to him by the Vidya Peeth but has stuck in the minds of the people as part of his name.

More than thirty years of dedicated service were behind Lal Bahadur Shastri. In the course of this period, he came to be known as a man of great integrity and competence. Humble, tolerant, with great inner strength and resoluteness, he was a man of the people who understood their language. He was also a man of vision who led the country towards progress. Lal Bahadur Shastri was deeply influenced by the political teachings of Mahatma Gandhi. "Hard work is equal to prayer," he once said, in accents profoundly reminiscent of his Master. In the direct tradition of Mahatma Gandhi, Lal Bahadur Shastri represented the best in Indian culture.

After the Chinese aggression of 1962, India faced another aggression from Pakistan in 1965 during Shastri's tenure. Shastri showing his mettle, made it very clear that India would not sit and watch. While granting liberty to the Security Forces to retaliate, he said, "Force will be met with force".

The Indo-Pak war ended on 23 September 1965 after the United Nations passed a resolution demanding a ceasefire. The Russian Prime Minister, Kosygin, offered to mediate and on 10 January 1966, Lal Bahadur Shastri and his Pakistan counterpart Ayub Khan signed the Tashkent Declaration.

But the controversy about the death of Prime Minister Lal Bahadur Shastri in Tashkent (now in Uzbekistan) is in a different league altogether. Mystery surrounds Shastri's death due to several reasons — foremost being the absence of a proper medical report stating the cause of death. It is all the more puzzling because Shastri's personal physician had accompanied him to Tashkent, then in the USSR. But he did not ensure a proper medical investigation. It is rumoured that he was drunk at that time. Though a post-mortem report was given by the Soviet authorities at Tashkent, nothing was done in India to determine the exact cause of the Prime Minister's death despite tell-tale signs of poisoning.

Lal Bahadur Shastri, who had earlier suffered two heart attacks, died of a third cardiac arrest on 11 January, 1966. He is the only incumbent Indian Prime Minister to have died overseas. Lal Bahadur Shastri was awarded the Bharat Ratna, India's highest civilian award posthumously in 1966.

—*Editor*

Contents

1

Biography

Lal Bahadur Shastri (October 2, 1904-January 11, 1966) was the third (second, and acting, being Gulzarilal Nanda) Prime Minister of independent India and a significant figure in the Indian independence movement.

INTRODUCTION

Small of stature, simple and soft-spoken, Lal Bahadur proved to be one of the heroes of the history of India. A great general in Gandhi's army of peaceful soldiers of freedom. He became the symbol of India's valor and self-respect.

Early Life

Lal Bahadur was born in the year 1904 in Mughalsarai, Uttar Pradesh as Lal Bahadur Srivastava. His father Sharada Prasad was a poor school teacher, who later became a clerk in the Revenue Office at Allahabad. When Lal Bahadur was three months old, he slipped out of his mother's arms into a cowherd's basket at the ghats of the Ganges. The cowherd, who had no children, took the child as a gift from God and took him home. Lal Bahadur's parents lodged a complaint with the police, who traced the child, and returned him to his parents.

Lal Bahadur's father died when he was only a year and a half old. His mother Ramdulari Devi took him and his two sisters to her father's house and settled down there. Lal Bahadur stayed at his grandfather Hazari Lal's house till he was ten. Since there was no high school in their town, he was sent to Varanasi where he stayed with his maternal uncle and joined the Harischandra High School. While in Varanasi, Shastri once went with his friends to see a fair on the other bank of the Ganges. On the way back he had no money for the boat fare. Instead of borrowing from his friends, he jumped into the river and swam to the other bank.

As a boy, Lal Bahadur loved reading books and was fond of Guru Nanak's verses. He revered Bal Gangadhar Tilak, the Indian nationalist, social reformer and freedom fighter. After hearing a speech of Mahatma Gandhi at Varanasi in 1915, he dedicated his life to the service of the country. He also dropped his surname, as it indicated his caste and he was against the caste system. During the non-cooperation movement of Mahatma Gandhi in 1921, he joined processions in defiance of the prohibitory order. He was arrested but let off as he was a minor. He then enrolled at the nationalist Kashi Vidyapeeth in Varanasi. During his four years there, he was greatly influenced by the lectures of Dr. Bhagawandas on philosophy. Upon completion of his course at Kashi Vidyapeeth in 1926, he was given the title *Shastri* ("Scholar"). The title was a bachelor's degree awarded by the Vidya Peeth, but it stuck as part of his name. He also enrolled himself as a life member of the Servants of the People Society and began to work for the upliftment of the Harijans at Muzaffarpur. Later he became the President of the Society.

In 1927, Shastri married Lalita Devi of Mirzapur. In spite of the prevailing hefty dowry tradition, Shastri accepted only a *charkha* and a few yards of *khadi* as dowry. In 1930, he threw himself into the freedom struggle during Mahatma Gandhi's Salt Satyagraha. He was imprisoned for two and a half years. Once, while he was in prison, one of his daughters fell seriously ill. He was released for fifteen days, on the condition that he not take part in the freedom movement. However, his daughter died before he reached home. After performing the funeral rites, he voluntarily returned to prison, even before the expiry of the period. A year later, he asked for permission to go home for a week, as his son had contracted influenza. The permission was given, but his son's illness was not cured in a week. In spite of his family's pleadings, he kept his promise to the jail officers and returned to the prison.

Later, he worked as the Organizing Secretary of the Parliamentary Board of U.P. in 1937. In 1940, he was sent to prison for one year, for offering individual Satyagraha to support the freedom movement. On August 8, 1942, Mahatma Gandhi issued the Quit India speech at Gowalia Tank in Mumbai, demanding that the British leave India. Shastri, who had just then come out after a year in prison, travelled to Allahabad. For a week, he sent instructions to the freedom fighters from Jawaharlal Nehru's home, Anand Bhavan. A few days later, he was arrested and imprisoned until 1946. Shastri spent almost nine years in jail in total. During his stay in prison, he spent time reading books and became familiar with the works of western philosophers, revolutionaries and social reformers. He also translated the autobiography of Madam Curie into Hindi language.

In Government

Following India's independence, Shastri was appointed Parliamentary Secretary in his home state, Uttar Pradesh. He became the Minister of Police and Transport under Govind Ballabh Pant's Chief Ministership. As the Transport Minister, he was the first to appoint women conductors. As the minister in charge of the Police Department, he ordered that Police use jets of water instead of lathis to disperse unruly crowds.

In 1951, he was made the General Secretary of the All-India Congress Committee, with Jawaharlal Nehru as the President. He was directly responsible for the selection of candidates and the direction of publicity and electioneering activities. He played an important role in the landslide successes of the Congress Party in the Indian General Elections of 1952, 1957 and 1962.

In 1951, Nehru nominated him to the Rajya Sabha. He served as the Minister of Railways and Transport in the Central Cabinet from 1951 to 1956. In 1956, he offered his resignation after a railway accident at Mahbubnagar led to 112 deaths. However, Nehru did not accept his resignation. Three months later, he resigned accepting moral and constitutional responsibility for a railway accident at Ariyalur in Tamil Nadu that resulted in 144 deaths. While speaking in the Parliament on the incident, the then Prime Minister, Jawaharlal Nehru, stated that he was accepting the resignation because it would set an example in constitutional propriety and not because Shastri was in any way responsible for the accident. Shastri's unprecedented gesture was greatly appreciated by the citizens.

In 1957, Shastri returned to the Cabinet following the General Elections, first as the Minister for Transport and Communications, and then as the Minister of Commerce and Industry. In 1961, he became Minister for Home. As Union Home Minister he was instrumental in appointing the Committee on Prevention of Corruption under the Chairmanship of K. Santhanam.

PRIME MINISTER

Shastri worked by his natural characteristics to obtain compromises between opposing viewpoints, but in his short tenure was ineffectual in dealing with the economic crisis and food shortage in the nation. However, he commanded a great deal of respect in the Indian populace, and he used it to advantage in pushing the Green Revolution in India; which directly led to India becoming a food-surplus nation, although he did not live to see it. During the 22-day war with Pakistan, Lal Bahadur Shastri created the slogan of "Jai Jawan Jai Kisan" ("Hail the soldier, Hail the farmer"), underlining the need to boost India's food production. Apart from emphasizing the Green Revolution, he was instrumental in promoting the White Revolution. Greatly impressed by a visit to the Kaira district in October 1964, he urged the rest of the country to learn from the successful experiment at Anand. The National Dairy Development Board was formed in 1965 during his tenure as Prime Minister.

Though he was Socialist, Shastri stated that India cannot have a regimented type of economy. During his tenure as Prime Minister, he visited Russia, Yugoslavia, England, Canada and Burma in 1965.

War with Pakistan

The chief problem for Shastri's administration was Pakistan. Laying claim to half of the Kutch peninsula, Pakistan sent incursion forces in August 1965, which skirmished with Indian tank divisions. In his report to the Lok Sabha on the confrontation in Kutch, Shastri stated:

"In the utilization of our limited resources, we have always given primacy to plans and projects for economic development. It would, therefore, be obvious for anyone who is prepared to look at things objectively that India can have no possible interest in provoking border incidents or in building up an atmosphere of strife... In these circumstances, the duty of Government is quite clear and this duty will be discharged fully and effectively... We would prefer to live in poverty for as long as necessary but we shall not allow our freedom to be subverted."

Under a scheme proposed by the British PM, Pakistan obtained 10%, in place of their original claim of 50% of the territory. But Pakistan's aggressive intentions were also focused on Kashmir. When armed infiltrators from Pakistan began entering the State of Jammu and Kashmir, Shastri made it clear to Pakistan that force would be met with force. Just in September 1965, major incursions of militants and Pakistani soldiers began, hoping not only to break-down the government but incite a sympathetic revolt.

The revolt did not happen, and India sent its forces across the Ceasefire Line (now Line of Control) and threatened Pakistan by crossing the International Border near Lahore as war broke out on a general scale. Massive tank battles occurred in the Punjab, and while Pakistani forces made some gains, Indian forces captured the key post at Haji Pir, in Kashmir, and brought the Pakistani city of Lahore under artillery and mortar fire.

On 17 September 1965, while the Indo-Pak war was on, India received a letter from China. In the letter, China alleged that the Indian army had set up army equipment in Chinese territory, and India would face China's wrath, unless the equipments are pulled down. In spite of the threat of aggression from China, Shastri declared "China's allegation is untrue. If China attacks India it is our firm resolve to fight for our freedom. The might of China will not deter us from defending our territorial integrity." The Chinese did not respond, but the Indo-Pak war resulted in great personnel and material casualties for both Pakistan and India.

The Indo-Pak war ended on September 23, 1965 with a United Nations-mandated ceasefire. In a broadcast to the nation on the day the of ceasefire, Shastri stated:

> *"While the conflict between the armed forces of the two countries has come to an end, the more important thing for the United Nations and all those who stand for peace is to bring to an end the deeper conflict... How can this be brought about? In our view, the only answer lies in peaceful coexistence. India has stood for the principle of coexistence and championed it all over the world. Peaceful coexistence is possible among nations no matter how deep the differences between them, how far apart they are in their political and economic systems, no matter how intense the issues that divide them."*

THE SHASTRI SAGA

DURING THE 1930s Lala Lajpat Rai's Servants of the Society provided financial assistance to families of freedom fighters in distress. When Lal Bahadur Shastri was in jail, he wrote to his mother asking if she was getting money regularly and able to meet family requirements. She replied she was getting Rs.50 out of which she spent 40 and saved the rest. Shastri then wrote a letter of thanks to the Servants of the Society and asked them to send his family only Rs.40 from next time and send the money saved to someone else needy.

Today as his 100th birth anniversary is celebrated by the Ministry of Culture and Lal Bahadur Shastri Institute of Management, his sons Anil and Sunil Shastri reflect on different aspects of this frail yet powerful man.

Great Self-respect, Remembered Sunil Shahtri

"I was in the last year of my school at St. Columba's when Babuji became Prime Minister. It was only after he became the PM that he bought a car on loan," recalls elder son Anil, a Congressman and Chairman of LBSIM. "Since I am post-Independence born, I did not see the days of his freedom struggle but I saw him as a father who would idealise his mother for being a woman behind his success. He had great self-respect. So much so that he would swim across the Ganges if he did not have money to pay the boatman," he says.

Anil, who joined politics "to carry on the lineage" reveals, "He wouldn't mingle with family members much. We used to have a respectable distance from him. He wasn't a great movie buff but he saw Manoj Kumar's *Shaheed* and old *Mirza Ghalib* and relished them. He loved eating potatoes, salad and green vegetables but did not have a sweet tooth."

Sunil Shastri, who belongs to the BJP, recalls, "We hardly got to have meals together because of his hectic schedule but whenever he called us for meals, it used to be like a festival. Once he called all the family members for dinner and said, `*Kal se ek hafte tak sham ko chulha nahin jalega.* Kids will get milk and fruits only, others will fast.' After a week he called us again and explained, `I just wanted to see if my family can sacrifice one meal every day, my larger family (the nation) can definitely stay hungry at least once a week.' It was in response to the U.S.'s PL-480 pressure. He refused to pay for PL-480 saying we can stay hungry but will not compromise with our self-respect. After this incident he appealed to the public on All India Radio not to cook one meal at least once a week. All dhabas, restaurants and families followed it religiously."

Has Shastriji been sidelined today? Anil defends, "I don't think so. In all AICC meetings his name is being mentioned, his portrait forms the backdrop, there are talks of a stamp release on him on the Centenary."

A Tough Ideal

Sunil is forthright. "Because present politicians cannot live up to his ideology which demands shunning glamorous life, he has been sidelined."

Both brothers, despite being in different political parties "do not have personal differences".

While Anil is now monitoring the transformation of the Shastri Memorial Hall into a museum to exhibit his belongings-the pandal where he got married, his car, etc.-Sunil is in the final stages of another book on him, "Shastriji as a Political Leader". Sunil also hopes to bring one of his three sons into politics.

On the Congress Treatment of Shastri

I don't think India has forgotten Lal Bahadur Shastri. Whatever he did is remembered even today. I must say since Sonia Gandhi has taken charge Shastri*ji*'s portraits are displayed in all the annual sessions of the party.

Many people have observed that there was a conspiracy to underplay Shastri's legacy within the Congress. This serious charge is untrue for the simple reason that due to his untimely death his contribution to the nation was confined to those 18 to 19 months when he was PM.

Nehru ruled the country for 17 years, Indira Gandhi for 16 years and Rajiv Gandhi for 5 years. Obviously the Nehru-Gandhi contribution is unparalleled because nobody got this opportunity. And remember Shastri*ji* considered him as a protege of Pandit Nehru. He was never outside the sphere of the Nehru ideology which is the Congress ideology.

Our nation is going to celebrate his birth centenary throughout the year. The committee is formed under the chairmanship of Prime Minister Manmohan Singh. Even in Tashkent, Uzbekistan, celebrations have been organised on a big scale. E Ahmed, minister of state for external affairs, was in Tashkent to participate in the celebrations.

Shastri*ji* who represented a certain value system is more relevant today than before because a majority of us today have no value systems. I feel difficult to contest elections. I feel a little out of place but for my lineage I have survived in politics.

His Father

I still miss him although I was just 16 years old when he died. If he would have lived 10 more years he would have done much more for the country.

He was down to earth. A real son of the soil. His grounding was from the grassroots level. He was a practical man too. He strongly believed the laws of the land should be changed because the British formed them to rule over India. He did make an attempt by constituting the administrative reforms commission and made Morarji Desai its chairman. But after he died the idea was shelved.

The most cherished memory I have is the verses of Guru Nanak, which were displayed on his table. As Nehru kept Robert Frost's lines — 'Miles to go before I sleep', on his desk, my father kept Nanak's quotes in Gurmukhi.

When translated into English they mean — 'O Nanak! Be tiny like the grass, for other plants will whither away, but grass will remain ever green.' When under the PL 480 programme, America was going to send inferior quality of wheat to India, he opposed it. He asked the nation to go hungry once a day than accept poor quality food from US.

Before making this announcement he asked my mother not to cook evening meals. He himself followed what he recommended.

1965: THE OTHER STORY

Lal Bahadur Shastri saw that the economic policies India had been following since independence needed to be changed. The past few weeks have seen intense discussions about the 1965 war with Pakistan. Less attention has been paid to an intriguing possibility: the surge in popularity for the diminutive Lal Bahadur Shastri after the war could have given him the political heft to pursue the sort of radical economic reforms that India eventually embraced in 1991.

Shastri was a practical man. He saw early in his tenure that the economic policies India had been following since independence needed to be changed: the emphasis on physical controls rather than prices, the neglect of agriculture because of the focus on heavy industry, and the growing web of controls spun by central planners. But Shastri had to face stiff opposition from within the Congress party, which quite naturally considered it sacrilegious to retreat from the path laid down by Jawaharlal Nehru so soon after his death.

"The victory in the 1965 war had made him very popular in his own right. During the brief period of his stewardship he had acquired his own popular political support that would, I believe, have given him added confidence to pursue an agenda of economic reform of the kind that was taken up only twenty-five years later, in 1991," economist P.N. Dhar later wrote of Shastri in *Indira Gandhi, the 'Emergency' and Indian Democracy,* his insightful book on his years as a policy advisor.

Independent India started off with a belief that the state should take the lead in industrialization. Nehru is most closely identified with this development strategy, but several other leaders had also held similar views: B.R. Ambedkar, V.D. Savarkar and Subhas Chandra Bose. They all argued in favour of quickly building an industrial base, not just to create jobs outside agriculture, but also to give a country emerging out of colonial rule more strategic depth in a hostile world. I had earlier written a more detailed essay on the good, bad and ugly of Nehruvian economics.

What India did in those years was in tune with what most development economists of the time believed in, ever since Paul Rosenstein-Rodan wrote his landmark paper in 1943 about the need for a big push towards industrialization. There were only a few dissenters who stood outside the development economics consensus of the day. One of them was Peter Bauer. Most major developing countries tried some variant of the strategy India had chosen.

Independent India saw economic growth accelerate in its first decade of planning, after almost two centuries of economic stagnation. The initial success of the Nehruvian plans soon petered out. B.R. Shenoy had warned in his famous dissent note to the second Five-Year Plan that the aggressive investment push through deficit financing would lead to inflation as well as balance of payments pressures. India stumbled into a balance of payments crisis in 1957, and the system of import controls was put into place to ration foreign exchange. This bizarre system soon grew large enough to strangle the Indian economy.

Dhar says that Shastri saw what needed to be done. "Lal Bahadur Shastri, the unassuming prime minister who had succeeded the charismatic Nehru, seemed an unlikely person to face up to the (economic) situation. But in his own quiet way he did initiate a series of steps which would have not only brought the economy out of the existing crisis but possibly put it on a high-growth path in the long run. He wore no ideological blinkers; he saw facts as they were in all their starkness. Chronic food shortages made him shift investment from basic industries to agriculture. Roaring black markets persuaded him to make a relative shift from controls to incentives, and the glaring inefficiency of the public sector made him accept a larger role for the private sector and foreign investment. He also took measures to shift the locus of economic decision-making from the Planning Commission to the ministries and from the Centre to the states. These measures reduced the influence of the Planning Commission—which had developed a rigid, almost doctrinaire outlook on economic policies—and at the same time decentralized decision-making."

Shastri died before he could begin the course correction. This was broadly the time when several countries in East Asia had begun to shift their policy focus to internal liberalization plus exports. South Korea is a classic example. Indira Gandhi, on the other hand, responded to the mounting problems in the country with political mobilization rather than with economic reforms. Her response was a sharp turn to the left after 1969.

India began to retreat from that position in baby steps: 1975, 1981 and 1985. The tentative policy changes of those years reduced some of the restrictions on the private sector within the existing system of controls. The old system was decisively junked only in 1991, 25 years after Shastri prematurely died in Tashkent.

INDIA FOUND A LEADER, BUT LOST A STATESMAN

Reading through the archives of The Hindu from September 23, 1965, you get a sense of the relief and euphoria of a nation, now united around a leader who braved immense criticism and led from the front in its time of crises. An excerpt reads: "Tributes to Shastri's leadership: The Prime Minister's announcement in Parliament today of a cease-fire in the fighting between

India and Pakistan had an electrifying effect on the Members of Parliament and on the people.(...) (...) Members belonging to all political parties (...) praised the PM for the firm, determined and able manner in which he handled the worsening India-Pakistan relations, which finally erupted in an undeclared war."

It is interesting then that narratives often understate the tragically short-lived Prime Minister Lal Bahadur Shastri's significant contribution to the handling of >the 1965 conflict. It is ironic that he's often accused of "losing the war on the diplomatic table at Tashkent" or remembered for the intrigue surrounding his death. Apart from political appropriation, very little ink seems to have been spent on examining his diplomatic and political acumen which made India stronger domestically and helped regain its international stature post the 1965 crises.

Quiet strength

Shastri's mandate was not an easy one. There was a fractured consensus within the Congress party around his ability to lead the nation after Pandit Jawaharlal Nehru's demise. India was demoralised after the 1962 defeat and battling an acute food crisis. Pakistan's adventurism in 1965, historians argue, wanted to take advantage of this alleged "weakness in leadership".

In hindsight, Shastri's handling of the war has many lessons for contemporary leaders. His biographer C.P. Srivastava, in " *A Life of Truth in Politics*", recalls that Shastri's slight build was often mistaken for a lack of ability, but really concealed a very sharp mind.

This plays out from the first meeting between Prime Minister Shastri and Pakistani President Ayub Khan, says former ambassador M. K. Rasgotra, who was a war book officer at that time.

The former diplomat recalled a conversation between Gen. Khan and his Foreign Minister Z.A. Bhutto soon after meeting Shastri in Karachi in October 1964. Gen. Khan had reportedly remarked, "This little man. What will I speak to him?" This was "a total miscalculation as time would prove," Mr. Rasgotra says. Shastri's observations, however, were quite astute. He assessed Khan as practical, but described Bhutto as "someone who could throw the spanner in the works for Indo-Pak relations," records his biographer. A prophetic observation given how 1965 played out.

Firm stand

Contrary to expectations, Shastri had responded to Pakistani provocations on the border through speeches in Parliament from the very beginning, making

India's red lines clear, says Srivastava. He was determined to convince President Khan that 'India had no desire whatsoever to acquire even one square inch of Pakistani territory [...] [but] would never allow any interference by Pakistan in Kashmir which was an integral part of India.'

During the Rann of Kutch incident, a probing exercise by the Pakistani forces in early 1965, Shastri withstood immense pressure from the opposition to resolving the issue through an international tribunal. Having agreed to the ceasefire, his government survived a no-confidence motion to defend the decision of arbitration. Very few knew, reveals Srivastava, that Army Chief J.N. Chaudhuri and Air Chief Marshal Arjan Singh were against escalating the conflict, as the terrain was unsuitable for large-scale operations by India.

Politically, arbitration was seen as capitulation and many demanded its rollback. Shastri stood his ground, arguing India would not be a 'irresponsible nation", reneging on an "international commitment", records Srivastava — a stance that would later bolster India's position in the UNSC ceasefire dialogues.

Shastri's ability to lead and carry the nation in the face of surprise attacks was exemplified during the failed attempt by Pakistan to stir an uprising in Kashmir in August 1965. Shastri responded with a clear policy response: India would not approach the UNSC and defend its territorial integrity; no interference from Pakistan would be tolerated; contingency plans — especially vis a vis China — would be prepared; and the nation would be kept abreast of all government decisions. He articulated this in a public address on August 13, 1965, which assured the nation that 'force will be met with force'. There was no room for speculation.

Indian forces had to capture the Haji Pir Pass and the Kishen Ganga bulge, the two supply routes for infiltration into the valley to thwart the attacks. This operation required crossing the Cease Fire Line. In another bold first for India, the forces were assured of the firm backing of the Prime Minister and told the government would handle the consequences, records Srivastava.

The boldest decision came in September 1965, when Pakistani Patton tanks rolled into Chambh in J&K, aiming to capture Amritsar and more. When advised that to defend Kashmir, a diversionary attack in West Pakistan was needed to push enemy forces on the defensive, Shastri's iron will came into play.

Srivastava, then joint secretary to the Prime Minister, recalls Shastri pacing up and down in his office on September 1, 1965. He says "All I heard him say was: *ab toh kuch karna hi hoga* (now something has to be done)". He then convened an emergency cabinet meet "to carry his colleagues with him in his decision" and prepare for repercussions to India's stand. On September 3, Shastri asked the Indian forces to march to Lahore, the first time that India would take the battle to the invader's territory.

Through all of this, Shastri had ensured India's able representation in the UNSC and convinced the big powers of India's response as proportionate to Pakistani aggression, was briefed constantly by military commanders, consulted the opposition, and even organised regular press briefings to inform the people and instil confidence in the leadership.

Even his much-criticised decision to "return Haji Pir pass" during the Tashkent Conference, it is argued, was not done under pressure. His biography reveals that Shastri knew international opinion would shift if India refused, as it was a pre-requisite to the UNSC ceasefire resolution.

He was also aware that giving up Haji Pir would invite scathing accusations of betrayal domestically. Before Tashkent, records Srivastava, the military chiefs had told Shastri that while they would not want to vacate, "it could not come at the cost of peace in the subcontinent". Perhaps Prime Minister Shastri became the fall guy to circumstance.

1965 clearly has lessons for conduct of government and diplomacy for the present day establishment. We both found a leader and lost a statesman, perhaps a little too soon.

LAL BAHADUR SHASTRI SYMBOLIZED THE 'IDEA OF INDIA'

Lal Bahadur Shastri's death in Tashkent half a century ago robbed India and his party, the Congress, of many cherished possibilities which might have led the country and the party to greater glory.

From this aspect, his life which was tragically cut short at the age of 61 can be regarded as one of unfulfilled expectations.

The time of his ascent to the prime minister's position after Jawaharlal Nehru's death provided the first inklings of his own high capabilities and the assurance of a smooth succession in a nascent democracy.

The uneventful transition, brokered by the strong, silent man of Indian politics at the time, K Kamaraj, provided the much-needed sense of continuity which was necessary after years of speculation in India and abroad about "After Nehru, who?"

As The Statesman wrote in an editorial/obituary, quoting a Tagore poem, that just as earthen lamps were lit in the gathering darkness after the sun had set, Shastri was "India's earthen lamp in an hour of destiny". The imagery reflected Shastri's quiet, earthy, soothing, understated personality in contrast to Nehru's dazzling flamboyance. It took time for the ordinary people to become accustomed to the fact that Nehru's successor was not an Oxbridge man, but an unassuming person from Kashi Vidyapith. In the newsreels of the time, people used to burst into laughter as the meek, short-statured Shastri appeared on the cinema hall screens.

But it did not take long for the ridicule to turn into admiration after the 1965 war against Pakistan which saw the Indian Army advancing towards Lahore. After the humiliation of the 1962 conflict with China during which Shastri and other Congressmen had compelled Nehru to remove VK Krishna Menon from the defence minister's post, the 1965 war raised the new prime minister's prestige sky high.

His "Jai jawan, Jai kisan" slogan of the time is still remembered, as is his decision to resign as the railway minister in 1956 following an accident which claimed 144 lives. Nehru described the resignation as an act of "constitutional propriety", which hasn't been emulated by any other railway minister since then.

The 1965 war was however not the only time when Shastri revealed the steeliness of his personality. This side of his character could be seen within days of his assuming office when he dropped the acerbic Morarji Desai from the cabinet for insisting on the No.2 position. Shastri also constituted the prime minister's secretariat, which is the precursor of today's Prime Minister's office (PMO).

For the Congress, Shastri was the ideal man for enabling the party to retain not only its primacy of position in politics but also for reinvigorating the ideals of Gandhian simplicity and honesty which the party was gradually beginning to lose.

In this respect, Shastri's down-to-earth nature revived the Congress at the grassroots level by making the ordinary people remember the sterling qualities which had marked the party during the independence movement.

Had he lived, there is little doubt that the Congress would have retained its influence for a longer period than it has been able to do.

Not only that, the greatest service which a normal spell of life would have enabled Shastri to render to his party was to nullify the dynastic factor by creating a big enough gap in terms of years between Nehru's death and the succession of his progeny.

It is even possible that Nehru's descendants might not have made it to the top at all if the party had developed in a normal way instead of turning into a "feudal oligarchy", as prime minister Rajiv Gandhi said on the occasion of the Congress's centenary celebrations in 1985.

Unfortunately, there was a gap of a mere year-and-a-half between Nehru's death in May 1964 and Shastri's in January 1966. Moreover, Indira Gandhi's ascent as prime minister in January 1966 and her long tenure as well as that of her son, Rajiv, ensured that Congressmen began to associate their party so closely with the Nehru-Gandhis that the latter retained the whiphand even when the party was not in power.

The ill-effects of this association between the dynasty and its sycophants have undermined the Congress's idealism and political health.

Shastri took charge at a time when the country's morale was at a low ebb after the 1962 setback. It would sink even lower after his death with the Congress experiencing its first major electoral defeats in the 1967 assembly elections.

But, unknown to Shastri, the 1965 war had set in motion the process of Pakistan's disintegration as it led to Ayub Khan's ouster, Yahya Khan's installation and the liberation of Bangladesh.

Of the two prime ministers from outside the Nehru-Gandhi clan who will be remembered by history, Shastri will be held in high esteem because he represented the "idea of India" as a secular, multicultural nation governed by high-minded leaders.

As a believer in a "socialist democracy", he was different from PV Narasimha Rao, who followed another path of development by opening up the economy. But the two together underline their party's potential for adapting to the exigencies of varying periods when it is not stifled by feudal norms.

THE 1965 WAR WITH PAKISTAN

He appeared very modest but was a man of steel. He had the ability to take quick decisions. It was demonstrated on August 31, 1965. On that day he came home for an early dinner. One of his secretaries told him that the three chiefs of the defence services had come to see him. He immediately left for his office next door at 10, Janpath.

The three chiefs visited him to inform him that the Pakistan army had crossed the international border with 100 battle tanks in the Chamb sector of Jammu. They told him that in a short span of time the Pakistan army would cut off Kashmir from the rest of India.

Without losing time he asked for the opening of a new front including Lahore. Retaliate with full force, he said. What I remember is that the historic meeting lasted less than five minutes. Arjan Singh, the then chief of the air force was present. He is the only surviving member from that meeting.

He told them, "Be prepared for war." He called Defence Minister Y B Chavan and informed him of the decision. He responded positively and expressed his support. He didn't wait for international reactions.

The next day, newspapers reported that the Indian army was marching towards Lahore. It was a big morale booster for the country.

During those tense days, in his address to the nation from Red Fort on Independence day, he said: "*Hathiyaron ka jawab hathiyaron se denge.* (Force will be met with force.) *Hamara desh rahega to hamara tiranga rahega.* (Our flag will survive only if our country does)"

On Shastri and the Nehru-Gandhi Family

Pandit Nehru was very found of him. Shastri*ji* was around 15 years younger but he trusted him fully. In 1956, when a train accident killed 144 passengers near Ariyalur in Tamil Nadu, Shastri*ji* resigned. Pandit*ji* refused to accept the resignation but he prevailed upon Pandit*ji* to accept it.

On the following day in Parliament, Nehru said no one could wish for a better comrade than Lal Bahadur. A man of the highest integrity and devoted to ideas is called Lal Bahadur, said Nehru.

Once he was sent to Kashmir by Nehru to help resolve the theft in the Hazaratbal shrine. Nehru asked him whether he had enough woollens for the trip.

"Are you aware Kashmir must be having snowfall at this time?" asked Nehru.

Shastri showed him the jacket he was wearing and Nehru immediately gave his own mink overcoat. My father was short in stature so he told Nehru the coat was quite long. But Nehru said woollen overcoats were always longer. That no one would know it was a borrowed one.

On his return from Kashmir when father went to him to return the overcoat, Nehru asked him to keep it. The next day newspapers reported: Nehru's Mantle Falls on Shastri.

Shastri*ji* and Indira*ji* also enjoyed a close relationship. She had the highest personal regard for him. After Nehru's death in 1964, the Congress chose him as a consensus candidate. He did make an attempt to persuade Indira Gandhi to take over as prime minister. He went to see her and asked her to become prime minister. She put her foot down and said no. "You become PM and I'll totally support you," she said. When he was PM he would drop by at 1, Safdarjung Road (*Indira Gandhi's home*) without intimation just to chat with her.

DEATH AT TASHKENT

After the declaration of ceasefire, Shastri and Pakistani President Muhammad Ayub Khan attended a summit in Tashkent (former USSR, now in modern Uzbekistan), organised by Kosygin. On January 10, 1966, Shastri and Khan signed the Tashkent Declaration.

The next day Shastri, who had suffered two heart attacks earlier, died of a heart attack at 1:32 AM. He is the only Indian Prime Minister, and indeed probably one of the few heads of government, to have died in office overseas. Some conspiracy theories allege his death to be of unnatural causes.

Memorial

All his lifetime, Shastri was known for honesty and humility. He was the first person to be posthumously awarded the Bharat Ratna, and a memorial "Vijay Ghat" was built for him in Delhi. Several educational institutes, roads, public squares and monuments in India are named after him. The Lal Bahadur Shastri Stadium in Hyderabad, Andhra Pradesh is an example.

In 2005, the Government of India opened the Lal Bahadur Shastri Memorial and set up a library in New Delhi, as part of the Lal Bahadur Shastri Centenary Celebrations. Doordarshan produced a docu-drama on his life, and a national award was instituted in his name. Also, a chair was created in his name in the field of democracy and governance in Delhi University.

2

Legacy of Lal Bahadur Shastri

Lal Bahadur Shastri (2 October 1904 – 11 January 1966) was the 2nd Prime Minister of the Republic of India and a leader of the Indian National Congress party.

Shastri joined the Indian independence movement in the 1920s. Deeply impressed and influenced by Mahatma Gandhi (with whom he shared his birthday), he became a loyal follower, first of Gandhi, and then of Jawaharlal Nehru. Following independence in 1947, he joined the latter's government and became one of Prime Minister Nehru's principal, first as Railways Minister (1951–56), and then in a variety of other functions, including Home Minister.

He led the country during the Indo-Pakistan War of 1965. His slogan of "Jai Jawan Jai Kisan" ("Hail the soldier, Hail the farmer") became very popular during the war and is remembered even today. The war formally ended with the Tashkent Agreement of 10 January 1966; he died the following day, still in Tashkent, the cause of death was said to be a heart attack but there are various reasons to think that it was a planned murder by the CIA.

EARLY YEARS (1904-1917)

Shastri was born at the house of his maternal grandparents in Mughalsarai, Varanasi in a Kayastha Hindu family, that had traditionally been employed as Highly administrators and civil servants. Shastri's paternal ancestors had been in the service of the *zamindar* of Ramnagar near Varanasi and Shastri lived there for the first one year of his life. Shastri's father, Sharada Prasad Shastri, was a school teacher who later became a clerk in the revenue office at Allahabad, while his mother, Ramdulari Devi, was the daughter of Munshi Hazari Lal, the headmaster and English teacher at a railway school in Mughalsarai. Shastri was the second child and eldest son of his parents; he had an elder sister, Kailashi Devi (b. 1900).

In April 1906, When Shastri was hardly one year old, his father, had only recently been promoted to the post of deputy tahsildar, died in an epidemic of bubonic plague. Ramdulari Devi, then only 23 and pregnant with her third child, took her two children and moved from Ramnnagar to her father's house in Mughalsarai and settled there for good. She gave birth to a daughter, Sundari Devi, in July 1906. Thus, Shastri and his sisters grew up in the household of his maternal grandfather, Hazari Lal. However, Hazari Lal himself died from a stroke in mid-1908, after which the family were looked after by his brother (Shastri's great-uncle) Darbari Lal, who was the head clerk in the opium regulation department at Ghazipur, and later by his son (Ramdulari Devi's cousin) Bindeshwari Prasad, a school teacher in Mughalsarai. Thus, the greatness of the traditional Indian joint family system, and the traditions of family responsibility and kinship, are deeply evident in Shastri's case, where the orphan child of a penniless widow was raised by his distant relatives in a manner which enabled him to become Prime Minister of India.

In Shastri's family, as with many Kayastha families, it was the custom in that era for children to receive an education in the Urdu language and culture. This is because Urdu/Persian had been the language of government for centuries, before being replaced by English, and old traditions persisted into the 20th century. Therefore, Shastri began his education at the age of four under the tutelage of a *maulvi* (a Muslim cleric), Budhan Mian, at the East Central Railway Inter college in Mughalsarai. He studied there until the sixth standard. In 1917, Bindeshwari Prasad (who was now head of the household) was transferred to Varanasi, and the entire family moved there, including Ramdulari Devi and her three children. In Varanasi, Shastri joining the seventh standard at Harish Chandra High School. At this time, he decided to drop his caste-derived surname of "Verma" (which is a traditional optional surname for all Kayastha families).

The young *satyagrahi* (1921–1945)

While Shastri's family had no links to the independence movement then taking shape, among his teachers at Harish Chandra High School was an intensely patriotic and highly respected teacher named Nishkameshwar Prasad Mishra, who gave Shastri much-needed financial support by allowing him to tutor his children. Inspired by Mishra's patriotism, Shastri took a deep interest in the freedom struggle, and began to study its history and the works of several of its noted personalities, including those of Swami Vivekananda, Bal Gangadhar Tilak, Gandhi and Annie Besant. In January 1921, when Shastri was in the 10 standard and three months from sitting the final examinations, he attended a public meeting in Benares hosted by Gandhi and Pandit Madan

Mohan Malaviya. Inspired by the Mahatma's call for students to withdraw from government schools and join the non-cooperation movement, Shastri withdrew from Harish Chadra the next day and joined the local branch of the Congress Party as a volunteer, actively participating in picketing and anti-government demonstrations. He was soon arrested and jailed, but was then let off as he was still a minor. Shastri's immediate supervisor was a former Benares Hindu University lecturer named J.B. Kripalani, who would become one of the most prominent leaders of the Indian independence movement and among Gandhi's closest followers. Recognising the need for the younger volunteers to continue their educations, Kripalani and a friend, V.N. Sharma, had founded an informal school centered around "nationalist education" to educate the young activists in their nation's heritage. With the support of a wealthy philanthropist and ardent Congress nationalist, Shiv Prasad Gupta, the Kashi Vidyapith was inaugurated by Gandhi in Benares as a national institution of higher education on 10 February 1921. Among the first students of the new institution, Shastri graduated with a first-class degree in philosophy and ethics from the Vidyapith in 1925. He was given the title *Shastri* ("scholar"). The title was a bachelor's degree awarded by the Vidyapith, but it stuck as part of his name.

Shastri enrolled himself as a life member of the Servants of the People Society (Lok Sevak Mandal), founded by Lala Lajpat Rai, and began to work for the betterment of the Harijans under Gandhi's direction at Muzaffarpur. Later he became the President of the Society.

Independence activism

In 1928 shastri become an active member of congress at the call of gandhiji. Shastri participated in the Salt Satyagraha in 1930. He was imprisoned for two and a half years. Later, he worked as the Organizing Secretary of the Parliamentary Board of U.P. in 1937. In 1940, he was sent to prison for one year, for offering individual Satyagraha support to the independence movement.

On 8 August 1942, Mahatma Gandhi issued the Quit India speech at Gowalia Tank in Mumbai, demanding that the British leave India. Shastri, who had just then come out after a year in prison, travelled to Allahabad. For a week, he sent instructions to the independence activists from Jawaharlal Nehru's home, Anand Bhavan. A few days later, he was arrested and imprisoned until 1946. Shastri spent almost nine years in jail in total. During his stay in prison, he spent time reading books and became familiar with the works of western philosophers, revolutionaries and social reformers.

POLITICAL CAREER (1947-64)

State minister

Following India's independence, Shastri was appointed Parliamentary Secretary in his home state, Uttar Pradesh. He became the Minister of Police and Transport under Govind Ballabh Pant's Chief Ministership on 15 August 1947 following Rafi Ahmed Kidwai's departure to become minister at centre. As the Transport Minister, he was the first to appoint women conductors. As the minister in charge of the Police Department, he ordered that police use jets of water instead of lathis to disperse unruly crowds. His tenure as police minister (As Home Minister was called prior to 1950) saw successful curbing of communal riots in 1947, mass migration and resettlement of refugees.

Cabinet minister

In 1951, Shastri was made the General Secretary of the All-India Congress Committee with Jawaharlal Nehru as the Prime Minister. He was directly responsible for the selection of candidates and the direction of publicity and electioneering activities. His cabinet consisted of the finest business men of India including Ratilal Premchand Mehta. He played an important role in the landslide successes of the Congress Party in the Indian General Elections of 1952, 1957 and 1962. In 1952, he successfully contested UP Vidhansabha from Soraon North cum Phulpur West seat and won getting over 69% of vote. He was believed to be retained as home minister of UP, but in a surprise move was called to Centre as minister by Nehru. Shastri was made Minister of Railways in First Cabinet of Republic of India on 13 May 1952.

PRIME MINISTER OF INDIA (1964-66)

Jawaharlal Nehru died in office on 27 May 1964 and left a void. Then Congress Party chief Minister K. Kamaraj was instrumental in making Shastri Prime Minister on 9 June. Shastri, though mild-mannered and soft-spoken, was a Nehruvian socialist and thus held appeal to those wishing to prevent the ascent of conservative right-winger Morarji Desai.

In his first broadcast as Prime Minister, on 11 June 1964, Shastri stated:

"There comes a time in the life of every nation when it stands at the cross-roads of history and must choose which way to go. But for us there need be no difficulty or hesitation, no looking to right or left. Our way is straight and clear—the building up of a secular mixed-economy democracy at home with freedom and prosperity, and the maintenance of world peace and friendship with select nations."

Domestic policies

Shastri retained many members of Nehru's Council of Ministers. T. T. Krishnamachari was retained as the Finance Minister of India, as was Defence Minister Yashwantrao Chavan. He appointed Swaran Singh to succeed him as External Affairs Minister. He also appointed Indira Gandhi, daughter of Jawaharlal Nehru and former Congress President, as the Minister of Information and Broadcasting. Gulzarilal Nanda continued as the Minister of Home Affairs.

Lal Bahadur Shastri's tenure witnessed the Madras anti-Hindi agitation of 1965. The government of India had for a long time made an effort to establish Hindi as the sole national language of India. This was resisted by the non-Hindi speaking states particularly Madras State. To calm the situation, Shastri gave assurances that English would continue to be used as the official language as long the non-Hindi speaking states wanted. The riots subsided after Shastri's assurance, as did the student agitation.

Economic policies

Shastri discontinued Nehru's socialist economic policies with central planning. He promoted the White Revolution – a national campaign to increase the production and supply of milk – by supporting the Amul milk co-operative of Anand, Gujarat and creating the National Dairy Development Board.

He visited Anand on 31 October 1964 for inauguration of the Cattle Feed Factory of Amul at Kanjari. As he was keenly interested in knowing the success of this co-operative, he stayed overnight with farmers in a village, and even had dinner with a farmer's family. He discussed his wish with Mr Verghese Kurien, then the General Manager of Kaira District Co-operative Milk Producers' Union Ltd (Amul) to replicate this model to other parts of the country for improving the socio-economic conditions of farmers. As a result of this visit, the National Dairy Development Board (NDDB) was established at Anand in 1965

While speaking on the chronic food shortages across the country, Shastri urged people to voluntarily give up one meal so that the food saved could be distributed to the affected populace. However he ensured that he first implemented the system in his own family before appealing to the country. He went on air to appeal to his countrymen to skip a meal a week. The response to his appeal was overwhelming. Even restaurants and eateries downed the shutters on Monday evenings. Many parts of the country observed the "Shastri Vrat". He motivated the country to maximize the cultivation of food grains by ploughing the lawn himself, at his official residence in New

Delhi. During the 22-day war with Pakistan in 1965, On 19 October 1965, Shastri gave the seminal 'Jai Jawan Jai Kishan' ("Hail the soldier, Hail the farmer")slogan at Urwa in Allahabad that became a national slogan.

Underlining the need to boost India's food production. Shastri also promoted the Green Revolution. Though he was a socialist, Shastri stated that India cannot have a regimented type of economy.

The Food Corporation of India was set up under the Food Corporation's Act 1964. Also The National Agricultural Products Board Act.

Jai Jawan Jai Kisan

For the outstanding slogan given by him during Indo-Pak war of 1965 Ministry of Information and Broadcasting (India) commemorated Shastriji even after 47 years of his death on his 48th martyr's day:

Former Prime Minister Lal Bahadur Shastri was one of those great Indians who has left an indelible impression on our collective life. Shri Lal Bahadur Shastri's contribution to our public life were unique in that they were made in the closest proximity to the life of the common man in India. Shri Lal Bahadur Shastri was looked upon by Indians as one of their own, one who shared their ideals, hopes and aspirations. His achievements were looked upon not as the isolated achievements of an individual but of our society collectively.

Under his leadership India faced and repulsed the Pakistani invasion of 1965. It is not only a matter of pride for the Indian Army but also for every citizen of the country. Shri Lal Bahadur Shastri's slogan Jai Jawan! Jai Kisan!! reverberates even today through the length and breadth of the country. Underlying this is the inner-most sentiments 'Jai Hind'. The war of 1965 was fought and won for our self-respect and our national prestige. For using our Defence Forces with such admirable skill, the nation remains beholden to Shri Lal Bahadur Shastri. He will be remembered for all times to come for his large heartedness and public service.

Foreign policies

Shastri continued Nehru policy of non-alignment but also built closer relations with the Soviet Union. In the aftermath of the Sino-Indian War of 1962 and the formation of military ties between the Chinese People's Republic and Pakistan, Shastri's government decided to expand the defence budget of India's armed forces.

In 1964, Shastri signed an accord with the Sri Lankan Prime minister Sirimavo Bandaranaike regarding the status of Indian Tamils in the then

Ceylon. This agreement is also known as the Sirima-Shastri Pact or the Bandaranaike-Shastri pact.

Under the terms of this agreement, 600,000 Indian Tamils were to be repatriated, while 375,000 were to be granted Sri Lankan citizenship. This settlement was to be done by 31 October 1981. However, after Shastri's death, by 1981, India had taken only 300,000 Tamils as repatriates, while Sri Lanka had granted citizenship to only 185,000 citizens (plus another 62,000 born after 1964). Later, India declined to consider any further applications for citizenship, stating that the 1964 agreement had lapsed.

India's relationship with Burma had been strained after the 1962 Military coup followed by the repatriation of many Indian families in 1964 by Burma. While the central government in New Delhi monitored the overall process of repatriation and arranged for identification and transportation of the Indian returnees from Burma, it fell under the responsibilities of local governments to provide adequate facilities to shelter the repatriates upon disembarkation on Indian soil. Particularly in the Madras State the Chief Minister during that time, Minjur K. Bhaktavatsalam, showed care in rehabilitation of the returnees. In December 1965 Shastri made an official visit with his Family to Rangoon, Burma and re-established cordial relations with the country's military government of General Ne Win.

War with Pakistan

Shastri's greatest moment came when he led India in the 1965 Indo-Pak War.

Laying claim to half the Kutch peninsula, the Pakistani army skirmished with Indian forces in August, 1965. In his report to the Lok Sabha on the confrontation in Kutch, Shastri stated:

In the utilization of our limited resources, we have always given primacy to plans and projects for economic development. It would, therefore, be obvious for anyone who is prepared to look at things objectively that India can have no possible interest in provoking border incidents or in building up an atmosphere of strife... In these circumstances, the duty of Government is quite clear and this duty will be discharged fully and effectively... We would prefer to live in poverty for as long as necessary but we shall not allow our freedom to be subverted.

In September 1965, major incursions of militants and Pakistani soldiers began, hoping not only to break down the government but incite a sympathetic revolt. The revolt did not happen, and India sent its forces across the Ceasefire Line (now Line of Control) and threatened Pakistan by crossing the International

Border near Lahore as war broke out on a general scale. Massive tank battles occurred in the Punjab, and while the Pakistani forces made gains in the northern part of subcontinent, Indian forces captured the key post at Haji Pir, in Kashmir, and brought the Pakistani city of Lahore under artillery and mortar fire.

On 17 September 1965, while the Indo-Pak war was on, India received a letter from China alleging that the Indian army had set up army equipment in Chinese territory, and India would face China's wrath, unless the equipment was pulled down. In spite of the threat of aggression from China, Shastri declared "China's allegation is untrue".The Chinese did not respond, but the Indo-Pak war resulted in some 3–4,000 casualties on each side and significant loss of material.

The Indo-Pak war ended on 23 September 1965 with a United Nations-mandated ceasefire. In a broadcast to the nation on the day of the ceasefire, Shastri stated:

"While the conflict between the armed forces of the two countries has come to an end, the more important thing for the United Nations and all those who stand for peace is to bring to an end the deeper conflict.... How can this be brought about? In our view, the only answer lies in peaceful coexistence. India has stood for the principle of coexistence and championed it all over the world. Peaceful coexistence is possible among nations no matter how deep the differences between them, how far apart they are in their political and economic systems, no matter how intense the issues that divide them."

During his tenure as Prime Minister, Shastri visited many countries including Russia, Yugoslavia, England, Canada, Nepal, Egypt and Burma. Incidentally while returning from the Non Alliance Conference in Cairo on the invitation of then President of the Pakistan, Mohammed Ayub Khan to have lunch with him, Shastri made a stop over at Karachi Airport for few hours and breaking from the protocol Ayub Khan personally received him at the Airport and had an informal meeting during October 1964. After the declaration of ceasefire with Pakistan in 1965, Shastri and Ayub Khan attended a summit in Tashkent (former USSR, now in modern Uzbekistan), organized by Alexei Kosygin. On 10 January 1966, Shastri and Ayub Khan signed the Tashkent Declaration.

Death

Shastri died in Tashkent, at 02:00 on the day after signing the Tashkent Declaration, reportedly due to a heart attack, but people allege conspiracy behind the death. He was the first Prime Minister of India to die overseas.

He was eulogised as a national hero and the Vijay Ghat memorial established in his memory. Upon his death, Gulzarilal Nanda once again assumed the role of Acting Prime Minister until the Congress Parliamentary Party elected Indira Gandhi over Morarji Desai to officially succeed Shastri.

FAMILY AND DESCENDANTS

On 16 May 1928, Shastri married Lalita Devi a lady from Mirzapur. The marriage, which was arranged by their parents in the traditional Indian way, was harmonious and conventional. The couple were blessed with four sons and two daughters, namely

1. Kusum Shastri, the eldest daughter
2. Hari Krishna Shastri, eldest son, who was married to Vibha Shastri
3. Suman Shastri, second daughter, married to Vijay Nath Singh. Her son, Siddharth Nath Singh, is a spokesman of the Bharatiya Janata Party
4. Anil Shastri. He is married to Manju Shastri. Alone in his family, he remains a member of his father's Congress Party. His son Adarsh Shastri gave up his corporate career with Apple Inc to contest the General elections of 2014 from Allahabad on an Aam Aadmi Party ticket. He lost that election.
5. Sunil Shastri. He is married to Meera Shastri. He is a member of the Bharatiya Janata Party.
6. Ashok Shastri, the youngest son. He worked in the corporate world before his untimely death at the age of 37. His wife Neera Shastri and his son Sameep Shastri are members of the Bharatiya Janata Party.

LEGACY

Ramachandra Guha argued that Shastri shared little in common with his predecessor Jawaharlal Nehru. While Shastri preferred peace with Pakistan, writing to a friend after the Indo-Pakistani War in 1965 that the problems between both countries should be settled amicably, he had previously displayed a knack for taking quick and decisive actions during the war. He swiftly took the advice of his commanders, and ordered a strike across the Punjab border. This was in stark contrast to Nehru who in a similar situation in 1962, had refused to call in the air force to relieve the pressure on the ground troops. At the end of the conflict, Shastri flamboyantly posed for a photograph on top of a captured US-supplied Pakistani M48 Patton tank.

However, in common with Nehru, Shastri was a secularist who refused to mix religion with politics. In a public meeting held at the Ram Lila grounds in Delhi, a few days after the ceasefire, he complained against a BBC report which claimed that Shastri's identity as a Hindu meant that he was ready for a war with Pakistan. He stated:

"While I am a Hindu, Mir Mushtaq who is presiding over this meeting is a Muslim. Mr. Frank Anthony who has addressed you is a Christian. There are also Sikhs and Parsis here. The unique thing about our country is that we have Hindus, Muslims, Christians, Sikhs, Parsis and people of all other religions. We have temples and mosques, *gurdwaras* and churches. But we do not bring all this into politics. This is the difference between India and Pakistan. Whereas Pakistan proclaims herself to be an Islamic State and uses religion as a political factor, we Indians have the freedom to follow whatever religion we may choose, and worship in any way we please. So far as politics is concerned, each of us is as much an Indian as the other."

Kuldip Nayar, Shastri's media advisor from 1960 to 1964, recalls that, during the Quit India Movement, his daughter was ill and he was released on parole from jail. However, he could not save her life because doctors had prescribed costly drugs. Later on in 1963, on the day when he was dropped from the cabinet, he was sitting in his home in the dark, without a light. When asked about the reason, he said as he no longer is a minister, all expenses will have to be paid by himself and that as a MP and minister he didn't earn enough to save for time of need.

Although Shastri had been a cabinet minister for many years in the 1950s, he was poor when he died. All he owned at the end was an old car, which he had bought in instalments from the government and for which he still owed money. He was a member of Servants of India society (which included Gandhi, Lala Lajpat Rai, Gopal Krishna Gokhle) which asked all its members to shun accumulation of private property and remain in public life as servants of people. He was the first railway minister who resigned from office following a major train accident as he felt moral responsibility.

The foundation stone of Bal Vidya Mandir, a distinguished school of Lucknow, was laid by him during his tenure as the Prime Minister, on 19 November 1964.

He inaugurated the Central Institute of Technology Campus at Tharamani, Chennai, in November 1964.

He inaugurated the Plutonium Reprocessing Plant at Trombay in 1965. As suggested by Dr. Homi Jehangir Bhabha, Shastri authorized the development of nuclear explosives. Bhabha initiated the effort by setting up the nuclear explosive design group Study of Nuclear Explosions for Peaceful Purposes (SNEPP).

He inaugurated the Andhra Pradesh Agricultural University at Hyderabad on 20 March 1965 which renamed as Acharya N. G. Ranga Agricultural University in 1996 and was separated into two universities after formation Telangana State. The University in Telangana was named in July 2014 as Professor. Jayashanker Agricultural University.

Shasstriji also inaugurated the National Institute of Technology, Allahabad.

Lal Bahadur Shastri inaugurated the Jawahar Dock of the Chennai Port Trust & starts the construction work of Tuticorin Port (Now VOC Port Trust) in November 1964.

He inaugurated Sainik School Balachadi, in State of Gujarat. He laid the foundation stone of Almatti dam during the year ———— . Now the commissioned dam bears his name.

Memorials

Shastri was known for his honesty and humility throughout his life. He was the first person to be posthumously awarded the Bharat Ratna, and a memorial "Vijay Ghat" was built for him in Delhi.

Several educational institutes, Lal Bahadur Shastri National Academy of Administration (Mussorie, Uttarakhand) is after his name.

Lal Bahadur Shastri Institute of Management was established in Delhi by the 'Lal Bahadur Shastri Educational Trust' in 1995 as is one of the top business schools in India.

The Shastri Indo-Canadian Institute was named after Shastri due to his role in promoting scholarly activity between India and Canada.

Lal Bhadur Shastri Memorial run by Lal Bahadur Shastri National Memorial Trust, is situated next to 10 Janpath his residence as Prime Minister, at 1, Motilal Nehru Place, New Delhi. In 2011, on Shastri's 45th death anniversary, Uttar Pradesh Government announced to renovate Shastri's ancestral house at Ramnagar in Varanasi and declared plans to convert it into a biographical museum. Varanasi International Airport is named after him.

Lal Bahadur Shastri Centre For Indian Culture with a Monument and a street is named after him in the city of Tashkent, Uzbekistan.

Few stadiums are named after him in the cities of Hyderabad, Andhra Pradesh Ahmadabad in Gujarat and another one at Kollam, Kerala. Shastri Road in Kottayam, Kerala

The Almatti Dam is renamed as Lal Bahadur Shastri Sagar in Northern Karnataka built across the River Krishna. The foundation stone was laid by him. MV Lal Bahadur Shastri a Cargo Ship is named after him. RBI released coins in the denomination of Rs.5 during his birth century celebrations.

All India Lal Bahadur Shastri Hockey tournament is held every year since 1991 a major tournament in the field of Hockey.

The Left Bank Canal form the Nagarjuna Sagar Dam in AP is named Lal Bahadur Shastri Canal which is 295 km in Length.

Life size statues of Shastri are erected at Mumbai, Bangalore(Vidhana Soudha), New Delhi(CGO Complex), Almatti Dam Site, Ramnagar-UP, Hisar, Vizagapattinam, Nagarjuna Dam site,Warangal.

Life size bust of Shastri are erected at Thiruvandram, Pune, Varanasi(Airport), Ahmedabad (lake side), Khrushetra, Shimla, Kasargod, Indore, Jalandar, Mhow, Uran.

Some major roads in the cities of New Delhi, Mumbai, Pune, Puduchery, Lucknow, Warangal and Allahabad bearing the name of the legend.

Lal Bahadur Shastri Medical College in Mandi, Himachal Pradesh.

Shastri Bhavans in Newdelhi, Chennai, Lucknow

In 2005, the Government of India created a chair in his honour in the field of democracy and governance at Delhi University.

PREMIERSHIP OF LAL BAHADUR SHASTRI

The premiership of Lal Bahadur Shastri extended from 9 June 1964 to 11 January 1966. Formerly the Minister of External Affairs, Shastri became the Indian Prime Minister after the death of Jawaharlal Nehru, India's first Prime Minister, on 27 May 1964. Shastri's tenure as Prime Minister lasted only nineteen months due to his sudden death in Tashkent (then Soviet Union).

Taking office

After the death of Nehru, several leaders of the ruling Indian National Congress nominated Shastri due to his socialist background, to stand against the conservative Morarji Desai. With the backing of Congress President Kumaraswami Kamaraj, Shastri became the party's choice for Prime Minister. Shastri was sworn in on 9 June 1964 taking over from the Acting Prime Minister Gulzarilal Nanda. Commanding a strong majority in the Indian Parliament that it had won in the Indian general election, 1962 Shastri and the Congress party did not call fresh elections. In his first broadcast as Prime Minister, Shastri said:

"There comes a time in the life of every nation when it stands at the cross-roads of history and must choose which way to go. But for us there need be no difficulty or hesitation, no looking to right or left. Our way is straight and clear – the building up of a socialist democracy at home with freedom and prosperity for all, and the maintenance of world peace and friendship with all nations."

Domestic affairs

Shastri continued Nehru's socialist economic policies with central planning. He promoted the White Revolution – a national campaign to increase the production and supply of milk – by supporting the Amul milk co-operative of Anand, Gujarat and creating the National Dairy Development Board. While speaking on the chronic food shortages across the country, Shastri urged people to voluntarily give up one meal so that the saved food could be distributed to the affected populace.

Security and foreign affairs

Shastri also continued Nehru's policy of non-alignment but also built closer relations with the Soviet Union. In the aftermath of the disastrous Sino-Indian War of 1962 and the formation of military ties between the Chinese People's Republic and Pakistan, Shastri's government considerably expanded the defence budget and strengthened India's armed forces.

Tashkent Declaration

Shastri and Pakistan's Ayub Khan agreed to a cease-fire mandated by the United Nations. Shastri won great popularity for taking a firm stand against Pakistani aggression. In a broadcast to the nation on the day of the ceasefire, Shastri stated:

"While the conflict between the armed forces of the two countries has come to an end, the more important thing for the United Nations and all those who stand for peace is to bring to an end the deeper conflict... How can this be brought about? In our view, the only answer lies in peaceful coexistence. India has stood for the principle of coexistence and championed it all over the world. Peaceful coexistence is possible among nations no matter how deep the differences between them, how far apart they are in their political and economic systems, no matter how intense the issues that divide them."

Shastri accepted mediation from the Soviet Union and signed the Tashkent Declaration on 10 January 1966 with Pakistani president Ayub Khan in the presence of Alexei Kosygin, the Premier of the Soviet Union. Both nations agreed to withdraw their forces to pre-war lines, normalise diplomatic relations and use dialogue to resolve disputes.

Death and succession

Prime Minister Shastri died in Tashkent due to a heart attack the day after signing the Tashkent Declaration. He was eulogised as a national hero and the Vijay Ghat memorial established in his memory. Upon his death, Gulzarilal Nanda once again assumed the role of Acting Prime Minister until the Congress Parliamentary Party elected Indira Gandhi over Morarji Desai to succeed Shastri.

LAL BAHADUR SHASTRI, THIRD PRIME MINISTER OF INDIA

He was the third Prime Minister of independent India and a significant figure in the Indian independence movement.

Early Career of Lal Bahadur Shastri

Lal Bahadur was born in the year 1904 in Mughalsarai, Uttar Pradesh as Lal Bahadur Srivastava. His father Sharada Prasad was a poor school teacher. When Lal Bahadur was three months old, he slipped out of his mother's arms into a cowherd's basket at the ghats of the Ganga. The cowherd, who had no children, took the child as a gift from God. Lal Bahadur's parents lodged a complaint with the police, who traced the child, and returned him to his parents.

Lal Bahadur's father died when he was only a year and a half old. His mother Ramdulari Devi took him and his two sisters to her father's house and settled down there.

Since there was no high school in their town, he was sent to Varanasi where he stayed with his maternal uncle and joined the Harischandra High School. While in Varanasi, Shastri once went with his friends to see a fair on the other bank of the Ganges. On his way back he had no money for the boat fare so Instead of borrowing money, he jumped into the river and swam to the other side.

As a boy, Lal Bahadur loved reading books and was devoted to Guru Nanak's verses.

He idolized Bal Gangadhar Tilak, the Indian nationalist, social reformer and freedom fighter.

After hearing a speech of Mahatma Gandhi at Varanasi in 1915, he dedicated his life to the service of the country. He also dropped his surname, as it indicated his caste and he was against the caste system. During the non-cooperation movement of Mahatma Gandhi in 1921, he joined processions by taking a bold step against the restrictive order.

Achievements of Lal Bahadur Shastri

Upon completion of his course at Kashi Vidyapeeth in 1926, he was given the title Shastri ("Scholar"). The title was a bachelor's degree awarded by the Vidya Peeth, but it remained as part of his name. He also enrolled himself as a life member of the Servants of the People Society and began to work for the upliftment of the Harijans at Muzaffarpur.

In 1927, Shastri married Lalita Devi of Mirzapur. In spite of the prevailing dowry tradition, Shastri accepted only a charkha and a few yards of khadi as dowry. All his lifetime, Shastri was known for his honesty and humility. He was the first person to be awarded the Bharat Ratna after his death, and a memorial "Vijay Ghat" was built for him in Delhi. Several educational institutes, roads, public squares and monuments in India are named after him. The Lal Bahadur Shastri Stadium in Hyderabad, Andhra Pradesh is an example of this.

Political Achievements of Lal Bahadur Shastri

Following India's independence, Shastri was appointed as Parliamentary Secretary in his home state, Uttar Pradesh. He became the Minister of Police and Transport under Govind Ballabh Pant's Chief Ministership. As the Transport Minister, he was the first one to appoint women conductors. As the minister in charge of the Police Department, he ordered that Police use jets of water instead of lathis to drive off unruly crowds. In 1951, he was made the General Secretary of the All-India Congress Committee, with Jawaharlal Nehru as the President.

In 1951, Nehru nominated him to the Rajya Sabha. From 1951 to 1956 Shastri served as the Minister of Railways and Transport in the Central Cabinet. However Shastri resigned accepting moral and constitutional responsibility for a railway accident at Ariyalur that resulted in 144 deaths.

Prime Minister, Jawaharlal Nehru, stated that he was accepting the resignation because it would set an example in constitutional decorum and not because Shastri was in any way responsible for the accident. Shastri's unprecedented gesture was greatly appreciated by the Indian citizens. In 1957, Shastri returned to the Cabinet, first as the Minister for Transport and Communications, and then as the Minister of Commerce and Industry. In 1961, he became Minister for Home.

As Union Home Minister he was instrumental in appointing the Committee on Prevention of Corruption under the Chairmanship of K. Santhanam. After Jawaharlal Nehru died in office on May 27, 1964 Shastri was made the Prime

Minister. Shastri worked by his natural characteristics to obtain compromises between opposing viewpoints. However, he commanded a great deal of respect in the Indian citizens, and he used it to advantage in pushing the Green Revolution in India, which directly led to India becoming a food-surplus nation, although he did not live to see it. During the 22 day war with Pakistan, Lal Bahadur Shastri created the slogan of "Jai Jawan, Jai Kisan" ("Hail the solider, Hail the farmer"), emphasising the need to boost India's food production.

Apart from emphasizing the Green Revolution, he was instrumental in promoting the White Revolution. He is the only Indian Prime Minister, and indeed probably one of the few heads of government, to have died in office outside the country. Some conspiracy theories alleges his death to be of unnatural causes.

LAL BAHADUR SHASTRI : INDIA'S GREATEST PMS

Exactly 50 years ago on this day, India's second prime minister Lal Bahadur Shastri, or beloved Shastriji of the nation died an untimely death. Although he remains a prime minister who died in office serving for one of the shortest spans of just about 18 months, there are still many things to his credit.

He restored the confidence of the Indian armed forces that had experienced a humiliating defeat in 1962 following the Chinese aggression. More importantly, he very successfully filled the post-Nehru void as during the last year or so of the Nehru era, the political atmosphere in India was agog with the question "Who after Nehru?"

When Shastriji was unanimously elected as the leader of the Congress parliamentary party, there were many doubting Thomases who openly expressed their reservations about Shastriji's selection. Within months, Shastriji silenced them. Once he had famously and very rightly said, "I am not as simple as I look."

A man of unimpeachable character, Lal Bahadur Shastri displayed rare qualities like the highest level of integrity and ownership of responsibility, emotional connect with the people and above all, leadership required for crisis management.

Many may not know that Shastriji was responsible for ending disparity in passenger amenities in different classes prevalent in the railways during those days. He abolished the luxury class and the most neglected third class. As the railway minister he improved amenities for the poor and deprived sections of the passenger community.

Known for his soft, accommodative approach, Shastriji very adroitly handled the anti-Hindi agitation and accepted that English too would continue as one of the official languages. He, very successfully, doused the fires of linguistic conflict.

In so far as his visionary policies are concerned, he laid the foundation of the Green Revolution and gave impetus to the Operation Flood campaign that ultimately led to the strengthening of our dairy industry and eventually the White Revolution as well. It was his brief tenure that saw the foundation of the National Dairy Development Board (NDDB).

However, his governance, more than anything else, always had an indelible mark of complete accountability and ownership of responsibility. While he was railway minister, in 1956, there were two railway mishaps, the first in September 1956, at Mahbubnagar that led to 112 deaths. Accepting complete responsibility, he tendered resignation which was rejected by prime minister Nehru.

Three months later, he resigned accepting moral and constitutional responsibility for a railway accident at Ariyalur in Tamil Nadu that resulted in 144 deaths. What Nehru said while accepting his resignation is noteworthy. Nehru stated in Parliament that he was accepting the resignation because it set an example in constitutional propriety and not because Shastri was in any way responsible for the accident.

Being extremely down to earth, simplicity was Shastri's greatest strength. Perhaps, it was this simplicity that earned him not only deep respect but also a very crucial emotional connect with the people. Post-Nehru, this was of great importance.

In 1965, while facing severe shortage of rice and other foodgrains, he easily prepared popular mindset to give up evening meals on Mondays. This was his way of making people participate in the government's efforts to achieve national goals. While the nation was facing challenges on the economic front, a simple appeal by him to women worked wonders and many offered their gold ornaments for the cause of the nation.

His slogan, "Jai Jawan, Jai Kisan" caught the imagination of the people as it underscored the need for involvement of people in both defence preparedness and food security. No wonder, years later, in 1998, the then prime minister Atal Bihari Vajpayee built on the same slogan and added a suffix "Jai Vigyan".

Shastri's leadership was put to test during the 1965 war with Pakistan and later while negotiating peace with Pakistan, from a position of strength.

Without mincing words, he told Pakistan that misadventures will cost her dearly.

Without his visionary statesmanship, our issues with Sri Lanka concerning the Tamil population there would have been far too complicated. Provisions of the Srimavo-Shastri pact were remarkable for his quest to find a permanent solution to the Tamil question.

Today, when the Congress finds the going tough, it can take a couple of leaves out of Lal Bahadur Shastri's politics as well as policies. This is relevant as the Grand Old Party of India almost completely lacks emotional connect with the people, leadership and more importantly, faces a grave crisis of ownership as well.

3

Shastri and the Congress

Shastri has been forgotten by the nation. He has been pushed into the background. I have no doubt that there was a Congress conspiracy to underplay Shastri after his death.

The Congress is the party that should have put him to the fore but I remember visiting a Congress meeting where Shastri's portrait was not even displayed with respect.

He simply didn't fit in. Mrs Gandhi was strongly against the Congress old guard. When he died there was a strong resistance against his cremation in the area where Gandhi and Nehru had been laid to rest. Most Congressmen wanted his body taken to Allahabad. When Mrs Lalita Shastri said she would go public only then did the Congressmen relent.

They even protested against inscribing the slogan — *Jai Jawan, Jai Kisan* on his *samadhi*. Then again, only when

Mrs. Shastri threatened to go on a hunger strike was it was allowed. After leaving the Press Information Bureau I became a reporter. Wherever I went to meet Congress leaders, I was labelled as *'Shastri ka aadmi'* [Shastri's man].

Now, a committee has been set up by the Congress-led government to celebrate his birth centenary but it seems like an afterthought. I think after the death of Shastri, the Congress did not know where to fit him. When Mrs Gandhi succeeded him, the Congress didn't know where to put his legacy in the scheme of things then.

Shastri stands for austerity.

Shastri stands for simplicity and consensus.

Shastri represents an ideology that was right of Centre but not left of Centre. After all, he is the man who said we need the five-year plan but let us have a one year holiday from plan.

I remember vividly a small incident that brought out the stark difference between the two (*Shastri and Indira Gandhi*) leaders.

During Shastri's tenure his home in Janpath was upgraded quite a bit to suit the status of a PM.

After his death, while searching for a suitable home Mrs Gandhi went to see Shastri's home. She entered the home, had a round inside and said, "middle class!"

THE MAKING OF SHASTRI

Shastri was selected by veteran Congress leaders K Kamaraj, Neelam Sanjeeva Reddy and S Nijalingappa to lead the nation. Moments after Nehru's death I asked him who should become PM, he said it should be the unanimous decision of the Congress.

He gave two names in order. First, Jayaprakash Narayan and second, Indira Gandhi. He told me he wanted a unanimous decision over the selection. "But if there is a contest (*which Morarji Desai contemplated*) then I can defeat Morarji Desai but not Indira Gandhi," he told me. Probably he was right. However, the question didn't arise because Kamaraj was asked to talk to members informally. Shastri was made PM but Morarji*bhai* never accepted the decision.

After Shastri became PM he had to face the war with Pakistan. When the Chamb border was attacked Shastri was asked to take a tough decision whether to cross the international border. The army chief said it would be difficult to hold on for long at Chamb. Shastri gave the order saying — before they can capture Chamb you should capture Lahore.

After the war was over, I asked Indira Gandhi if Nehru would have allowed the crossing of the international border. Mrs Gandhi said, 'Whatever the generals would have advised him he would have followed."

But I wonder.

A Slight man Made of Steel

After the war, Shastri's name was all over. Before the war many people laughed at him for his softness but not after the war. He came out as a tough hero.

His toughness was evident at Tashkent. When Russian Prime Minister Alexei Kosygin wanted Shastri to sign the agreement for peace with General Ayub Khan of Pakistan after the 1965 war, Shastri insisted on adding the assurance, "never again will weapons be used to sort out problems between India and Pakistan."

Ayub was maintaining a vague stance by quoting UN resolutions. "Then you will have to find another PM," said Shastri during the arguments. In the final agreement General Ayub Ḳhan had not mentioned those words but Shastri continued to press for it.

Ayub finally wrote it at the very last moment. General Ayub's handwritten assurance is still preserved in the Indian archives. Shastri was a slight person but with a strong mind.

SHASTRI CAN'T BE REVIVED

If the Congress wants to celebrate Shastri, it will have to re-emphasis the honesty of Shastri. He stood for the small men of India.

But the Congress has changed completely. Since Mrs Gandhi said that corruption is a world phenomenon, Congressmen are not losing sleep over it. Neither can I imagine Shastri imposing the Emergency.

All those Congressmen seen active during the Emergency are part of this government. Ambika Soni is a confidante of Sonia Gandhi, Pranab Mukherjee, Arjun Singh, Kamal Nath all were part of the establishment then.

How can these leaders bring in the values of Shastri?

The Nehru-Gandhi dynasty culture has also played a role in minimising Shastri's legacy. When Shastri was made a minister without portfolio in the Nehru's Cabinet, he was uncomfortable. Once in a huff he told me, "I shall quit and retire to Allahabad."

While cajoling him not to entertain an such idea I said, "Nehru has you in his mind."

Shastri said, "*Unke dimag main to unki putri hai. (He has his daughter in his mind as successor.)*"

As soon as Shastri died the dynasty culture returned to the Congress. Shastri's message of life was that if he could become PM anybody could because he was a common man. As the Bible says the meekest shall inherit the earth, he proved it.

In 1942 (*during the Quit India Movement*), when he was in a jail, his daughter was ill and he was released on parole. But he could not save her life because doctors had recommended costly drugs.

Shastri never made money. In 1963, on the day when he was dropped under the Kamaraj plan I went to meet him. He was sitting in his home without a light. "Why are you sitting in the dark?" I asked. He said, "From today all expenses will be borne by me." He told me as a MP and minister he didn't earn enough to save for his rainy day.

On that evening, I told him to turn a columnist to earn some money. So he wrote a column on Lala Lajpat Rai. That was the first syndicated column in India.

I syndicated it to four newspapers and collected Rs 500 from each. Quite a hefty sum!

The second column was on Nehru but before he could write more he was recalled to the Cabinet.

I don't see the revival of the values Shastri stood for. A day before his first press conference after becoming PM I asked him what will be your message tomorrow?

He said: "I'll tell them that during my tenure there will not be any increase in food price and as PM of India I would ask members of the Planning Commission to have one more column in their charts to show me how many jobs will be created after spending thousands of crores of rupees."

He was a man concerned about the common man of India. Can these values return to this country?

I don't think so.

Lal Bahadur Shastri was born in Moghalsarai, which is also spelt as Mughalsarai, on October 2, 1904. His parents were Sharada Prasad and Ramdulari Devi. Though his parents were Srivatsavas, Shastri dropped his caste identity in his early years. His father died when he was only a year old. His mother with the help of her father took care of the children. Lal Bahadur acquired virtues like boldness, love of adventure, patience, self-control, courtesy, and selflessness in his childhood.

His abandoned his studies to take part in the non-cooperation movement started by Gandhi in 1921. He was given the title 'Shastri' at Kashi Vidya Peetha in 1926. During his four years' stay there, he was very much influenced by the lectures of Dr. Bhagawandas on philosophy. In his later life, Shastri displayed poise in the midst of conflict and confusion which he learnt from his teacher, Bhagawandas.

After coming out from Kashi Vidya Peeth, he became the life-member of The Servants of the People Society which was started by Lala Lajpat Rai in 1921. The aim of the society was to train youth who were prepared to dedicate their lives to the service of the country. Shastri earned the love and affection of Lajpat Rai by his earnestness and hard work. Later he became the President of the society. In 1927, Shastri married Lalitha Devi who was from Mırzalyur.

Lal Bahadur Shastri took a leading role in 'Salt Satyagraha' which was intensified by 1930. He also advised people not to pay land revenue and taxes to the British government. He was sent to prison for two and half years for doing so. From this time onwards prison became his second home. He was sent to prison seven times and was forced to spend nine long years in various prisons on different occasions.

Going to prison became a blessing in disguise for him. He spent time reading number of books. He became familiar with the works of western philosophers, revolutionaries, and social reformers. He translated the autobiography of Madam Curie, a French scientist who discovered Radium, into Hindi. He was a ideal prisoner. The greatness of Shastri was that he maintained his self-respect even in prison.

A SELFLESS LEADER

When he was the Railway Minister, he owned moral responsibility for a train accident in south India and resigned, in 1956. He did not have a house of his own, even when he was the Home Minister and people used to tease him the "homeless Home Minister".

That was Lal Bahadur Shastri, who shares his date of birth with Mahatma Gandhi and was a staunch follower of the latter's path of truth and non-violence. In the first general elections of the Indian Republic, the Congress was returned to power with a huge majority.

Shastri, who was the general secretary of the party at that time, had complete control over the selection of partry candidates. But he did not contest the elections.

The Prime Minister, Jawaharlal Nehru, however, did not wish to leave such an able and honest man outside the government. He persuaded him to seek election to the Rajya Sabha. He won the election and was appointed the Railway Minister.

At that time there were four classes in the railways: first, second, inter and third. The first class compartments offered extreme luxury while the travails of passengers in the third class was beyond description. Shastri made relentless efforts to remove the wide disparity between the first and third class compartments. The first class, which offered royal comfort, was abolished. The old second class was converted into first class and the inter class was turned into second class. His idea was to have only two classes in course of time.

He provided greater facilities to passengers in third class compartments. It was during his time that fans were provided in third class compartments. He resigned as Railway Minister owning moral responsibility, when an accident occurred in Ariyalur in Tamil Nadu in 1956 in which 144 persons were killed. In fact, he had put in his papers when an accident had occurred in Mahboobnagar three months earlier, killing 112. But Nehru had not accepted it. He refused to continue in the post after the Ariyalur accident.

He became Home Minister after the death of Govind Ballabh Pant in 1961. He had rented a small house in Allahabad. Whenever he went to Allahabad, he used to stay in that house. After some time, the house owner had let it out to another family. When Shastri resigned as minister, he vacated the Government quarter and he did not have a place to live in.

Born at Mughalsarai in Uttar Pradesh on October 2, 1904, Lal Bahadur Shastri had spent his early childhood at his maternal uncle, Raghunath Prasad's house. His father, Sharada Prasad, died when Shastri was hardly one-and-a-half years old, leaving his mother, Ramdulari Devi, to take care of their three children. After the death of her husband, Ramdulari Devi shifted to her father's house in Mirzapur. She played a vital role in shaping Shastri's life by imbibing the right values in him.

After completing his primary education at Mirzapur, Shastri went to Benaras for further studies. He joined the Harish Chandra Vidyalaya, where he was deeply influenced by his mathematics teacher, Nishkameswar Prasad Misra, who inspired his students by telling them stories of great leaders like Guru Gobind Singh, Rana Pratap and Chhatrapati Shivaji.

He graduated from the nationalist university, Kashi Vidyapeeth, in 1925 and was given the title, 'Shastri', meaning one who is learned in the scriptures. The next year, he joined the 'Servants of the People Society' started by Lala Lajpat Rai and plunged into the freedom movement. Shastri married Lalita Devi, the youngest daughter of Ganesh Prasad, in 1928. He did not believe in the dowry system and refused to take dowry. However, on the insistence of his father-in-law he took five yards of khadi cloth as dowry.

Inspired by his political guru, Bapu Purushottamdas Tandon, Shastri joined the Congress Party. He became the City Congress secretary and the president of the Allahabad Congress Committee in 1930. He participated in all national movements between 1921 and 1942 and went to jail seven times. He was elected to the UP Legislative Assembly in 1937.

Once when Shastri was in jail, he received the news that his daughter fell ill. He requested the jailor to release him on parole to attend to his daughter. The jailor granted him 15 days parole.

On reaching home, he learnt that his daughter had died. He performed the last rites of his daughter and told his family members that he was going back to the jail. When they reminded him that he was granted 15 days parole, he said, "That was to attend to my sick daughter. But when she is no more, there is no reason for me to take leave."

He became the Prime Minister after the death of Jawaharlal Nehru. He tackled several problems like food shortage, unemployment and poverty. To overcome the acute food shortage, he initially imported food grains and distributed them throughout the country. Later, he drew long-term plans to make the country self-sufficient in food production.

He showed his mettle during the Indo-Pak war, which broke out in 1965. He made it clear to Pakistan and the world that India would not take it lying down, if Pakistan continued to encourage cross-border terrorism. He gave full freedom to the Armed Forces to retaliate and the military bases in Lahore and Sialkot were attacked.

The war had established the supremacy of India and brought Ayub Khan on to his feet. The United Nations passed a resolution demanding a ceasefire. The Russian Prime Minister, Kosygin, offered to mediate and Shastri and Ayub Khan started negotiations at Tashkent. A 'no-war' agreement was signed between the two countries on January 10, 1966, and peace was restored. Shastri suffered a fatal heart attack the same night.

He was awarded the highest civilian award, the Bharat Ratna, posthumously in 1966.A statue of this great little man has been installed in a corner at the park opposite the Municipal Corporation office.

India's second Prime Minister, he assumed office at a time of turmoil in the country. Pandit Nehru had just expired and Pakistan's hostility towards the Indians led to a war in 1965. The country was under heavy pressure due to drought and other internal problems. Quite a tough task for a new Prime Minister to handle.

But as he had been tempered by the freedom struggle and had served in Nehru's cabinet, he took it all in his stride.

CONGRESS AND NON-COOPERATION MOVEMENT.

The most significant event that unfolded in Indian politics in 1919 was the rise of Mohandas Karamchand Gandhi, known to the world as Mahatma

Gandhi. Gandhi's emergence on the Indian political scenario inaugurated the third phase of Indian Nationalism, during which the country witnessed the launch of a number of nationalist movements under his leadership. His unique political ideologies that basically represented an extension of his spiritual doctrines revolutionized Indian politics and played a major role in awakening the political consciousness of the masses. The National Movements launched under Gandhi's aegis gave expression to his celebrated political ideologies like satyagraha and ahimsa, and saw the country unifying to fight the single cause of India's independence.

The three important milestones of India's pre independence history, namely the Non-Cooperation Movement, the Civil Disobedience Movement and the Quit India Movement, were launched and gathered momentum under the leadership of Mahatma Gandhi. The first among these was the Non-Cooperation Movement. Before proceeding to an analysis of Gandhi's role in the Non-Cooperation Movement, it is pertinent to delineate the circumstances that shook Gandhi's confidence in the fairness of the British Government and transformed him into a non-co-operator.

When Gandhi returned to India in the year 1915, he did not directly enter the political scenario, following the advice of his political mentor Gopal Krishna Gokhle. However, in the period between 1917 and 18, he rendered leadership to some local disputes and thus rose to prominence. He supported the cause of the oppressed cultivators of Champaran district of Bihar, associated himself with the campaign of the peasants of the Kheda district in Gujarat and also backed the textile workers of Ahmedabad, who were fighting for their wages. During this phase, Gandhi was loyal to the colonial government and even volunteered for the recruitment of soldiers to fight on behalf of the English, during the First World War. However, the Gandhi's role as a co-operator of the British government did not last long. The Rowlatt Act, followed by the Jallianwallah Bagh massacre and the Khilafat issue embittered Gandhi's feelings towards the British government. Gandhi stance changed to that of a non-co-operator of the British government and he soon after launched the Non-Cooperation Movement. When Gandhi realized that there was no prospect of getting any fair treatment at the hands of British, he planned to withdraw the nation's co-operation from the government and thereby mar the administrative set up of the country.

In this initiative, he expected to garner the support of the Muslims, who were nurturing anti British sentiments, on the Turkey-issue. Gandhi's main objective was to procure justice for the Muslims, through his method of passive resistance; satyagraha.

In August, 1920, a hartal was organized in the entire country. The formal launch of the Non-Cooperation Movement in the August of 1920 followed the expiry of the notice that was sent to the Viceroy by Gandhi. He returned to the Viceroy, all the medals he had received in recognition of his war services from the British government.

Gandhi urged the Congress to launch a Non-Cooperation Movement on three issues, which were; redressal of the wrongs committed in Punjab that entailed the Jallianwala Bagh massacre and the atrocities related to the marital laws, the Khilafat wrong and accomplishment of swaraj. In September, 1920, a special session of the Congress, presided by Lala Lajpat Rai was convened at Calcutta that sought to approve the scheme.

Several legislations were passed by the delegates, wherein the British government was criticized and condemned for its incapability of protecting innocent lives in Punjab and failing to keep its promise in the Khilafat issue. In one of the resolutions, it was declared by the Congress that the people of India had no other option but to approve and endorse the non violent, non-cooperation policy inaugurated by Gandhi, till the wrongs were rectified and swaraj established. The Non-Cooperation resolution garnered mixed responses. Pt. Motilal Nahru and Anil Ali Brothers supported the resolution, whereas Mrs Annie Besant, Pt. Malaviya and Shri C. R Das vehemently opposed. They feared that large scale mass action against the British government would lead to violence on a wide scale, as occurred during Rowlatt satyagraha.

In December 1920, at the Nagpur Congress, the resolution on Non-Cooperation was repeated again. This session garnered greater support in favour of the resolution. The Congress redefined the resolution as the procurement of Swaraj by the use of peaceful and legitimate means. According to Gandhi, swaraj meant establishment of self rule within British Empire with complete freedom to secede any time. The program and policies of the Non-Cooperation Movement that was adopted at the special session of the Congress in Calcutta and restated at the Nagpur session included; promotion of swadeshi and boycott of foreign made articles, surrender of honorary posts and titles, rejection of official Durbars, progressive rejection by lawyers of British courts, boycott of elections appointing new Councils, refusal by clerks and soldiers to serve in Mesopotamia and boycott of Government run and state assisted schools.

Gandhi played an active role in propagating the policies and programs of the Non-Cooperation Movement throughout the country. He along with other loyalists toured around the country in a bid to gather public support and mobilize the masses in favour of the movement. Following the persuasion of Gandhi to withdraw from state institutions and join national schools, several students left their schools. This period also witnessed the coming into being of numerous national educational institutions for the benefit of the students. Noteworthy among them were Jamia Milia University, Aligarh University and National College, Lahore. In contradiction to the approach of non violence championed by Mahatma Gandhi, the Non-Cooperation Movement sparked off an incident of mob violence in Chauri Chaura in the United Provinces. A few police constables were killed, following an attack of a police outpost on February 5th, 1922. Disillusioned by this incident, Gandhi called for the suspension of the movement in 1922. This sudden suspension of the movement was not welcomed by the radical section of the Congress, like Jawaharlal Nehru and Subhas Chandra Bose. Against the background of widespread dissatisfaction that was generated by Gandhi's decision to withdraw the movement, Motilal Nehru and Chitta Ranjan Das formed the Swaraj Party. The motif of the Swaraj Party was to enter the Council and then destroying the constitution from inside. Although, Gandhi initially opposed the policy of the Swaraj Party, he later gave the Congressmen the choice to affiliate or not with the British institutions.

It can be said without any doubt that The Non Cooperation Movement and the role played by Gandhi in it took the Indian freedom movement to new heights. It ushered in a new political fervour among the people and taught the Indians fearlessness. Under the leadership of Mahatma Gandhi, Swarajya found popular expression and a patriotic zeal gripped the entire nation. The weapon of passive resistance or satyagraha, that Gandhi gave to the nation, emerged as the greatest asset of the Indians. An important program of The Non-Cooperation Movement was the promotion of khadi. Under the guidance of Gandhi, charkha and Indian handloom products gained back their glory. Many weavers were employed. The contribution of Gandhi to this movement and eventually to Indian Nationalism was that for the very first time he coasted the entire country bound by a single ethos. The freedom struggle assumed an all India character under his impeccable leadership.

The beginning of the non-cooperation movement was marked with the withdrawal of the native members from the councils and the boycott of law courts and schools, established by the British colonizers. Congress embraced this program of non-cooperation at a special session conducted on August 20,1920. Mohandas Karamchand Gandhi inspired the Indian womanhood with the mantra of "Swadeshi" and religion of Satyagraha i.e. nonviolent resistance. Sarojini Naidu, the outstanding female leader, guided politically inclined female minds to the formation of a political body.

Meanwhile, Rashtriya Stree Sangha (RSS), an independent women's organization, asked its members to merge with the District Congress Committee. Urmila Devi, the widowed sister of the eminent lawyer and Congress nationalist, C.R.Das emerged to be a potential mass puller. She invited woman's participation in mainstream politics. By November, 1,000 women in the Presidency of Bombay were protesting against the Prince of Wales' visit to India.

In Bengal, C. R. Das advocated the selling of khaddar (homespun cloth). The female members of his family, his wife, Basanti Devi, his sister, Urmila Devi, and his niece, Miss Suniti Devi, came down to the streets exhibit their resentment. History reports, the activities of the women from the Das family, "They resumed picketing cloth shops and selling khaddar joined by numerous lady volunteers, especially Sikh ladies." The three respectable women underwent arrest on December 8, 1921. The news of their arrest set the city on huge protest. A tumultuous crowd of "Marwaris, Muslims, Bhattias, Sikhs, coolies, mill-hands and school boys" It was surprising to find that on that very day, 170 protesters were arrested.

Gandhi, the venerated Bapu or Father of the nation welcomed this phenomenal arrival of women into politics. His article, published in Young India, communicated his wish to make the entire breed of Indian women proceed along the lines of the progressive Bengali women. 6,000 women crowded at the All-Indian Ladies Conference in Ahmedabad, presided over by Bi Amma, the mother of Shaukat Ali and Muhammad Ali, leaders of the All-India Khilafat Committee. Bi Amma persuasively insisted women to serve as Congress activists and, help the arrested male volunteers through picketing and flag raising.

Madras had her women catered to the ideology of Gandhi. In East Godavari District, Smt. Duwuri Subbamam, tried her best to create a group of the socially marginal devasevikas (god-devoted female servants). Again, Durgabai, a twelve year old enthusiast, utilized, the opportunity of Gandhi's trip to the Kakinada in East Godavari District, during April of 1921. She motivated the Devdasis to collect a fund of Rs. 5,000 for Gandhi's enterprise. Gandhi met this band of budding women nationalists and had his speeches interpreted to them, through the interpreter, Durgabai. Women donated even jewelry to the nationalist cause.

The so-called social outcasts, the public woman, i.e. prostitutes lent their support to the nationalist campaign. Manada Devi Mukhopadhyay describes in Sikshita Patitat Atmarcharit ("Autobiography of an Educated Fallen Woman,"

1929), endeavour of the Bengali prostitutes to raise money for Congress in 1922 and in 1924. They also joined C. R. Das` satyagraha movement. These women gathered the courage to fight against the vicious corruption of the Mahant of Tarakeshwar Temple.

Saraladevi Chaudhurani, Muthulakshmi Reddy, Amrit Kaur, voiced the feminist's demands for franchise. Gandhi's glorification of the Indian heritage of womanhood, added a lot of impetus to the females contact with patriotic spirit. He exhibited to the Indian women, the golden examples of ideal womanhood, illustrated by the idealized figures of Sita, Draupadi, and Damayanti. Sita, remained committed to Ram, her husband's will till the last breath in her, in the epic, Ramayana. Damayanti, was able to identify her husband, Nala, in any disguise. And, Draupadi, endured the extremes of suffering, on the behalf of her husbands, the Pandavas, in Mahabharata. Gandhi, traversed through the entire country, convincing women about the potentials inherent in them. Women's rise to prominence over the tide of nationalism became the order of the day, during the non-cooperation movement. Swarup Rani, Motilal's wife, and Neheru's mother, Rajkumari Amrit Kaur, Mrs. Vijay lakshmi Pandit, began to establish their sway since, the Non-cooperation Movement.

THE SWARAJIST STRATEGY

The return of elite politics to its old constitutional track was both a consequence and a cause of the underclass retreat. As the promise of *swaraj* faded and as it became clear that the Surtis were gradually dissociating themselves from noncooperation, many of the Congress leaders began to reconsider their political options. Often they felt the need to resume bargaining with their rulers too compelling to continue their efforts to undermine the institutions of local self-government. And as they reentered the politics of legislative councils and municipalities, they often pursued their claims to justice through the idiom of public politics, reproducing conventional civic discourse through their political practice. They now became only representatives of the people, losing their identities as *chelas* and *sannyasis.* Abandoning the hard line of noncooperation in turn indicated clearly to the larger population that the achievement of some alternative to the colonial order was unlikely in the near future and that continued participation in the most conspicuous forms of nationalist resistance would probably not bear much more fruit.

The emergence of the Swarajya party during early 1923 opened the first cracks in the Gandhian strategy of noncooperation. Led in the Bombay

Presidency by Vithalbhai Patel and M. R. Jayakar, the Swarajists proposed entering the reformed legislative council to pursue a policy of obstructing government from within. When Patel visited Surat from Bombay in early May to solicit support for his party, a number of local politicians, including some who had been the staunchest supporters of noncooperation only two years earlier, quickly jumped on board. Surat suddenly became the centre of Swarajist activity in Gujarat. Dr. Dixit, Dr. Mehta, and Maganlal Vidyarthi, all local noncooperators with sufficient education and professional training to make the shift to a politics based upon the idiom of constitutionalism and progress, assumed important positions in the Gujarat Provincial Swarajya party. All three planned campaigns to run for provincial office. Opposition to the Swarajya program came largely from activists who had been arrested and their supporters. In Surat, however, this opposition was muted owing to the intervention of Dayalji Desai, now president of the District Congress Committee. Fearing the potential for a major rupture between local nationalists, Dayalji attempted to cultivate mutual respect among the two factions. With his encouragement, "NoChangers" and Swarajists both appeared in the same public meetings to present their views on entry into the councils while confirming their shared commitment to Gandhi's constructive program, to agitation against the local municipality, and to the national schools. Dayalji even encouraged Vithalbhai Patel to address Surat's citizens from a Congress platform just before the elections.

In recent years, historians have tended to view the willingness of Congress politicians to back the Swarajya party after 1923 as evidence of a materialistic concern with gaining access to networks of patronage controlled by the provincial legislatures. Evidence from Surat certainly indicates that an interest in personal political influence was important, but it also suggests that scholars might need to probe further into the question of why this influence was sought. In Surat local Gandhians of all stripes were genuinely flustered by the ability of Liberal politicians to frustrate the Congress cause. Many felt that Chunilal Gandhi, the city's representative in the Bombay council, was partly responsible for the suspension of the noncooperating municipality, the appointment of the Committee of Management, and a variety of other government efforts to suppress the cause of *swaraj*. As long as persons with little commitment to the Congress program remained in control of the legislatures, they reasoned, government could easily thwart their activities. In entering the Bombay legislature, Dixit, Mehta, and Vidyarthi sought not only to paralyze the colonial government of the province but also to restore the municipality to Congress hands. By gaining control of the council, they believed that they could reinvigorate such efforts essential to attaining independence as nationalizing local schools. They by no means wished to abandon other aspects of the Congress constructive program such as the promotion of *khadi* and of Hindu-Muslim unity.

But once they decided to reenter legislative politics, the Swarajists found themselves compelled to adhere to political conventions quite different from those that had governed noncooperation. They defended their actions largely in terms of the principles of public discourse, in part because these principles allowed them best to dismiss the claims of their opponents. In the election campaign of September and October 1923, none of the Swarajya party's candidates used Gandhian rhetoric extensively. Each stressed the violations of citizen rights that had occurred under their opposition's tenure of office. According to their arguments, a coterie of Liberals such as Chunilal Gandhi, voted in by tiny minorities of the population during the boycotted elections of 1920, had frustrated the true will of the people. M. M. Mehta, running for Surat's single urban seat, contended that as a result of moderate cooperation with the British in the legislative councils, "the whole country has had to accept increases in the salt tax; citizens in the municipalities of Surat, Ahmedabad and Nadiad have had their rights of self-government taken from them; the birthright of mothers and fathers to educate their children as they wish has been trampled upon; reputable householders have been prosecuted and fined under the compulsory education law; and national schools have been locked up under various government schemes."

"It is a duty of the representatives of the people," he insisted, "... to attempt to prevent such disastrous developments," thus criticizing the moderates for failing to perform their responsibilities as legislators while claiming that he, if elected, would certainly fulfill his obligations to his voters. Dixit, running in the rural constituency of South Gujarat, promised in his speeches that the Swarajists would try to regain popular control over municipalities, to free Mahatma Gandhi and other political prisoners from jail, and to fight for independence and other political rights. For the most part, the rhetoric of both candidates was devoid of the religious allusions they had employed just a year or so earlier. The language of representative government was clearly beginning to reestablish its preeminence in the civic arena.

Such appeals, however, were by themselves hardly sufficient to ensure election Vietories. After all, the public meetings of the Swarajist candidates, often attended by no more than fifty people, could not hope to reach the entire urban electorate of Surat, now more than seven thousand voters, or the even larger rural constituency. To a great extent the election of 1923 relied on techniques that had often been used in the campaigns of prewar Surat but that had been abandoned during the noncooperation years. Candidates again secured the support of agents—that is, men of local influence—to canvass neighborhoods of the city and persuade voters to attend the polls. On the day of the election, these agents intensified their personal methods of contacting citizens. With a number of private motor cars and carriages at their disposal, the Swarajists ferried many voters to the polling station at the city castle individually. The district magistrate's remarks that there had been "a great deal of improper influence used in the town," while obviously reflecting a heavy bias against the Congress, confirmed the existence of a second, more personal, idiom of politics operating alongside and supplementing civic discourse, one that the Swarajists used more effectively than the Liberals. During the next provincial campaign, in 1926, the *Gujarat Mitra* would remark that these electoral practices had become so engrained that even "a voter only a hundred yards away from the polling station... expects a car to be near his door before he thinks of leaving his place for the purpose of voting." English-educated politicians of every party tended to agree that these methods were necessitated by an electorate "ignorant of the value of the vote" which required further "training" in the proper exercise of democratic government. No doubt the inaccessibility of constitutional rhetoric for the local population inhibited plebeian participation in the exercise of public power. But no one gave voice to the possibility that the language of liberal representative politics could be as responsible for that as any deficiency in the political education of the Surtis.

As a result of their effective use of this bilingual campaign, the Swarajists won a resounding success in the 1923 election. In Surat City, Dr. Mehta won easily, with 2,433 votes to Chunilal Gandhi's 407 and Jamshedji Antia's 302. Dr. Dixit won one of the two rural seats. Vidyarthi finished far down in the polling, but H. B. Shivdasani, a former assistant collector who had recently resigned his post and who had won the tacit backing of Dayaiji when he signed up as a Congress member, was the leading vote getter in the countryside. Shivdasani immediately became one of the most vocal and effective members of the Bombay Swarajists in the legislature. Even the old home ruler Kanaiyalal Desai, who finished third in the rural voting, signed the Congress pledge just before the election.

Once in the councils, Mehta, Dixit, and Shivdasani found themselves bound by severe constraints, some of which they had never anticipated. Within the Bombay council, colonial authority was still strong. Under the system of dyarchy that had been created by the Montagu Chelmsford reforms of 1919, wide areas of policy were entirely excluded from discussion by the elected legislators. But even in those spheres of policy designated as appropriately within the council's domain, government and its Indian allies retained considerable informal influence. Owing to unevenness in support for the Swarajists elsewhere in the Bombay Presidency and to the abundance of separate electorates and reserved seats for Muslims, non-Brahmans, and a variety of special interests, the nationalists captured only a minority of the positions on the council. Only persons with "loyal" inclinations—including one Britisher and two Muslims—were selected as ministers. Of course, Dixit, Mehta, and Shivdasani could have chosen—as the all-India program of their party suggested—to resign from the council, but this would again leave them with no influence in such matters as the restoration of Surat Municipality. On issues that concerned them most, their best option seemed to lie in alliance with Bombay Independents and, on occasion, the Moderates. Any partnership in the council, however, required at the very least a relatively civil demeanor, that is, a renewed adherence to the conventions and idiom of parliamentary politics. In the end, to paraphrase David Arnold's work on Madras politics, it was not the Swarajists who captured the legislature but the legislature which captured the Swarajists.

Members of the new party continued to espouse the ideal of obstruction in principle. Dixit and particularly Shivdasani pestered the governor's ministers with endless questions, which usually had to be sent off to the departments of government for answers; they made long tirades on the budget and on other issues that came before the legislature, whether or not these issues genuinely engaged their interest. And, for a brief period in 1926, they joined the other Swarajists in boycotting the council. But when matters they considered to be vital arose, such as municipal affairs, they made sure their voices were heard. In March 1924, only a few months after the council began its sessions, Dixit petitioned Gulam Hussein Hidayatullah, the minister of local selfgovernment, to allow new municipal elections in Surat and to bring the Committee of Management's administration to an end. In July he fought a municipal bill giving government the power to dissolve municipalities and call new elections in addition to the powers of supercession it already possessed. In both cases, he reminded government of its own avowed commitments to the devolution of power. In the July debates, for instance, he argued: "We are now working the new reforms; the ultimate aim of the British government is to give self-government to India, and if you go on adding further powers to the power already possessed by government in dealing with the municipalities which they consider as defaulting, I do not think it will be consistent in spirit so far as the present reforms are concerned."

This sort of constitutional argument was obviously a major departure from the rhetoric noncooperators had used three years earlier when they had claimed that it was a sinful or *adharmik* act to participate in the legislature and that boycott of the councils embodied the Hindu ideal of renunciation and self-sacrifice.

But now the Congress leaders were addressing a different audience and with different purposes. The need to influence provincial ministers and to win the support of Independents and Moderates required use of an idiom more at home in the halls of the legislature than on the streets of Surat. Ironically, representation of the people now involved using symbolic skills that uneducated citizens could not hope to master: knowledge of legislative rituals and procedures, familiarity with parliamentary traditions, the ability to speak and think quickly in English and to manipulate legal rules and statistics in debate.

In following the conventions of public debate, even for the purpose of contesting colonial policy, the Swarajists in essence conceded that the major issues of provincial politics were going to be fought on the terrain of constitutional and devolutionary principle. At a more implicit level, they agreed to strive for the same kind of polity that their British overlords were now themselves attempting to forge: a liberal, representative order that would pursue the objective of political and economic progress.

POST-INDEPENDENCE CONGRESS

After Indian independence in 1947, the Congress became the dominant political party in the country. In the first general election in 1952 held after Independence, the party swept to power at the centre as well as in most state legislatures. The Congress was continuously in power until 1977, when it was defeated by the Janata Party. It returned to power in 1980 and ruled until 1989, when it was once again defeated. It formed the government in 1991 at the head of a coalition, as well as in 2004 and 2009, when it led the United Progressive Alliance. During this period it has remained centre-left in its social policies, while steadily shifting from a socialist to a neoliberal economic outlook.

1947-66

From 1951 until his death in 1964, Jawaharlal Nehru, the paramount leader of the Indian independence movement under the tutelage of Mahatma Gandhi dominated the Congress Party, which won overwhelming victories in the elections of 1951–52, 1957, and 1962. During his tenure, Nehru implemented policies based on import substitution industrialisationand advocated a mixed economy where the government controlled public sector would co-exist with the private sector.

He believed that the establishment of basic and heavy industry was fundamental to the development and modernisation of the Indian economy. The Nehru government therefore directed investment primarily into key public sector industries – steel, iron, coal, and power – promoting their development with subsidies and protectionist policies. Nehru embraced secularism, socialistic economic practices based on state driven industrialization, and a non-aligned and non-confrontational foreign policy, which became the hallmark of the modern Congress party. The policy of non-alignment during the Cold War meant that Nehru received financial and technical support from both power blocs in building India's industrial base from scratch. There were four known assassination attempts on Nehru. The first attempt on his life was during partition in 1947 while he was visiting North-West Frontier Province (now Khyber Pakhtunkhwa in Pakistan) in a car. The second one was by a knife-wielding rickshaw-puller in Maharashtra in 1955. The third one happened in Bombay (now in Maharashtra) in 1956. The fourth one was a failed bombing attempt on train tracks in Maharashtra in 1961. Despite threats to his life, Nehru despised having too much security around him and did not like to disrupt traffic due to his movement. In 1964, Nehru died due to an aortic dissection and signalled the first time the party's future came into question.

In 1964 after Nehru's death, K. Kamaraj became the president of the All India Congress Committee. Kamalraj was also involved in the Indian independence movement and remembered for bringing school education to millions of the rural poor by introducing free education and the free Midday Meal Scheme during his tenure as chief minister of Tamil Nadu during 1954–63. Being part of a group of leaders in the Congress known as "the syndicate", he proposed the Kamaraj Plan (six Congress chief ministers and six senior Cabinet ministers to resign to take up party work). Kamaraj was widely credited as the "kingmaker" in Indian politics for bringing Lal Bahadur Shastri to power in 1964. As no other leader had Nehru's popular appeal, other than the gentle, soft-spoken and Nehruvian Lal Bahadur Shastri. Kamaraj stepped down as AICC president in 1967. Shastri as Prime Minister continued Nehru's policies of non-alignment and socialism. He became a national hero following the victory in the Indo-Pakistan War of 1965. His slogan of *Jai Jawan Jai Kisan* (*Hail the soldier, Hail the farmer*) became very popular during the war. Shastri retained many members of Nehru's Council of Ministers. T. T. Krishnamachari was retained as the Finance Minister of India, as was Defence

Minister Yashwantrao Chavan. He appointed Swaran Singh to succeed him as External Affairs Minister.

Shashtri appointed Indira Gandhi, daughter of Jawaharlal Nehru and former Congress President, as the Minister of Information and Broadcasting. Gulzarilal Nanda continued as the Minister of Home Affairs. Shashtri continued Nehru's policy of non-alignment but also built closer relations with the Soviet Union. In the aftermath of the Sino-Indian War of 1962 and the formation of military ties between the Chinese People's Republic and Pakistan, Shastri's government decided to expand the defence budget of India's armed forces. He also promoted the White Revolution – a national campaign to increase the production and supply of milk by creating National Dairy Development Board. Shastri's tenure witnessed the Madras anti-Hindi agitation of 1965. On 11 January 1966, Prime Minister Shastri died in Tashkent, the day after signing the Tashkent Declaration, reportedly due to a heart attack but circumstances of his death still remain a mystery.

1966-84

In 1966, after Shastri's death, the Congress party elected, Nehru's daughter, Indira Gandhi, over the Morarji Desai as their leader. Once again, Kamaraj was instrumental in achieving this result. In 1967, following a poor showing in the general election, Indira Gandhi started progressively moving to the left in the political spectrum. In 1969, after falling out with senior party leaders on a number of issues, the party president S. Nijalingappa expelled Indira Gandhi from the party. Gandhi, in turn floated her own faction of the Congress party and managed to retain most of the Congress MPs on her side with only 65 on the side of Congress (O). In the mid-term parliamentary elections held in 1971, the Gandhi-led Congress (R) Party scored a landslide victory on a platform of progressive policies such as poverty elimination (Garibi Hatao). The progressive policies of the Congress under Indira Gandhi, prior to the 1971 elections, also included proposals for the abolition of Privy Purse to former rulers of the Princely states and the 1969 nationalization of the fourteen largest banks in India.

In the mid-1970s, the New Congress Party's popular support began to fracture. From 1975, Gandhi's government grew increasingly more authoritarian, and unrest among the opposition grew. On 12 June 1975, the High Court of Allahabad declared Indira Gandhi's election to the Lok Sabha void on grounds of electoral malpractice. However, Gandhi rejected calls to resign and announced plans to appeal to theSupreme Court. Gandhi moved to restore order by ordering the arrest of most of the opposition participating in the unrest. Her cabinet and government then recommended that President Fakhruddin Ali Ahmed declare a state of emergency, because of the disorder and lawlessness. Accordingly, Ahmed declared a State of Emergency caused by internal disorder, based on the provisions of Article 352 of the Constitution, on 25 June 1975. The 19 months of the Emergency saw widespread oppression and abuse of power by Gandhi's unelected younger son, Sanjay Gandhi and his close associates., This period of oppression ended when on 23 January 1977, Gandhi called fresh elections to the Lok Sabha for March and released all political prisoners.

The Emergency officially ended on 23 March 1977. In the parliamentary elections held in March 1977, the opposition Janata Party scored a landslide victory over the Congress Party, winning 295 seats in the Lok Sabha (the lower house of India's parliament) against 153 for the Congress; Gandhi herself lost to her Janata opponent, Raj Narain. On January 2, 1978, she and her followers seceded and formed a new opposition party, popularly called Congress (I)—the *I* signifying Indira. Over the next year, her new party attracted enough members of the legislature to become the official opposition.

In November 1978, Gandhi regained a parliamentary seat, and in January 1980, following a landslide victory for the Congress (I), she was once again elected prime minister. In 1981, the national election commission declared Congress (I) the real Indian National Congress.

In 1996, the *I* designation was dropped. In her new term as Prime minister, Gandhi faced the personal loss of the death of her younger son and political heir, Sanjay Gandhi, in a plane crash in June 1980. This led her to induct her elder pilot son, Rajiv Gandhi to enter politics.

Gradually, Indira Gandhi grew moreauthoritarian and autocratic in her policies and outlook and became the central figure of the Indian National Congress party. As Prime Minister, Gandhi became known for her political ruthlessness and unprecedented centralisation of power. Gandhi's term as Prime Minister also witnessed increasing turmoil in Punjab with demands for Sikh autonomy by Jarnail Singh Bhindranwale and his militant followers.

In 1983, they headquartered themselves in the Golden Temple and started accumulating weapons. After several futile negotiations, Gandhi, in June 1984, ordered the Indian army to enter the Golden Temple in order to establish control over the temple complex in Amritsar, Punjab and remove Jarnail Singh Bhindranwale and his armed followers from the complex buildings. This event was known as Operation Blue Star. On 31 October 1984, two of Gandhi's bodyguards, Satwant Singh and Beant Singh, shot her with their service weapons in the garden of the Prime Minister's residence, in response to her actions in authorising Operation Blue Star. The shooting occurred as she was walking past a wicket gate guarded by Satwant and Beant. She was to have been interviewed by the British actor Peter Ustinov, who was filming a documentary for Irish television. Beant Singh shot her three times using his side-arm, and Satwant Singh fired 30 rounds. Later, the 1984 anti-Sikh riots took place over the assassination of Indira Gandhi where more than 3000 people were killed.

In 1984, Indira Gandhi's son, Rajiv Gandhi became nominal head of the party and, upon her assassination in October 1984, he became prime minister. In December, he led the Congress Party to a landslide victory in which it secured 401 seats in the legislature. His administration took vigorous measures to reform the government bureaucracy and liberalise the country's economy.

Gandhi's attempts to discourage separatist movements in Punjab and Kashmir backfired, however, and after his government became embroiled in several financial scandals, his leadership became increasingly ineffectual. Gandhi was regarded as a nonabrasive person who consulted other party members and refrained from hasty decisions. The Bofors scandal shattered his image as an honest politician; however he was posthumously cleared over this allegation in 2004. On 21 May 1991, Gandhi was killed by a bomb concealed in a basket of flowers carried by a woman associated with the Tamil Tigers.

He was campaigning in Tamil Nadu for upcoming parliamentary elections. In 1998, an Indian court convicted twenty six people in the conspiracy to assassinate Gandhi. The conspirators, who consisted of Tamil militants from Sri Lanka and their Indian allies, had sought revenge against Gandhi because the Indian troops he sent to Sri Lanka in 1987 to help enforcea peace accord there had ended up fighting the Tamil separatist guerrillas.

Rajiv Gandhi was succeeded as party leader by P.V. Narasimha Rao, who was elected prime minister in June 1991. His ascendancy to the prime ministership was politically significant in that he was the first holder of this office from South India.

He led an important administration, overseeing a major economic transformation and several home incidents affecting national security of India. Rao who held the Industries portfolio was personally responsible for the dismantling of the Licence Raj as this came under the purview of the Ministry of Commerce and Industry. He is often referred to as the *"Father of Indian Economic Reforms"*. Future prime ministers Atal Bihari Vajpayee and Manmohan

Singh continued the economic reform policies pioneered by Rao's government. Rao accelerated the dismantling of the Licence Raj, reversing thesocialist policies of the previous governments. He employed future prime minister, Manmohan Singh as his | Finance Minister to embark on a historic economic transition.

With Rao's mandate, Singh launched India's globalisation angle of the reforms that involved implementing the International Monetary Fund (IMF) policies to rescue the almost bankrupt nation from economic collapse. Rao was also referred to as *Chanakya* for his ability to steer tough economic and political legislation through the parliament at a time when he headed a minority government. By 1996, however, the party's image was suffering from various allegations of corruption, and in elections that year the Congress Party was reduced to 140 seats, its lowest number in the Lok Sabha to that point, becoming parliament's second largest party. Rao subsequently resigned as prime minister and, in September, as party president. He was succeeded as president by Sitaram Kesri, the party's first non-Brahmin leader.

CONGRESS AND CONGRESSISM IN INDIAN POLITICS

The Congress has, by any standards, remarkable political accomplishments to its credit. As the Indian National Congress, its guidance fashioned a nation out of an extraordinarily heterogeneous ensemble of peoples. The party has played an important role in establishing the foundations of perhaps the most durable democratic political system in the developing world. As scholars Francis Robinson and Paul R. Brass point out, the Congress constituted one of the few political organizations in the annals of decolonialization to "make the transition from being sole representative of the nationalist cause to being just one element of a competitive party system." The Congress dominated Indian politics from independence until 1967.

Prior to 1967, the Congress had never won less than 73 percent of the seats in Parliament. The party won every state government election except two—most often exclusively, but also through coalitions—and until 1967 it never won less than 60 percent of all elections for seats in the state legislative assemblies. There were four factors that accounted for this dominance. First, the party acquired a tremendous amount of good will and political capital from its leadership of the nationalist struggle. Party chiefs gained substantial popular respect for the years in jail and other deprivations that they personally endured. The shared experience of the independence struggle fostered a sense of cohesion, which was important in maintaining unity in the face of the party's internal pluralism.

The second factor was that the Congress was the only party with an organization extending across the nation and down to the village level. The party's federal structure was based on a system of internal democracy that functioned to resolve disputes among its members and maintain party cohesion. Internal party elections also served to legitimate the party leadership, train party workers in the skills of political competition, and create channels of upward mobility that rewarded its most capable members.

A third factor was that the Congress achieved its position of political dominance by creating an organization that adjusted to local circumstances rather than transformed them, often reaching the village through local "big men" (*bare admi*) who controlled village "vote banks."

These local elites, who owed their position to their traditional social status and their control over land, formed factions that competed for power within the Congress. The internal party democracy and the Congress's subsequent electoral success ultimately reinforced the local power of these traditional elites and enabled the party to adjust to changes in local balances of power. The nonideological pragmatism of local party leadership made it possible to coopt issues that contributed to opposition party success and even incorporate successful opposition leaders into the party. Intraparty competition served to channel information about local circumstances up the party hierarchy.

Fourth, patronage was the oil that lubricated the party machine. As the state expanded its development role, it accumulated more resources that could be distributed to party members. The growing pool of opportunities and resources facilitated the party's ability to accommodate conflict among its members. The Congress enjoyed the benefits of a "virtuous cycle," in which its electoral success gave it access to economic and political resources that enabled the party to attract new supporters. The halcyon days of what Indian political scientist Rajni Kothari has called "the Congress system" ended with the general elections in 1967. The party lost seventy-eight seats in the Lok Sabha, retaining a majority of only twenty-three seats. Even more indicative of the Congress setback was its loss of control over six of the sixteen state legislatures that held elections.

The proximate causes of the reversal included the failure of the monsoons in 1965 and 1966 and the subsequent hardship throughout northern and eastern India, and the unpopular currency devaluation in 1966. However, profound changes in India's polity also contributed to the decline of the Congress. The rapid growth of the electorate, which increased by 45 percent from 1952 to 1967, brought an influx of new voters less appreciative of the Congress's role in the independence movement. Moreover, the simultaneous spread of democratic values produced a political awakening that mobilized new groups and created a more pluralistic constellation of political interests. The development of new and more-differentiated identities and patterns of political cleavage made it virtually impossible for the Congress to contain the competition of its members within its organization. Dissidence and ultimately defection greatly weakened the Congress's electoral performance.

It was in this context that Indira Gandhi asserted her independence from the leaders of the party organization by attempting to take the party in a more populist direction. She ordered the nationalization of India's fourteen largest banks in 1969, and then she supported former labour leader and Acting President Varahagiri Venkata Giri's candidacy for president despite the fact that the party organization had already nominated the more conservative Neelam Sanjiva Reddy. After Giri's election, the party organization expelled Indira Gandhi from the Congress and ordered the parliamentary party to choose a new prime minister. Instead, 226 of the 291 Congress members of Parliament continued to support Indira Gandhi. The Congress split into two in 1969, the new factions being the Congress (O)—for Organisation—and Mrs. Gandhi's Congress (R)—for Requisition. The Congress (R) continued in power with the support of non-Congress groups, principally the Communist Party of India (CPI) and the Dravida Munnetra Kazhagam (DMK—Dravidian Progressive Federation). With the Congress (O) controlling most of the party organization, Indira Gandhi adopted a new strategy to mobilize popular support.

For the first time ever, she ordered parliamentary elections to be held separately from elections for the state government. This delinking was designed to reduce the power of the Congress (O)'s state-level political machines in national elections. Mrs. Gandhi travelled throughout the country, energetically campaigning on the slogan "*garibi hatao*" (eliminate poverty), thereby bypassing the traditional Congress networks of political support. The strategy proved successful, and the Congress (R) won a dramatic Vietory. In the 1971 elections for the Lok Sabha, the Congress (R) garnered 44 percent of the vote, earning it 352 seats. The Congress (O) won only sixteen seats and 10 percent of the vote. The next year, after leading India to Vietory over Pakistan in the war for Bangladesh's independence, Indira Gandhi and the Congress (R) further consolidated their control over the country by winning fourteen of sixteen state assembly elections and Vietories in 70 percent of all seats contested.

The public expected Indira Gandhi to deliver on her mandate to remove poverty. However, the country experienced a severe drought in 1971 and 1972, leading to food shortages, and the price of food rose 20 percent in the spring of 1973. The decision by the Organization of the Petroleum Exporting Countries (OPEC) to quadruple oil prices in 1973-74 also led to inflation and increased unemployment. Jayaprakash (J.P) Narayan, a socialist leader in the preindependence Indian National Congress who, after 1947, left to conduct social work in the Sarvodaya movement (*sarvodaya* means uplift of all), came out of retirement to lead what eventually became widely known as the "J.P. movement."

Under Narayan's leadership, the movement toppled the government of Gujarat and almost brought down the government in Bihar; Narayan advocated a radical regeneration of public morality that he labelled "total revolution."

THE DEATH OF A PRIME MINISTER

Mystery surrounds the fate of not only Subhas Chandra Bose, but also the death of former Prime Minister Lal Bahadur Shastri.

Diplomat's Diary

India is one rare country where mysteries continue to shroud the deaths of top political leaders. In a way, it is not surprising that a definite conclusion is still eluding the Netaji disappearance controversy. Subhas Chandra Bose's disappearance occurred at the end of second world war when India was under the British rule. Subhas had engaged himself with the Japanese and later in August 1945 he had escaped to the Soviet Union. So, the mystery about his disappearance is understandable — because the sources of information available at that time, and thereafter in the Soviet Union, were few and far between.

But the controversy about the death of Prime Minister Lal Bahadur Shastri in Tashkent (now in Uzbekistan) is in a different league altogether. Mystery surrounds Shastri's death due to several reasons — foremost being the absence of a proper medical report stating the cause of death. It is all the more puzzling because Shastri's personal physician had accompanied him to Tashkent, then in the USSR. But he did not ensure a proper medical investigation. It is rumoured that he was drunk at that time. Though a post-mortem report was given by the Soviet authorities at Tashkent, nothing was done in India to determine the exact cause of the Prime Minister's death despite tell-tale signs of poisoning.

It was very baffling indeed why such indifference was shown when three Cabinet Ministers — Jagjivan Ram, Y.B. Chavan and Swarn Singh — were present in January 1966 at Tashkent, where Shastri breathed his last.

According to the Soviet sources, a glass of milk was bought for Shastri by personal servant of Indian Ambassador T.N. Kaul. This personal servant, Jan Mohammad, was never questioned or interrogated by any one in the Soviet Union or in India despite his being the prime suspect. This is indeed mystifying, because just after consuming milk Shastri complained of "pain in the chest" and "difficulty in breathing." Thereafter the Prime Minister slipped into coma. The Soviet doctors were called in and they pronounced him dead.

At present, it appears that no headway can be made in inquiring into the death of Lal Bahadur Shastri. Nonetheless the incident warrants a through inquiry so that adequate measures can be taken to safeguard the Prime Minister during his/her visits abroad.

Lal Bahadur Shastri was born in Moghalsarai, on October 2, 1904. His parents were Sharada Prasad and Ramdulari Devi. His father died when he was only a year old. His mother with the help of her father took care of the children.

His abandoned his studies to take part in the non-cooperation movement started by Gandhi in 1921. He was given the title 'Shastri' at Kashi Vidya Peetha in 1926. During his four years' stay there, he was very much influenced by the lectures of Dr. Bhagawandas on philosophy. After coming out from Kashi Vidya Peeth, he became the life-member of The Servants of the People Society which was started by Lala Lajpat Rai in 1921. The aim of the society was to train youth who were prepared to dedicate their lives to the service of the country. He became the President of the society. In 1927, Shastri married Lalitha Devi who was from Mirzalyur.

Lal Bahadur Shastri took a leading role in 'Salt Satyagraha' which was intensified by 1930. He also advised people not to pay land revenue and taxes to the British government. He was sent to prison for two and half years for doing so. He was sent to prison seven times and was forced to spend nine long years in various prisons on different occasions. Going to prison became a blessing in disguise for him. He spent time reading number of books. He became familiar with the works of western philosophers, revolutionaries, and social reformers. He translated the autobiography of Madam Curie, a French scientist who discovered Radium, into Hindi. He was a ideal prisoner. The greatness of Shastri was that he maintained his self-respect even in prison.

After Independence, he became the Minister of police in the ministry of Govind Vallabh Panth. In 1951, he was appointed as the General Secretary of Lok Sabha before regaining a ministerial post as Railways Minister. He resigned following a rail disaster near Ariyalur. He returned to the Cabinet following the general elections, first as Minister of Transport, and then in 1961, he became the Home Minister

Nehru died in office on May 27, 1964, and left something of a vaccum. Though eclipsed by such stalwarts of the congress party as Kamaraj, and Morarji Desai, the Finance Minister in Nehru's government, Shastri emerged as the consensus candidate in the midst of the party warfare. The ruling congress party Shastri unanimously as its leader. He became the Prime Minister on June 9, 1964.

The first problem he had to face after becoming the P.M was the one caused by Pakistan. After the Chinese aggression, when India's confidence in her strength had been shaken, Pakistan was creating trouble along the borders. But Shastriji would not yield to the wickedness of Pakistan. He first tried to earn the goodwill and support from the other nations for India. He attended a meeting of non-aligned nations and explained India's position. Pakistan was awaiting to swallow Kashmir into its territory. She pushed her forces across the eastern border into the Rann of Kuch in Gujarat in 1965. Shastri faced the problem with great tact. But later there was a large scale invasion of the territory by Pakistani soldiers which lead to the break out of war along the cease-fire line on the Kashmir border. Addressing the Nation on 13th August 1965, Shastri referred to Pakistan threats and said, "Force will be met with force".

Some big Nations feared that if India won a total victory over Pakistan, it would lower their prestige. The Security Council of the United Nations Organization called on India and Pakistan to stop fighting. On the invitation of Kosygin, the Premier of Soviet Russia, Shastri and Ayub Khan met in Tashkent on January 4, 1966. Shastri wished to give one more chance to Pakistan to live in peace and friendship with India. So he signed the treaty of friendship.

Shastriji had suffered heart attacks twice before and during the period of Pakistan war and the following days his body had to bear a very heavy strain. He signed the Joint Declaration on 10th January 1966. He died the same night. Gone was the war hero and the messenger of peace, gone was the great statesman who restored to India her honour and self-respect in the assembly of nations.

He was posthumously awarded the Bharat Ratna and a memorial was built for him in Delhi. The slogan, 'Jai jawan, Jai kisan' is attributed to Shastri. Lal Bahadur Shastri was a star of great brightness in the history of India.

Shri Lal Bahadur Shastri was born on October 2, 1901 at Mughalsarai, a small railway town seven miles from Varanasi in Uttar Pradesh. His father was a school teacher who died when Lal Bahadur Shastri was only a year and half old. His mother, still in her twenties, took her three children to her father's house and settled down there.

Lal Bahadur's small town schooling was not remarkable in any way but he had a happy enough childhood despite the poverty that dogged him. He was sent to live with an uncle in Varanasi so that he could go to high school. Nanhe, or 'little one' as he was called at home, walked many miles to school without shoes, even when the streets burned in the summer's heat.

As he grew up, Lal Bahadur Shastri became more and more interested in the country's struggle for freedom from foreign yoke. He was greatly impressed by Mahatma Gandhi's denunciation of Indian Princes for their support of British rule in India. Lal Bahadur Sashtri was only eleven at the time, but the process that was end day to catapult him to the national stage had already begun in his mind.

Lal Bahadur Shastri was sixteen when Gandhiji called upon his countrymen to join the Non-Cooperation Movement. He decided at once to give up his studies in response to the Mahatma's call. The decision shattered his mother's hopes. The family could not dissuade him from what they thought was a disastrous course of action. But Lal Bahadur had made up his mind. All those who were close to him knew that he would never change his mind once it was made up, for behind his soft exterior was the firmness of a rock.

Lal Bahadur Shastri joined the Kashi Vidya Peeth in Varanasi, one of the many national institutions set up in defiance of the British rule. There, he came under the influence of the greatest intellectuals, and nationalists of the country. 'Shastri' was the bachelor's degree awarded to him by the Vidya Peeth but has stuck in the minds of the people as part of his name.

In 1927, he got married. His wife, Lalita Devi, came from Mirzapur, near his home town. The wedding was traditional in all senses but one. A spinning wheel and a few yards of handspun cloth was all the dowry. The bridegroom would accept nothing more.

In 1930, Mahatma Gandhi marched to the sea beach at Dandi and broke the imperial salt law. The symbolic gesture set the whole country ablaze. Lal Bahadur Shastri threw himself into the struggle for freedom with feverish energy. He led many defiant campaigns and spent a total of seven years in British jails. It was in the fire of this struggle that his steel was tempered and he grew into maturity.

When the Congress came to power after Independence, the sterling worth of the apparently meek and unassuming Lal Bahadur Shastri had already been recognised by the leader of the national struggle. When the Congress Government was formed in 1946, this 'little dynamo of a man' was called upon to play a constructive role in the governance of the country. He was appointed Parliamentary Secretary in his home State of Uttar Pradesh and soon rose to the position of Home Minister. His capacity for hard work and his efficiency became a byeword in Uttar Pradesh.

He moved to New Delhi in 1951 and held several portfolios in the Union Cabinet-Minister for Railways; Minister for Transport and Communications; Minister for Commerce and Industry; Home Minister; and during Nehru's illness Minister without portfolio.

He was growing in stature constantly. He resigned his post as Minister for Railways because he felt responsible for a railway accident in which many lives were lost. The unprecedented gesture was greatly appreciated by Parliament and the country.

The then Prime Minister, Pt. Nehru, speaking in Parliament on the incident, extolled Lal Bahadur Shastri's integrity and high ideals. He said he was accepting the resignation because it would set an example in constitutional propriety and not because Lal Bahadur Shastri was in any way responsible for what had happened.

Replying to the long debate on the Railway accident, Lal Bahadur Shastri said; "Perhaps due to my being small in size and soft of tongue, people are apt to believe that I am not able to be very firm. Though not physically strong, I think I am internally not so weak."

In between his Ministerial assignments, he continued to lavish his organising abilities on the affairs of the Congress Party. The landslide successes of the Party in the General Elections of 1952, 1957 and 1962 were in a very large measure the result of his complete identification with the cause and his organisational genius.

More than thirty years of dedicated service were behind Lal Bahadur Shastri. In the course of this period, he came to be known as a man of great integrity and competence. Humble, tolerant, with great inner strength and resoluteness, he was a man of the people who understood their language.

He was also a man of vision who led the country towards progress. Lal Bahadur Shastri was deeply influenced by the political teachings of Mahatma Gandhi. "Hard work is equal to prayer," he once said, in accents profoundly reminiscent of his Master. In the direct tradition of Mahatma Gandhi, Lal

Bahadur Shastri represented the best in Indian culture. Shastriji's life is one that has a million inspirational tales. The way he lived every moment of his life is a legend in it's own. Please go through the brief description of his life in the Hero of the Month section. Let us discuss here the things that inspire us the most and ask us to being in a change within.

The life of Lal Bahadur Shastri (1904-66), India's second Prime Minister and successor to Jawaharlal Nehru, is an absorbing saga of a little man who, while suffering the rigours of poverty in early life, rose to political eminence on the strength of moral principle. When Shastri died he left no house, no land, no money.

But he did leave behind an example which is morally inspiring. In an age riddled with political corruption, his career of exemplary integrity possesses a very special relevance for contemporary India as well as the world.

Although Lal Bahadur Shastri's tenure as Prime Minister lasted only nineteen months, it was a period of high excitement and drama. Under Shastri's leadership India successfully fought a major war against Pakistan. This came as a tremendous boost to India after the China debacle three years earlier. This Indo-Pak war was followed by successful peace negotiations between the two countries at the famous Tashkent Conference, where after the ink scarcely dry after all the momentous signatures, Shastri died of a heart attack.

Several social and political issues of national importance and international interest emerged or found successful resolution during the time that Shastri held political power in Nehru's cabinet, as well as when he took over the premiership of India.

Upon hearing the news of the death of Lal Bahadur Shastri, one of the most perceptive comments were made by one of the outstanding and respected figures of Indian journalism at that time-Frank Moraes, editor of the Indian Express. In an editorial, he observed:

"The drama of Tashkent has been cruelly heightened by its tragic denouement. The sudden death of Mr. Lal Bahadur Shastri is a grievous loss to India for never were his qualities of patience and persistence, of flexibility and firmness, more needed than today. Following in the wake of the incandescent figure of Jawaharlal Nehru, Shastriji's homely, homespun personality suffered by comparison in the early days of his prime ministership but with each successive month, as crisis followed crisis, he grew in confidence and strength until the last confrontation with Pakistan found him the country's prime minister in his own right. Tashkent added more than a cubit to his stature as a statesman. It revealed him as a diplomat of considerable finesse and skill.

Lal Bahadur had the wisdom which consists of commonsense in an uncommon degree, and this he revealed in growing measure in the brief nineteen months of his prime minstership. In that period he faced calmly and with resolution more successive crises than have come the way of most prime minsiters. Foodgrain scarcity with rising prices posed the first menacing problem in his early days in office, and this was followed by growing tensions in Kashmir, culminating the in the detention of Sheikh Abdullah. Then came the Pakistani incursion in Kutch and attack on Kashmir accompanied by Communist China's increasingly minatory postures on our northern frontier. Lal Bahadur had a rare capacity for remaining imperturbable but acutely vigilant through the most threatening times, and something of this calmness and confidence he was able to convey to his countrymen, more especially in the later months of his prime ministership.

He was a leader who because of his unusual attributes was ideally suited to guide his country in a time of crisis and fluidity, and it is no derogation of aspiring contestants to the prime ministership to observe that he will be difficult to replace. Although not unconscious of his qualities, Lal Bahadur was a man of real humility in so far as he did not regard his own opinions omnipotent and immutable was prepared to listen to others and surprisingly often to defer to them. Politicians are notoriously prone to dot the capital I but nobody could accuse Shastriji of being self-centred. He was outgiving by temperament and training".

The above comment aptly summarises the life of a great man.

Dr. Radhakrishnan said "Lal Bhadur Shastri's case is an illustration of the strength of democracy in this country. From humble beginnings, without any advantage of birth, position or wealth, he rose to the highest position in the Government of the country. It is due entirely to his force of character and integrity of life. These things enabled him to rise to the top".

The National Academy of Administration was renamed as the :Lal Bhadaur Shastri National Academy of Administration in 1972.

Writing a full-fledged biography of Lal Bahadur Shastri is a labour of love as well as a tribute this author offers to the memory of a unique and fascinating personality that bestrode the Indian political stage after Independence-a bright and shining meteor that flashed across India's Horizon.

For a long, long time to come, Indians, their children and their children's children will speak with gratitude of the great little man who so briefly, and yet indelibly, illumined the pages of modern India's history, in whose light physical frame, gentle nature, humility and strength of character, they saw embodied the Indian ideal of a public servant so completely dedicated to nishkamakarma. Shastri translated into real, crass political life the biblical phrase the meek shall inherit the earth. He combined a child's heart that was easily moved to tears by human suffering with a granite will that ordered the Indian Army to march across the international frontier into West Pakistan to punish the latter's perfidious activities in Jammu and Kashmir.

His great achievement was to have bolstered up the Indian people's sagging spirits during depressing years and restored self-confidence to them as a nation. He had taught a truculent neighbour to respect India and in the process won the confidence and personal regard of its arrogant dictator.

4

The Martyrdom of Shastri

There were some Russian cooks also, says the writer, but does not specify. A little later Ram Nath brought some milk and was with him till Shastriji slept at around 12.30 a.m. Though Shastriji walked quietly upto aides room to call his doctor after he had heart attack at around 1.20 a.m., he had started coughing continuously. As he turned back to his bed, he could not speak, he pointed to a flask, and was given some water. When the doctor gave him injection, Shastri "was still alive, but in acute pain, coughing and breathless but uttered the words, Arey baap, arey Ram (O my father, O Lord Rama). Probably this was his last gasp. Dr. Chugh now gave him artificial respiration but the PM passed away at 1.32 a.m. (January 11, 1966). To continue the account of the biographer further; he also says, perhaps Shastri had a premonition of death. On the morning of 10th January he had written the verse of a venerated Urdu poet, Saqib Lakhnavi on a piece of paper which Jagannath had picked up and kept with him for quite sometime. It was as follows :

Zamana bade shauq se sun raha tha Hamin so gaye daastan kehtay kehtay

(All the world was listening to me very eagerly; only I fell asleep while narrating the story.) Ironically, during all the last day of hectic activity, nobody saw any cause for worry about his health or asked him about it, not only because "Shastri was rather private and reticent on the question of his health, and regarded this as a matter strictly between himself and his physician, Dr. Chugh," but also because they always found him cheerful till the end. * * * Regarding the matter of blue patches on Shastriji's dead body, including nook and face which appeared at Tashkent when it was being put in a box, and were later clearly noticed while it was kept for public darshan at his residence in New Delhi, it naturally led to a widespread suspicious comments, but the author says the Russians explained it as due to the embalming material injected into his body consisting of "three litres of pure spirit, one litre of formalin and two hundred grammes of urotrophine introduced through an incision into femoral artery in the inguinal part of the body" by Soviet doctors to save it from degeneration.

The author further says that when he was later posted in UK as Secretary General of UN's International Maritime Organisation, he showed the medical reports by Soviet doctors and Dr. Chugh to two reputed medical practitioners of UK, Dr. David M. Spiro and Dr. Jan West, both of whom said blue patches are quite natural in such cases of heart attack due to removal of oxygen and the embalming process. However, he wonders why there was no post mortem at Tashkent or even in Delhi (much less an enquiry). This was perhaps because nobody including the Acting Prime Minister, Gulzari Lal Nanda asked for it. Which, in a way, is expression of suspicion and dissatisfaction. Perhaps, the intense politicking about his successor in Delhi, soon after his death were responsible for it. The Congress leaders were too busy in this more urgent business.

Significantly, the Soviet Premier Kosygin stayed on in Delhi for four days after the funeral to oversee the election of Indira Gandhi as successor. The Soviets were worried about the right-wing shift, which they had seen even in the election of Shastri, and had started appeasing Pakistan, inviting Ayub Khan to Moscow. Thus Shastriji passed away within twelve minutes of appearing at the door of the bedroom of his doctor and the two aides. Explaining away the lack of buzzer by his bedside, Srivastava says it was in the adjoining study room of the PM but perhaps he was too gentle to ring the alarm while walking through that room upto the aides' room to ask, "Where is the doctor?". Or perhaps, he did not think his condition too serious at that time, though it worsened within a minute or so later. Regarding the surmise of pressure of worry on his heart for having given away Haji Pir Pass and other infitration points snatched from Pakistan at great sacrifice, the author says Shri Shastri was quite cheerful and satisfied about the agreement till he left him three hours before his death. Earlier in the day he was cheerfully mixing with Soviet and Pakistani leaders after signing the agreement. He was confident of selling the agreement to the Indian people. However, at around 11 pm, he had a telephonic talk with his people in Delhi as well as with another P.A. Venkataraman who told Jagannath Sahai that the agreement had been well received except by a couple of opposition leaders, at which Shri Shastri said, "They are in the opposition and it is their right to be critical."

HOW difficult the parleys were till the end is revealed from the following last minute hitch: Everything had been agreed between Premiere Kosygin and President Ayub Khan at dinner the previous night between 9.30 p.m. to 11.30

p.m. (January 9, 1961) when Kosygin came to Shastri's villa with Gromyko, the Soviet foreign minister, beaming with a feeling of success, he told Shastri, "I have some good news on Kashmir and on the reaffirmation of the obligation under the UN charter not to use force in the settlement of disputes". It fulfilled Shastri's two main conditions—that India did not have to discuss Kashmir with Pakistan as it was an integral part of India and that if anything had to be discussed, it was vacation of the Pak-occupied part, whereas Pakistan was insisting on inclusion of a "self-executing mechanism" to settle the problem of Kashmir. Secondly, Shastri wanted Pakistan to commit to a 'No-War Pact' to bind Pakistan to firm commitment on non-use of force in future, before withdrawal to August 5, 1965 position, implying vacating of the points occupied by India beyond the cease-fire line including Hajipir Pass.

But Ayub, egged on by Bhutto, was resisting the non-use of force clause, Bhutto even saying that he would not mind a war of extermination to get Kashmir, (which Pakistan is still waging in proxy form). However, Ayub agreed to a No-War commitment indirectly by pledging non-use of force under the UN charter. "Ayub seemed to have been convinced that Bhutto's line of hatred, clandestine terrorism, use of force and threat of a thousand years' war against India was not going to enable Pakistan to seize Kashmir." But even when at 11.30 p.m. the 'good news' of Ayub's approval was conveyed to Shastri by Kosygin at Shastri's villa, a phone call was received from Bhutto to Gromyko, the Soviet foreign minister. 'It was chilling moment' when Gromyko lifted the receiver, heard Bhutto for a few moments and then exploded suddenly, "No, No, No, Mr. Bhutto, you are quite wrong, you had agreed to this, Ayub himself had agreed to this.

You cannot go back on it now. It will be very bad, very bad. Please convey this to your President immediately.... A few minutes later, Bhutto came back on the phone and withdrew whatever he had said." As Gromyko explained later, Bhutto had again raised objection to the clause of non-use of force for the settlement of disputes. The last hitch seemed to be over. Kosygin left at 12.45 a.m. (10 January). "Shastri had gone through another gruelling day in which despair and hope had alternated from hour to hour. He was naturally very pleased at the final outcome." The way was clear for signing the final agreement at 4 p.m. on January 10. On the morning of 10th January, "all was quiet and peaceful. The days of hectic parleys, of anxious moments, of intense arguments... were over all".

Shastriji spent half the day reclining against the pillows in bed reading papers, coming out into the garden for fresh air, collecting his thoughts for the day, discussing matters with aides, and then preparing to go for luncheon with Ayub Khan at 1.30 p.m., when they gave formal approval to the text of the agreement, three copies of which were prepared in two languages each—English and Russian. He returned at 3 p.m. and again left for the venue of the final signing ceremony at 4 p.m., exactly six days after the opening ceremony on January 4. There were speeches also by three leaders—Kosygin, Shastri and Ayub, followed by standing ovation and elasping of hands for photographs.

There were rumours of secret promise of economic and military aid and arm-twisting, as it was literally an eleventh hour decision—at 11 p.m. on 9th January when Ayub Khan finally agreed. There was one final engagement still or rather two—Shastri briefed the press before leaving for his villa and starting back again at 7.30 p.m. for Kosygin's reception cum cultural programme at 8 p.m., from which he came back to his suit at 10.15 p.m., shaking many hands of the present dignitaries and exchanging Khuda Hafiz with Ayub finally.

There were joyous scenes, well arranged by the Soviets, in the streets of Tashkent, as he drove back. Shastri had to leave for halt in Kabul next morning, before returning to India; his luggage was being packed up. There have been tributes galore to Shastriji's gentle, homespun, Swadeshi, realistic and daring leadership. One such by one of the Nehrus— In this context, the Cabinet Secretary of the Shastri era, Shri Dharmavira has pointed out in his Reminiscences, that while Pakistan's ammunition was almost totally exhausted in the 18-day war, obliging it to accept ceasefire, the Indian Government could have continued fighting for another week, but that it was misinformed that its stocks too were exhausted. The ministers and bureaucrats were very anxious that Lahore and Sialkot should be occupied or at least one of the two should be bagged, to create an impression of decisive victory.

However, this was not to be to make it look like a drawn match to the world, with Pakistan even claiming a victory. However, Shastriji's biographer, Shri C.P. Srivastava says that there was no intention to capture Lahore, as it would have led to international uproar. However, the question of capturing Sialkot was left to the Army Chief, General Chaudhuri. But Chaudhuri preferred to bypass it, though Indian troops were within two miles of Sialkot, as the cost of capturing it would be heavy loss of life, for something he knew would be surrendered after the war. However, both the cities started being deserted. In this context, B.K. Nehru relates two very interesting incidents. When sometime later, he happened to meet Begum Viqar-un-Nissa Noon, the Australian wife of Sir Feroz Khan Noon (like B.K. Nehru's own Australian wife Fori), a Pakistani Governor of West Punjab and pre-partition India's High Commissioner in London, told him during a visit to Delhi, that "while Bhutto had been raving and ranting about a thousand year war in UN Security Council, in Lahore the booming of Indian guns could be heard night and day and hospitals were full of wounded soldiers coming in from the front with the defeated troops close behind.

Another observation he gives is from Robert MacNamara, the US Defence Secretary, who was very much pro-Pakistan. McNamara told him at a dinner in Washington during the 1965 war, that "he feared for stability of Pakistan; the greatest danger to its internal stability was the return of a defeated army back from the front to their homes." Though Ayub was trying to convince his people that it was a victory, "but the Pakistani Army knew that they had been routed. McNamara further said that "something had to be done to restore the morale of the Pakistani Army." At this Nehru said, "Surely you are not going to arm them once again?" At this, "McNamara hummed and hawed and said, "Well, I don't know. Perhaps we shall have to." This was said three days before the ceasefire.

Which shows that how the Pentagon, the US defence establishment has been firmly committed to Pakistan's security and military parity with India. In this context, an eminent Indian defence expert, wrote in an article in a national daily, that the latest release of US classified information shows that the Pentagon had concluded on the basis of war exercise sometime before the 1965 war that Pakistan would beat India because of the supply to it of the latest armour like Patton tanks and star fighter and other U.S. planes. Obviously, Ayub Khan's appetite for aggression had been greatly sharpened because of this message

LAL BAHADUR SHASTRI

Lal Bahadur Shastri (*October 2, 1904-January 11, 1966*) was the second Prime Minister of independent *India* and a significant figure in the struggle for independence.

Lal Bahadur was born in Moghalsarai, also spelt as *Mughalsarai*. To take part in the non-cooperation movement of *Mahatma Gandhi* in *1921*, he began studying at the nationalist, non-government university in Kashi, and upon completion was given the title *Shastri*, or *Scholar, Doctor* at *Kashi Vidya Peetha* in *1926*. He spent almost nine years in jail in total, mostly after the start of the *Satyagraha* movement in *1940*, he was imprisoned until *1946*. Following India's independence, he was Home Minister under Chief Minister *Govind Vallabh Pant* of *Uttar Pradesh*. In *1951*, he was appointed General Secretary of the *Lok Sabha* before re-gaining a ministerial post as Railways Minister. He resigned as Minister following a *rail disaster* near Ariyalur, *Tamil Nadu*. He returned to the *Cabinet* following the General Elections, first as Minister for Transport, in *1961*, he became Home Minister.

Jawaharlal Nehru died in office on *May 27, 1964* and left something of a vacuum. The major figures of the *Congress Party* were unable to find enough support which allowed the lesser regarded Shastri to come through as the compromise candidate, becoming Prime Minister on *June 9*. Shastri, though mild-mannered and soft-spoken, was a Nehruvian socialist and thus held appeal to those wishing to prevent the ascent of conservative right-winger *Morarji Desai*.

Shastri worked by his natural characteristics to obtain compromises between opposing viewpoints, but was ineffectual in dealing with the economic crisis and food shortage in the nation. His administration began on a rocky turf.

The chief problem was *Pakistan*. Laying claim to half of the *Kutchch* peninsula, *Pakistan* sent incursion forces in August 1965, who skirmished with Indian tanks. Under a scheme proposed by the British PM, *Pakistan* obtained 10% of their original claim of 50%. But *Pakistan*'s main aggressive intentions were upon *Kashmir*. Just in September 1965, major incursions of militants and *Pakistan*i soldiers began, hoping not only to break-down the government but incite a sympathetic revolt. The revolt did not happen, and an angry India sent its forces across the *Line of Control*, and the war broke out on a general scale. Massive tank battles occurred in the *Punjab*, and while *Pakistan*i forces made some gains, Indian forces captured the key post at Haji Pir, in *Kashmir*, and brought the *Pakistan*i city of *Lahore* under artillery and mortar fire.

A ceasefire was declared, and the soft-spoken, mild-mannered Shastri, once butt of jokes was now a national hero. In January *1966* Shastri and Pakistani President *Muhammad Ayub Khan* attended a summit in *Tashkent* (former *USSR*), organised by *Kosygin*. Shastri signed a treaty with Pakistan on *January 10*, the *Tashkent* Declaration, but the next day he was dead of a heart attack. He is the only Indian Prime Minister to have died in office overseas, and indeed probably one of the few *heads of government* in history to do so. All his lifetime, he was known for his honesty and humbleness.

He was the first person to be posthumously awarded the *Bharat Ratna* and a memorial "*Vijay Ghat*" was built for him in Delhi. The slogan *Jai Jawan, Jai Kisan* (*Hindi* for "Hail the soldier, Hail the farmer") is attributed to Shastri.

If Pakistan has any ideas of annexing any part of our territories by force, she should think afresh. I want to state categorically that force will be met with force and aggression against us will never be allowed to succeed.

October 2 reminds us the birthday of other great son of India.

Yes it is Lal Bahdur Shastri. He was been on Oct 2,1994 at Moghalsarai in U.P. His father died when Shastri was a toddler. So, he was brought up by his maternal grandfather, Shastriji's childhood was spent in poverty.

Mr. Shastri was attracted toward freedom movement at the age of 17 He took part in the non-cooperation movement launched by Mahatma Gandhi. This was the time when he went to jail. After his release he joined Kashi Vidyapith. Here he studied at the feet of great Teachers like late Dr. Bhagwan Das from the Kashi Vidyapeeth he secured his Shastri degree which became a part of his name. Mr. Shastri took part in freedom movement. In 1926, he joined the servants of the People Society started by Late Lajpat Rai.

Between 1953 and 1964 Mr. Shastri was several times a member of India's council of ministers. After the death of Mr. Nehru in May 1926, he was unanimously chosen to succeed him as the Prime minister of India. Early in 1965, the south was shaken by a violent anti Hindu agitation. But with his tact patience and skill. Mr Shastri was successful in bringing the situation back to normal within a short time.

Those were testing times and they brought out the best in Mr. Shastri. In dealing with Pakistan, he gave proof of Statesmanship of a high order. He gave a chance to Pakistan to return to the path of peace. But two months later, Pakistan invaded Kashmir. Then Mr. Shastri hit backhard. The man of peace was forced to lead his people into a fierce conflict for saying.

During the conflict, Mr. Shastri displayed rare courage and combativeness. After the cease-fire, he was even more relentless in the cause of peace with honour. He agreed to meet President Ayub in Tashkent. There he signed an assignment.

He gave the last once of energy in his small frame to win the peace. But fate struck him, he died within a few hours of signing the agreement at Tashkent.

When he was the Railway Minster he was responsible for two-tire and three-tier. Sleeping accomdation for 3rd class passengers and electric fans filled in 3rd class compartments and that service was also introduced.

The Lal Bahadur Shastri Memorial Foundation was established in 1986, to commemorate the memory of the late Prime Minister of India. Lal Bahadur Shastri was a great patriot and a staunch nationalist. He was not just a great personality or a great individual but an institution in himself. His ideals of simple living and high thinking endeared him to the people and his remarkable qualities of leadership gave them hope.

Lal Bahadur Shastri was a man of the masses. He had a deep-rooted concern for the upliftment of the people of India especially the farmers and the rural poor. He believed the real industry for the rural areas was agriculture and every effort should be made to develop it. He also took keen interest in Khadi and village industries and had a vision of setting up a vast network of processing industries in the villages.

His leadership skills blossomed when he led the country to victory in the 1965 war against Pakistan. He gave the nation a soul-stirring slogan ' Jai Jaiwan-Jai Kisan'. He gave the country a new dynamism, a new impetus and a new hope. The Foundation embodies in its objectives his cherished dream of improving the fabric of life of the common man, thereby contributing to the strength and stability of the nation.

Indian National Congress : After Nehru's death in 1964, the party's future comes into question, no leader is competitive enough to touch Nehru's iconic status, so the second-stage leadership mustered around the compromise candidate, Lal Bahadur Shastri

1964-President : After Nehru's death in 1964, the party's future comes into question, no leader is competitive enough to touch Nehru's iconic status, so the second-stage leadership mustered around the compromise candidate, Lal Bahadur Shastri

1964-Prime Minister : 2nd June Appointed Prime Minister of India, India's 2nd Prime Minister

1965-Conference of Tashkent : Tashkent A settlement is reached with Pakistan over Kashmir during a meeting in Tashkent

1965-Declaration of War : War is declared over the rule of Kashmir

1965-Rule of Kashmir : Kashmir A settlement is reached with Pakistan over Kashmir during a meeting in Tashkent. Kashmir War is declared over the rule of Kashmir

1965-Rule of Rann of Kutch : April Rann of Kutch A clash between border patrols erupted into fighting in the Rann of Kutch. April Rann of Kutch India is forced to retreat after intense fighting

1966-Death : 11th Jan Tashkent Death of Lal Bahadur Shastri, at the Indo-Pakistan summit

1966-Summit : 11th Jan Death of Lal Bahadur Shastri, suffers a fatal heart attack

"Forging a Radical Centre: A Response to Extremism and Intolerance" because I believe it aptly reflects the philosophy of the late Prime Minister

Shastri and is very relevant in today's socio-political climate. When researching the life of Lal Bahadur Shastri, what I found remarkable was the resoluteness and the strength of his convictions in his political vision despite his simplicity which almost bordered on invisibility. Like Mahatma Gandhi, whose fearless stance on non-violence revolutionized the thinking of the early twentieth century, Lal Bahadur Shastri too was committed to the path of Ahimsa and non-violence. However, unlike the Mahatma, Shastriji was a practicing politician and what I find remarkable was his continued commitment to the Gandhian principles, even in the turbulent and expedient world of 'real politick.'

Lal Bahadur Shastri's simplicity was not a weakness or lack of vision. Rather, it was an, integral element of his unique, moderate, centrist style of governance that sprang from Shastri's personality, resoluteness and the courage of his convictions. He was indeed a 'Radical Centrist' by example, vehemently and vigorously committed to ahimsa, tolerance and moderation.

The achievements of Lal Bahadur Shastri and his fellow leaders in the Indian independence struggle are all the more remarkable because they formed their political philosophy at a time when the world was being torn between the competing ideologies of fascism and communism. In an era where revolutions, regional wars and armed conflicts was the norm, the Indian independence struggle's adoption of the Gandhian approach of non-violent civil disobedience and democracy as the means to achieve freedom was indeed a radical affirmation of centrist values.

With regard to my own country, an important milestone in Indo-Sri Lanka relations was the successful negotiation and conclusion of the Sirima-Shastri Pact signed by Prime Ministers Lal Bahadur Shastri and Madame Sirimavo Bandaranaike. This was an important step in addressing the issue of stateless persons of Indian origin that had been an irritant in Indo-Sri Lanka bilateral relations. Even today, the Sirima-Shastri pact has significant symbolism. It reflects the statesmanship of our leaders as well as the moderation and resilience that always underlies Indo-Sri Lanka relations. It is also an example of the spirit of flexibility and mutual accommodation needed when dealing with difficult bilateral issues. It was just a few years ago, after the end of the cold war and the fall of the Berlin Wall in the late eighties, that there was new hope that the world would be freed from destructively clashing ideologies. However, in the early years of the twenty first century, it is apparent that there continues to exist sharp divides of political visions and economic approaches.

On the one hand, we are experiencing a largely intolerant reaffirmation of ethnic, nationalistic and religious fundamentalism. On the other hand, the idea of the state commanding the sectors of the economy as well as the blind belief in the virtues of the free market, have proven to be greatly misplaced. I believe today, the global challenge is to forge a centrist alternative that is radically committed to resolving the ill consequences of those failed and negative extremes. In doing so, Shastriji's philosophy and lifework remains as a beacon of light.

Ladies & Gentlemen, I personally am not against globalization. But we do have to be cognizant of certain well founded reservations. In 1998, Dr. Mahathir Mohamad, at the 7th International Conference on the Future of Asia, in his inimitable style posed the question, "So what is there beyond globalism and globalization? There could be total oppression of the weak by the strong as capitalism runs riot. Or, there could be a world democracy where the resources of the world are combined with human ingenuity to create the greatest human civilization ever."

There are many who claim that in every country across the world, globalization, spurred by the rise of international corporations, has made the poor poorer while the rich have gotten richer. According to Nobel Laureate Joseph Stiglitz, during the last ten years, the world's total income has increased by an average of 2.5% per year. Yet the number of poor has increased by 100 million. The top 1% of the world earns as much as the bottom 57%. This disparity keeps increasing. It would be difficult, and indeed imprudent, to delink this growing chasm from civil unrest, which we see happening across the globe on a daily basis.

Arundhati Roy, one of the most outspoken and outstanding commentators today noted that civil unrest does not only mean marches, demonstrations and protests against globalization. Unfortunately, it also means a desperate downward spiral into crime and chaos and all kinds of despair and disillusionment. As we know from history and from events unravelling before our eyes, these gradually become a fertile breeding ground for terrible things – cultural nationalism, religious bigotry, fascism, and of course terrorism. Hence, the growth of intolerance and extremism that we face today.

As extremists from every part of the political spectrum – the evangelical right, the revolutionary left, fundamentalist zealots and separatist megalomaniacs monopolize the global media which thrives on sensationalism, many may wonder if moderation and tolerance are becoming bygone values of a distant and more civilized era. The loud and violent sounds of extremism make better news than the democratic pronouncements of the silent majority. The tyranny of the 'few' as opposed to the silence of the 'majority' is perhaps the biggest challenge many of our democracies have to face today.

Ladies & Gentlemen, this is why a 'radical centre' is needed to stop this slide towards open ended polarization and extremism. A vigorous reiteration of liberal values is the need of the hour. The 'Centre' should be home to a radical commitment to liberalism. The need is for a new political culture based on reviving the value systems drawn from Lord Buddha's middle path to Gandhi's path of non-violence, from Nehru to Martin Luther King, from Nelson Mandela to Bill Clinton; the liberal centre must strike back. Moderates all over, like brothers in arms must unite and stand up for a liberal ideology.

As I see it, the root causes of extremism are either economic, religious or socio-political in nature. Economic stereotypes have been thrust upon the developing countries under the guise of globalization. Many of the developed countries have reached the post-modern state of capitalism after several centuries of economic evolution and costly trials and errors, both in terms of human and social development. However, in many developing countries like ours, this form of capitalism is being thrust upon us without the slow learning curve the developed countries enjoyed in their evolution. This is why it is important that each country must evolve its own form of market economics if it is to get the most cost effective results.

As envisioned by Aristotle in his treatise 'Politics' in 350 BBC., the "middling element," was the substance that bridged the chasm between the rich and the poor. It is more relevant to us than ever before in this first decade of the 21st century. The middling element that Aristotle wrote about was what Lal Bahadur Shastri practiced. In his case, it included the strengthening of agriculture and the upliftment of the rural poor.

Neo-liberalism which has brought much confusion and confrontation in developing countries must be replaced by a renewal of the principles of consensual democracy that looks beyond the adversarial politics of the left and the right. As Anthony Giddens states in his book 'The Third Way', "a society where the market has free play may create large economic inequalities." And in doing so, it has been proven in many countries that a pro-poor, pro-growth approach to economics is a more successful model in meeting the demands of a developing nation. In fact, both the Indian and Sri Lankan electorates endorsed such policies in the general elections held in the two countries in 2004. Since then, India has averaged a growth rate between 8%-9% while Sri Lanka, despite its continuing struggle against terrorism recorded a growth rate of 7.5% in 2006.

The American Declaration of Independence in many ways is an example of classic liberalism as it views life, liberty and the pursuit of happiness as the key objective of a Government. Such a philosophical stance of course implies that politicians must essentially concern themselves in providing the means necessary for each individual's vision of happiness.

However, in countries like ours, where there still is a large underprivileged class, such facilitation should be combined with provisions for the State to look after the weak and the poor with an effective social safety net. This is necessary in order to ensure that the free market does not become 'gravitational fall' for those unable to survive the test of the fittest. In some instances, ignorance or the lack of knowledge about issues make people take extreme hard line positions. When I was the Minister of Telecommunications in Sri Lanka, a strategic decision was taken in 1994 to convert the state owned telephone corporation into a partnership with the private sector. There was strong opposition to this move by almost all the trade unions. When analyzing the reasons for this opposition, it was obvious that the primary reason was lack of knowledge about the proposed changes. Most of the employees did not understand what the changes meant and were opposed to it, primarily based on hearsay and misinformation provided by parties with a paucity of knowledge, and a bounty of vested interests.

In order to dispel the myths about the evils of this partnership as preached by some union leaders, we made a decision to send a direct mailing to every employee, their spouses and to every other stakeholder. The mailing explained the benefits of public/private partnership and helped stakeholders properly understand the issues. All employees were made shareholders of the new company. Thereafter the process went through smoothly and the telecom sector in Sri Lanka emerged to become one of the most successful enterprises in our country where consumers, investors and stakeholders have benefited greatly. Tele-density in Sri Lanka which was 0.7 in 1994 has now reached 19.2. The telecom partnerships are now the two top companies in the Colombo Stock Exchange in terms of market capitalization and profitability. This to me is a clear example of how the power of reason can win over the politics of economic extremism.

Ladies & Gentlemen, our contemporary world is distorted by covert and overt hatred. Modern crusaders of intolerance, like their predecessors from the middle ages, are wreaking havoc and destruction in different parts of the world. Extremists that deliberately misinterpret religious teachings and values have begun to spread their gospel of fear and intolerance to many corners of the world.

Adding fuel to this fire are various non-state entities, who under the pretext of bringing development to the poor and the underprivileged are engaged, in the process of converting the most vulnerable segments of society with financial and economic enticements. Exploiting poverty and ignorance, these new missionaries have become front organizations for induced mass scale conversions.

However, when responding to this threat, no Government in a modern, democratic society can try to counter this challenge by imposing anti-conversion legislation which will only serve to fuel further tensions. Those who engage in mass conversions should also understand that freedom to pursue ones religious beliefs, no matter how different they may be, is a fundamental right of all human beings. The state must remain aloof from interfering in the right of personal beliefs and must follow a policy of secularism, as India, to her credit, has done very successfully since independence.

With the rise of crime and corruption levels, which in many cases is the direct result of growing economic disparity, even ordinary people may see extreme measures as the only solution to society's ills. Citizens, being made helpless and frustrated by ever increasing levels of crime and violence ask for the return of capital punishment. Many politicians, wishing to be seen in tune with populist sentiment, do not dare state that capital punishment is not the answer to crime and violence. Sri Lanka has had a virtual moratorium on capital punishment for decades.

There has been no evidence that indicates that capital punishment reduces crime or violence in any country. Rather, successful investigation and fair and swift judicial process, remains the most effective deterrent. Countries where the rule of law and independence of the judiciary and the police are not firmly established are open to manipulation of the law by those in power. The weak and the ordinary go to the gallows while the powerful and well connected go scot-free.

It is in the face of such feelings of helplessness, that even good, decent and honest people begin to believe that extremism and intolerance might provide solutions to their problems. The recent execution of Saddam Hussein can be taken as an example. Regardless of the cruel and despotic nature of his rule, the question remains whether his execution will ultimately contribute to the healing process the people of Iraq so desperately require. As Mahatma Gandhi said, "An eye for an eye will only make the world go blind,"

The biggest challenge of our post-modern world is the scourge of terrorism. Those who have had to face the sorrows of terrorism in any part of the world must join hands in defeating this menace. Like poverty, terrorism anywhere is a threat to humanity everywhere. It must be fought vigorously and fearlessly. That it should be defeated if democracies are to survive, is beyond question. However, the debatable question is, how does one defeat terrorism?

Sometimes, Governments grappling with the scourge of terrorism respond to terrorist atrocities with equal amounts of brutality and violence. They seem to forget that democratically elected Governments must be above reproach at all times. Elected leaders do not have the option of resorting to terror tactics even when fighting some of the deadliest terrorists in the world. In fact, as Mr. Jaswant Singh wrote in his latest book, 'A Call to Honour', "the vital imperative of remaining 'civilized' is to avoid at all costs, the trap of becoming 'terrorists' to fight the terrorist. Our fight against terrorists must not convert us into a clone of their methods: unseeing, uncaring and totally unmindful of our civilizational and human norms."

Despite the challenge of having to battle one of the most ruthless terror machines in the world for three decades, Sri Lanka is constantly aware of the obligations to respect the rule of law and the need to address the grievances of the affected minorities. That is why we remain committed to a negotiated settlement to our ethnic question.

Despite having to respond to a brutal war, thrust upon us by an intransigent and murderous terrorist group, the solution is in how we gently nudge, or entice if you will, these extreme elements to move towards moderation and democratic methods without compromising our own integrity. The need today is how to find a durable and lasting peace without a craven surrender to a terrorist group.

There are those who think that the middle path is a philosophy of weakness and impotence. It may be seen as a recipe from bleeding heart liberals trying to find excuses for a situation where anything goes and where the rule of law doesn't exist. The Radical Centre as envisaged must not shy away from reasserting society's belief in the rule of law.

The middle path of the radical centre must be based on the courage of convictions based on the principals of decency, freedom and the rule of law. It must be a philosophy based on bringing the socio-economic extremists fearlessly and vigorously into a radically committed centre where the rule of law shall prevail. In doing so, it should engage civil society as its ally. At the same time, the radical centre must ready, whenever the need arises, to reassert society's belief in the rule of law with armed strength to protect the sovereignty of the nation.

Yet another personal example of how the rule of law played an important role in implementing a centrist vision occurred in 2001 when I was the Minister of Urban Development and Housing. I took a policy decision to clean up all the illegal and unauthorized structures which were not only an eyesore but a hazard to commuters in the centre of our capital city, Colombo. Hundreds, if not thousands of unauthorized businesses and some illegal dens of vice had sprouted making the sidewalks almost non-existent. Our policy was to remove every one of these illegal structures without any favouritism.

However, despite the illegality of the structures, this proposal was met with much opposition, even from my own parliamentary colleagues. Many of them accused me that I was going ahead with it only because my constituents were not affected by it. At this juncture, I went back to my own electorate, far to the South of Colombo, and made sure that all unauthorized and illegal structures were removed in my hometown of Matara. Many of these structures belonged to people who had supported me in the general election. Having completed that, my Ministry officials returned to Colombo and were able to remove the structures without much opposition. Subsequently, all bona fide businesses that were torn down were offered alternative locations while the slum dwellers were provided with alternate housing. The lesson to be drawn is that the rule of law, when applied to all fairly, can be a potent tool in development and progress.

I am of the opinion that the only way to resolve the conflict situation in Sri Lanka, or for that matter any of the myriad of other similar situations around the world, to a sustainable peace, is by developing the concept and practice of a "Radical Centre". This would entail the creation of a centrist middle way where dissenting voices and opinions from every part of the political spectrum would have a place within a democratic framework through the decentralization of governance and the devolution of power to all stakeholders. It would be a place where the years of deep mistrust would lose their sting within a non-violent, democratic system where pluralism and secularism flourishes. The radical centre should be a place where the intolerant find that those they hate are in fact, quite similar to themselves and have the same dreams and aspirations as well as fears and concerns.

In conclusion, Ladies & Gentlemen, I would re-emphasize my firm belief that a return to centrist values is the only possible path to ensure the survival of democracy whose credentials are tested today by the forces of anarchy and extremism. If we continue in our present path where even good people in desperation begin to feel that the only answer to extremism is more extremism, democracy as we know it today may surely be doomed to be confined to the pages of history as yet another tried, tested and failed political system. "God says I will quietly come with My armed forces at a time when no one will have the least inkling of the coming event. Most likely it will be in the small hours of the morning or after some part of the night or there-about."

It is now an open secret that only one day before making assault on the city of Lahore, the Indian Prime Minister Lal Bahadur Shastri made a prediction before his Assembly that he would be able to announce to them a good news within twenty-four hours.

It is also known that the Indian Defence Minister and Commander-in-Chief of their army had told their friends that same day, the September 5th 1965, that they would be having drinks in the Lahore Gymkhana the following day.

The frontal and repeated heavy assaults made on Lahore from three sides as well as the shelling of border villages nearby this area, were all certain evidences of the evil Indian design to take the provincial capital by the storm. But for 16 days of bitter and hardest struggle to capture the city of Lahore, the Indian forces ignominiously failed in their nefarious design. Moreover, these attacks and assaults were made all of a sudden and by surprise, without any formal declaration or ultimatum of war, contrary to all war ethics. The utter failure and foiling of this deliberate and determined Indian bid by the Pakistan Army is an amazing feat of performance, of heroism and valour. This story of the valiant fight put up by the Pakistan Army, small in size and comparatively scantily armed, is now being revealed during the "cease-fire" spell. However, before launching their offensive, the Indian war-lords headed by Mr. Shastri were so certain of the easy and rapid capture of Lahore that they had even supplied to the foreign news-agencies false reports of their victory and circulated the fictitious pictures of the entry of Indian Army in to the bazaars of Lahore. As the events turned out to be, the absolutely unexpected happened. Thus the awaited event of the announcement of a "good news" within twenty-four hours by Mr. Shastri to his Assembly proved to be wrong. How a much smaller Pakistani force, not so well-equipped and taken by surprise was not only able to resist a much larger, well-prepared and adequately-armed Indian Army so confident of their victory, is by itself surprising and strange a spectacle for the whole world.

What was shown in the vision to the Godly-Founder of the Ahmadiyya Movement, on the night of April 29th 1905, came actually to pass sixty years after in the early hours of the morning of September 6, 1965.

"*Shastri's* prediction has proved to be wrong."

There is not the shadow of a doubt that what Mr. Shastri and his war-lords considered to be so certain to happen turned out to be wrong.

That the disaster would be marked by the rocking of the earth was witnessed by the citizens of Lahore and Sialkot and especially by the country-side villages of these borders through heavy shelling and aerial bombing.

One of the signs of this happening related in the above vision is its nature of suddenness, the people having been taken unaware. So it happened, India attacked Pakistan suddenly without giving any notice of war. No one in the world ever suspected India to wage war and attack Pakistan in such a treacherous way. Even the time of its beginning has been so precisely foretold in the vision, i.e., it would be about dawn. And so it came about. The assault began at about 3 a.m. on the morning of September 6.

Modern man, in his little knowledge of the unbounded ocean of the secrets of life, may scoff at such spiritual phenomena as visions, clairvoyance, miracles and Divine intervention in human affairs. But the fact remains that these are the only windows through which man can have a glimpse of ultra-mundane realities, and establish some sort of firm contact with the Supreme Source of life.

Indeed the very institution of religion stands on these pillars. The prophets, sages and seers of all ages have testified to the existence of an ultra-mundane realm, these spiritual experiences being tele-communication waves, so to speak, from that realm, imprinted on the recipients' minds.

The Muslim *Umma,* throughout the centuries, was blessed with hundreds of such spiritual men who were the recipients of such communications from God. The Founder of the Ahmadiyya Movement claimed to be just such a one. Having drunk deep at the spiritual Fount of the Quran, and the Sunnah, he proclaimed, he had been blessed with the gift of communications from the Higher Realm about coming events, so that in this age of rank materialism, he should thereby bear personal witness to the existence of God and rehabilitate the fast dwindling values of Faith.

"Shastri's prediction turned out to be wrong," shown to the Founder as long ago as April 29, 1905, and recorded there and then, had stood as a mystery all these sixty years, till on September 6, when Indian forces gate-crashed into our borders, the words sparkled with the true content of this big historical event in this subcontinent's destinies.

As events showed, this Indian onslaught had been so thoroughly planned as to give a knock-out blow to Pakistan. The full armed might of the Indian forces had been hurled into this mad venture in such massive bulk that they had little doubt that in one sweep they would capture Lahore, the heart of Pakistan.

The Indian Prime Minister, Lal Bahadur Shastri was loudly applauded when he told Parliament that the attack against Pakistan had been launched and by the evening he would have for them the big news of the fall of Lahore.

The attack was launched at about 3 a.m., just the hour of early dawn, exactly the time described in the vision. It took Pakistan completely by surprise. There were no Pakistani forces to meet the foe. As shown in the vision, no one even had the least suspicion that India, regardless of all international laws, would stealthily cross into our borders. And the last link in the chain, the appearance of our forces on the scene, has been described in the vision as the coming of God Himself with His armed-forces.

And so indeed it turned to be. The deeds of valour which our Armed Forces performed were acclaimed by the foreign reporters as un-heard-of in the annals of warfare. The whole world stood amazed at their feats of dash and daring, defying death itself.

Those who had come to capture Lahore got the licking of their life. How a small army, one-fifth the size and strength of the enemy could inflict a crushing defeat on the invaders, no one could explain on any of the known laws of the science of war.

"A miracle has come to pass" – this was the expression on everybody's lips. 'God Himself came to the succour of Pakistan"– these were the words on the lips of the whole of the nation, men, women and children.

MYSTERY BEHIND LAL BAHADUR SHASTRI'S DEATH

Shastri's sudden death immediately after signing the Tashkent Pact with Pakistan raised many questions in the minds of Indian citizens. The Prime Minister of India going to Tashkent for a pact and never coming back has not been accepted easily by Indian citizens. His health was fit according to his doctor, R. N. Chugh, and he had no sign of heart trouble before.

Shastri's sudden death has led to persistent conspiracy theories that he was poisoned. The first inquiry into his death, conducted by the Raj Narain Inquiry, as it came to be known, however did not come up with any conclusions, and today no record of this inquiry exists with the Indian Parliament's library. It was alleged that no post-mortem was done on Shastri, but the Indian government in 2009, claimed it did have a report of a medical investigation conducted by Shastri's doctor and some Russian doctors. Furthermore, the Prime Minister's Office (PMO) revealed that there was no record of any destruction or loss of documents in the PMO having a bearing on Shastri's death. The Russian butler attending on Shastri at the time of his death was arrested for suspected poisoning but released later as per the news source. It was maintained that Shastri had died of cardiac arrest but his family insisted he was poisoned.

After Shastri's death, his wife Lalita Shastri had alleged he was poisoned. An epic poetry book in Hindi titled *Lalita Ke Aansoo* written by Krant M. L. Verma was published in 1978. In this book, the tragic story about the death of Shastri has been narrated by his wife Lalita Shastri. There are still serious doubts surrounding the nature of his death. His son, Sunil Shastri, asked the government to unravel the mystery behind Lal Bahadur Shastri's death.Raising doubts about the dark blue spots and cut marks on the abdomen of his father's body after his death in 1966, Sunil asked how the cut marks appeared if a post-mortem had not been conducted.

When Shastri went to the USSR for the Tashkent talks, he wanted a promise from Ayub Khan that Pakistan would never use force in the future. But the talks did not proceed and followed Shastri's death on the next day. The Indian Government released no information about his death, and the media then was kept silent. The possible existence of a conspiracy was covered in India by the *Outlook* magazine. A query was later posed by Anuj Dhar, author of *CIA's Eye on South Asia,* under the Right to Information Act to declassify a document supposedly related to Shastri's death, but the Prime Minister's Office refused to oblige, reportedly citing that this could lead to harming of foreign relations, cause disruption in the country and cause breach of parliamentary privileges. Another RTI plea by Kuldip Nayar was also declined, as PMO cited exemption from disclosure on the plea. The home ministry is yet to respond to queries whether India conducted a post-mortem on Shastri, and if the government had investigated allegations of foul play. The Delhi Police in their reply to an RTI application said they do not have any record pertaining to Shastri's death. The Ministry of External Affairs has already said no post-mortem was conducted in the USSR. The Central Public Information Officer of Delhi Police in his reply dated 29 July said, "No such record related to the death of the former Prime Minister of India Lal Bahadur Shastri is available in this district... Hence the requisite information pertaining to New Delhi district may please be treated as nil." This has created more doubts.

The PMO answered only two questions of the RTI application, saying it has only one classified document pertaining to the death of Shastri, which is exempted from disclosure under the RTI Act. It sent the rest of the questions to the Ministry of External Affairs and Home Ministry to answer. The MEA said the only document from the erstwhile Soviet Government is "the report of the Joint Medical Investigation conducted by a team comprising R. N. Chugh, Doctor in-Attendance to the PM and some Russian doctors" and added no post-mortem was conducted in the USSR. The Home Ministry referred the matter to Delhi Police and National Archives for the response pertaining to any post-mortem conducted on the body of Shastri in India. Sunil Shastri, son of the former Prime Minister, called the transferring of application as "absurd" and "silly joke". "He (Lal Bahadur Shastri) died as sitting Prime Minister. It sounds very silly that MHA is referring the matter of death of second Prime Minister of India to a district level police." He also demanded that "It should be looked into by highest authorities like President, Prime Minister and home minister."

Later, Gregory Douglas, a journalist who interviewed former CIA operative Robert Crowley over a period of 4 years, recorded their telephone conversations and published a transcription in a book titled *Conversations with the Crow*. In the book, Crowley claimed that the CIA was responsible for eliminating Homi Bhabha, an Indian nuclear scientist whose plane crashed into Alps, when he was going to attend a conference in Vienna; and Lal Bahadur Shastri. Crowley said that the USA was wary of India's rigid stand on nuclear policy and of then prime minister Lal Bahadur Shastri, who wanted to go ahead with nuclear tests. He also said that the agency was worried about collective domination by India and Russia over the region, for which a strong deterrent was required.

A HERO AFTER 1965

Within a year of taking office Shastri had proved himself capable of filling Jawaharlal Nehru's somewhat outsize shoes— this even Nehru's sister and daughter were now willing to recognise. But one who persisted in underestimating the little man was Field Marshal Ayub Khan of Pakistan. In August 1965, Pakistani-backed infiltrators began fomenting trouble in the Kashmir Valley.

When Indian army units chased them back over the border, Pakistan mounted a massive offensive in the Chamb sector of Jammu. The enemy tanks rolled menacingly on. Now Shastri pulled off a master-stroke, by asking the Indian Army to march into West Punjab. This at once relieved the pressure on the Jammu sector and took Indian troops tantalisingly close to the great city of Lahore. A cease-fire was called, to be followed by a peace agreement brokered by the Soviet Union, which mandated that both sides pull back to the positions they had held before August 5, 1965.

His conduct during the 1965 War made Shastri a hero — and justly so. His character comes through best in two speeches he made, one at the onset of the conflict, the other at its end. On August 13, after the evidence of mass infiltration into Kashmir had become manifest, the Prime Minister spoke to the nation on All India Radio. Now that the country's freedom and sovereignty were threatened, he said, Indians must set aside their partisan loyalties, those differences in policies and programmes that, in times of peace, were such "an essential part of our democratic set-up". And he issued this stern warning to the other side: "If Pakistan has any ideas of annexing any part of our territories by force, she should think afresh. I want to state categorically that force will be met with force and aggression against us will never be allowed to succeed".

The other speech was made at a public meeting at the Ram Lila grounds in Delhi on September 26, after hostilities had ceased. Here he took issue with a BBC report that claimed that "since India's Prime Minister Lal Bahadur Shastri is a Hindu, he is ready for war with Pakistan". Shastri said that while he was indeed a Hindu, "Mir Mushtaq who is presiding over this meeting is a Muslim.

Mr. Frank Anthony who has addressed you is a Christian. There are also Sikhs and Parsis here. The unique thing about our country is that we have Hindus, Muslims, Christians, Sikhs, Parsis and people of all other religions. We have temples and mosques, *gurdwaras* and churches. But we do not bring this all into politics... This is the difference between India and Pakistan. Whereas Pakistan proclaims herself to be an Islamic State and uses religion as a political factor, we Indians have the freedom to follow whatever religion we may choose (and) worship in anyway we please. So far as politics is concerned, each of us is as much an Indian as the other." Like Jawaharlal Nehru before him, Shastri upheld the idea of India as a multi-religious country where politics and faith were kept in separate compartments. However great the provocation, at least while he was around India would never become a Hindu Pakistan.

A War Leader

Lal Bahadur Shastri died on the night of January 10/11 1966, in the Uzbek city of Tashkent, hours after signing a peace agreement with Pakistan. He spent but 19 months in office, enough to show himself to advantage as a war leader. That, if at all, is how he is remembered today. But had he been lucky to enjoy a full term in office his legacy might have been more wide-ranging.

For he had interesting and (to this writer) innovative ideas in the fields of economic and foreign policy, among much else. He was keen to get rid of the sloth and waste in government, and to induct talent from outside — one of his suggestions, unfortunately never implemented, was to have top scientists inducted as cabinet ministers.

Lal Bahadur Shastri was a man of some considerable achievement and also, being a politician, of the odd failure as well. This column has saluted the achievements; the next one will highlight Shastri's one serious failure as Prime Minister.

Rich tributes paid to former Prime Minister at birth centenary celebrations.

The Government has decided to name the Alamatti dam in Bagalkot district and the proposed Bangalore Development Authority layout at Anjanapura here after the former Prime Minister the late Lal Bahadur Shastri.

Paying rich tributes to Shastri at his birth centenary celebrations at the Banquet Hall of the Vidhana Soudha, the Chief Minister, N. Dharam Singh, also announced that a statue of Shastri will be installed in the precincts of the Vidhana Soudha.

Foundation Stone

It was Shastri who laid the foundation stone for the Upper Krishna Project, of which the Alamatti dam is a part, in 1964.

The noted columnist Kuldip Nayyar, who delivered a lecture on Shastri's life and contribution to the nation, said the former Prime Minister had tried to resolve the Kashmir dispute between India and Pakistan by peaceful means.

In August 1965 heavy fighting broke out between the two countries, and a ceasefire was agreed upon in September 1965. Shastri and the then Pakistani President Ayub Khan signed the Tashkent agreement in the presence of the then Prime Minister of the erstwhile USSR, Alexei Kosygin, in January 1966, a few hours before Shastri's death. Shastri also accepted a unilateral ceasefire with China in 1962 and protected the country's borders, Mr. Nayyar said.

The life of the second Prime Minister of the country was the absorbing saga of a little man, who, while suffering the rigours of poverty in early life, reached political eminence through the strength of his character.

When Shastri died, he left behind no wealth or property; instead he left an example, which is morally inspiring in an age riddled with political corruption, the columnist said.

It was Shastri who for the first time conceived the idea of an ombudsman to eradicate corruption in public life, he said.

Shastri gave priority to boosting foodgrain production and generation of employment to tackle hunger and poverty. Although Shastri's tenure as Prime Minister lasted only 13 months (June 9, 1964 to January 11, 1966), it was a period of high drama during which several social and political issues of national importance and international interest, including a major war against

Pakistan, came up, Mr. Nayyar said. Shastri resigned as Minister for Railways in 1956 holding himself responsible for a railway accident in Tamil Nadu (Ariyalur) in which many lives were lost. The unprecedented gesture was greatly appreciated by Parliament and the country, he said.

The then Prime Minister Jawaharlal Nehru, speaking in Parliament on the incident, extolled Shastri's integrity and high ideals. He said he was accepting the resignation because it would set an example in constitutional propriety and not because Shastri was in any way responsible for what had happened. In between his ministerial assignments, he demonstrated organising abilities and figured in the Congress victories in the first three general elections, Mr. Nayyar said.

Man of Integrity

After more than 30 years of dedicated service, he came to be known as a man of great integrity and competence. Humble, tolerant, with great inner strength and resoluteness, he was a man of the people who understood their language. Shastri was deeply influenced by the political teachings of Mahatma Gandhi. His slogan "Jai Jawan, Jai Kisan" is popular even today, he said.

The Ministers M. Mallikarjun Kharge and R.V. Deshpande; the Speaker of the Legislative Assembly, Krishna; the former Chief Minister M. Veerappa Moily; Anil Shastri, son of Lal Bahadur Shastri; and Haranahalli Ramaswamy, former Law Minister, were present.

A SHIELD FOR INDIA'S HONOUR

Lal Bahadur Shastri was the Prime Minister of India at a crucial time in India's history. He was physically weak, but he faced the problems confronting the nation like a hero. The first problem that he had to face after he became the Prime Minister was one caused by Pakistan.

Pakistan took shape by eroding India's land, and was instigating Indian Muslims. After the Chinese aggression, when India's confidence in her strength had been shaken, Pakistan was creating trouble along the borders.

But Shastriji would not yield to the wickedness of Pakistan. He first tried to earn the goodwill and support of other nations for India. He visited Russia, Egypt, Canada and Britain and explained to the leaders of those nations India's stand. He attended a meeting of the non-aligned nations (nations which were neutral) and explained India's position. He even tried to reason with President Ayub Khan of Pakisthan. The wicked do not like advice. They can understand only one language, the language of war.

The Rann of Kutch

It had become Pakistan's habit to provoke India somehow and jump to arms. Pakisthan had been waiting to swallow Kashmir somehow. She pushed her forces across the eastern border into the Rann of Kutch in Gujarat State in April-May of 1965. Lal Bahadur was not unnerved by this unexpected attack. He faced the problem with great tact at that critical moment. The Indian Army forced the attackers to retreat. Then both countries agreed to stop fighting.

'Force will be met with force'

But friendly words cannot tame a serpent. There is but one way to do it-to remove the serpent's fangs.

Even before the ink with which they had signed the Kutch agreement dried up, Pakisthan raised its hood to strike again. Pakistani soldiers entered Kashmir in disguise. In September 1965 there was a large-scale invasion of the territory by Pakistani soldiers in the Chhamb area. War broke out all along the Cease-fire Line on the Kashmir border.

The enemies who had managed to enter Kashmir were cunning and mischievous. Pakistan also tried to incite Indian Muslims. The Pakisthan army was engaged in forcibly occupying areas, which belonged to India. There was the danger of the fighting spreading to the eastern border also. In addition to this, there was the threat posed by the Chinese on the northern borders of India. Lal Bahadur Shastri faced all these problems with a will of iron. It was at this time that the country understood the greatness of Lal Bahadur Shastri. He decided that was the time to teach Pakistan a lesson. He gave full freedom to the Commander of the Army. 'Go forward and strike' was Shastriji's command to the generals.

Addressing the nation on 13th August 1965 Shastriji referred to Pakistan's threats and said, "Force will be met with force." Two days later, during the celebration of Independence day, he declared from the ramparts of the Red Fort: "It does not matter if we are destroyed. We will fight to the last to maintain the high honour of the Indian nation and its flag."

'CHINA CANNOT FRIGHTEN US'

Just at this time another danger threatened India. China sent a letter, which said, "The Indian army has set up army equipment in Chinese territory. India should pull down this equipment. Otherwise it will have to face the wrath of China."

At that moment India was fighting against the Pakistani army equipped with the latest weapons supplied in plenty by the United States of America. And, at this very moment how was India to resist China?

China's allegations were a bundle of lies. If India removed the military equipment she would be admitting that China's charges were true. Also, that would mean India was afraid of China.

Even the big nations waited breathlessly to see what Lal Bahadur would say and what India would do.

Lal Bahadur did not take long to give a reply. The letter from China was received on the morning of 17th September 1965. He made a statement in the Parliament the same afternoon. He declared: "China's allegation is untrue. If China attacks India it is our firm resolve to fight for our freedom. The might of China will not deter us from defending our territorial integrity."

China kept quiet.

India's soldiers had no fear of death and fought most splendidly and heroically. The army and the air force functioned like the two arms of a single body. The invaders were beaten. The Pakistani army could not stand against the Indian army. It was then that, for the first time, the world came to realize the supremacy of the Indian army.

TASHKENT-TREATY

Some big nations feared that, if India won a total victory over Pakistan, it would lower their prestige. The Security Council of the United Nations Organization called on India and Pakistan to stop fighting. On the invitation of Kosygin, the Premier of Soviet Russia, Lal Bahadur Shastri and Ayub Khan met in Tashkent on January 4, 1966. The leaders agreed that their armies should withdraw to the old Cease-fire Line in Kashmir and that the two countries should live in peace and friendship.

Many people in India felt that we should not return the territory taken from Pakistan-occupied Kashmir. They argued that the entire Kashmir belonged to India. But Shastriji wished to give one more chance to Pakistan to live in peace and friendship with India. So he signed the treaty of friendship.

Shastriji is Immortal

Shastriji had suffered heart attacks twice before. And during the period of the Pakistan war and the following days, his body, already battered, had to bear a very heavy strain. He signed the joint Declaration on 10th January 1966. He died the same night.

The news of Lal Bahadur Shastri's death struck India like a bolt from the blue. The entire nation was plunged in grief. Some people suspected foulplay also. Gone was the war hero and the messenger of peace, gone was the great statesman who restored to India her honour and self-respect in the assembly of nations. A tiny, tidy figure. A soul that had lived in perfect purity of thought, word and deed. The very embodiment of selflessness, detachment and simplicity. Such was this man who had lived in our midst. He belongs to the race of the heroes of India. Lal Bahadur Shastri became the second Prime Minister of India after the death of Jawaharlal Nehru on 27 May 1964. He served the nation as Prime Minister for 19 months and two days i.e. from 9 June 1964 to 11 January 1966, at a very crucial period of independent India.

Shastri was born on 2 October 1904 at Mughalsarai, a railway colony about seven miles from Varanasi. At the age of ten he came to Benares to stay with his maternal uncle and started his studies. In 1921, responding to Gandhiji's call for non-cooperation he gave up his studies and joined the freedom struggle.

As a schoolboy, he had read the speeches of Tilak, Bipin Chandra Pal, Lajpat Rai and Gokhale. He enrolled himself as a life member of the Servants of the People Society and began to work for the upliftment of the Harijans at Muzaffarpur. In 1951 he was made the General Secretary of the A.I.C.C., with Jawaharlal Nehru as the President. From 1951 to 1956 he served as Minister of Railways and Transport in the Central Cabinet. He accepted moral and constitutional responsibility for the Aliyalur railway accident in 1956 and resigned. From 1957 to 1961 he was again in the Central Cabinet and held several portfolios successively as Minister of Transport and Communications, Minister of Commerce and Industry and Minister for Home.

Lal Bahadur Shastri was simple and unassuming in his behaviour, kind and gentle in his dealings and his ever-modest qualities endeared him to the masses of India. He was one of those few leaders, who, born in poverty, won recognition by their talent and sacrifice. Rising from the rank of an unknown worker, churning out cyclostyled copies of political leaflets at Anand Bhavan, to the position of highest authority as the Prime Minister of India.

Shastriji successfully led the nation during 22-day war with Pakistan in 1965. He gave the slogan of "Jai Jawan, Jai Kisan", which led to a rare display of unity in the country during Indo-Pak war. During 1965 he visited Russia, Yugoslavia, England, Canada and Burma. On January 10, 1966 he signed the historic Joint communique with President Agha Khan of Pakistan at Tashkent. Within few hours of the signing of the Declaration, the Hero of Tashkent passed away at Tashkent. The end came in the early hours at 1.32 a.m. on 11.1.1966. The great little man of masses died at the height of his career.

A great Indian patriot, a freedom fighter, a man of the people and a remarkable Prime Minister: the late Shri Lal Bahadur Shastri. While it is matter of coincidence that Shastriji shares a birthday with Mahatma Gandhi, his abiding commitment to the values and ideals of the Mahatma is truly significant.

Shastriji's life is aptly described as an illustration of the practical application of Gandhian principles. While in government, he abided by Gandhiji's dictum that when in office, "always sit light, never tight". Shastriji's innate sense of humility, sincerity and simplicity enabled him to establish a deep bond with people, and to easily strike a chord of understanding.

It is worth recalling that like many amongst his generation, Shastriji also gave up his studies to join the freedom struggle in response to Gandhiji's call to strengthen the non-cooperation movement. He was arrested for the first time at the age of seventeen, and again, like many of the stalwarts of our independence movement, prison was to become a second home. All told, Shastriji was sent to prison seven times, spending as many as nine long years in various prisons.

Despite his involvement in the freedom struggle, following the non-cooperation movement, Shri Lal Bahadur resumed and completed his studies at the Kashi Vidya Peeth. He was awarded the degree of "Shastri" in philosophy and the humanities, and this was the reason for the public at large to address him as "Shastriji". Those were also the years in which he joined the Servants of India society, which burnished his image as a man of simple habits, great commitment, diligence and sincerity. Shastriji was to participate in many landmark events of our freedom struggle, including the salt satyagraha and the Quit India movement. His organizational skills were noticed at an early stage. In an early recognition of his abilities, Shastriji was appointed as the Organizing Secretary of the Parliamentary Board of UP in 1937.

Subsequent to our independence, Shastriji graduated rapidly from state level politics to the national level. In the first General Elections of our Republic, Shastriji was General Secretary of the Congress Party. He was directly responsible for the selection of candidates and the direction of publicity and electioneering activities. In recognition of his abilities and his commitment to the values of the Congress Party, Pandit Nehru picked him for the Rajya Sabha, to utilize his talents in government.

Shastriji's first Ministerial term was as Railways and Transport Minister in the Union Cabinet in 1952. He worked to improve the functioning of the railways, guiding their transition out of the colonial era. Today, many of the younger generation may not be aware of these efforts, but most would have heard of Shastriji's resignation from the Ministerial post, taking moral responsibility for a major accident. In a tribute to his convictions, Panditji was to say that "no man can wish for a better comrade and better colleague in any undertaking". Despite this setback, Shastriji was to hold several other important portfolios in Panditji's cabinet, including the portfolios of Transport and Communications, Commerce and the Home Ministry.

Apart from his contributions to Panditji's Cabinet, Shastriji also contributed to the growth of the Congress Party. It was only natural, therefore, that when Panditji passed away in May 1964, a distraught country and Party turned to Shastriji for leadership. The choice of a successor was a major national concern in the early 1960s. "After Nehru Who?" was an oft-repeated question in the newspapers. Shri Lal Bahadur Shastri prove to the world that he was a worthy successor.

Shastriji's brief tenure of eighteen months as Prime Minister was testing times for our young Republic. And yet through crises such as war and privation, Shastriji's immense moral courage, character and great intuition were visible in his calm and effective leadership. In fact it would not be incorrect to say that few leaders of any democracy could have endured so many trials in such a short period of time. But the dexterity with which Shastriji braved complex challenges remains an inspiring episode in our recent history. It requires extraordinary courage and determination to have steered a vast and complex country like ours through such difficult times. The nation will always remember his slogan with which he captured the Nation's pride in our soldiers and our farmers: Jai Jawan, Jai Kisan. His sudden demise in Tashkent in 1966 was an enormous blow.

Today, as we launch the Birth Centenary celebrations of Shri Lal Bahadur Shastriji, we remember his sincerity of purpose and his commitment to integrity in public life. These qualities are the need of the hour, in our collective effort to steer our country through contentious times on the path of economic and social development. Whether it is the soldier, the farmer, the scientist, the worker, the entrepreneur, the teacher or the public official, each one of us plays a vital role in the process of nation building. Therefore, in the spirit of commitment exemplified by Shastriji, I wish to urge all of us to rekindle that sense of idealism, which inspired our freedom struggle. The best way for us to pay tribute to the memory of patriots like Shastriji is for us to live by the principles they cherished, of service to the Nation and pursuit of truth, with firm resolve, simple living and high thinking.

I would like to conclude with the hope that the National Committee of eminent persons with which the Government is consulting for activities to commemorate the centenary of Lal Bahadur Shastri will be able to develop suitable events to pay a truly fitting tribute to the memory of this great son of India.

Lal Bahadur Shastri was born in 1905 in Prayag. His father Sharada Prasad, a schoolteacher at the local school, passed away when Lal Bahadur was barely a year and a half. Growing up without a father forced Lal Bahadur to accept responsibility at an early age. He was sent by his uncle to Varanasi to pursue his studies.

After a short stay with a family that treated him unkindly, Lal Bahadur stayed with a teacher, Mishraji. Mishraji often sat and told stories about how India lost her freedom to the British to young Lal Bahadur. These conversations later inspired Lal Bahadur to join the struggle for Indian freedom

At about this time Gandhiji came to Varanasi and spoke of his non-cooperation movement. Lal Bahadur took a keen interest in the growing movement and when the time came to boycott the schools, he did so by not appearing for his examinations. With just one year left for his graduation, the news was not taken well at home. Neither his Uncle nor Mishraji supported Lal Bahadur's action, but his mother who had complete faith in him, supported his decision as long as he promised not to renege from the task later. With his mother's blessings, he became fully involved in the non-cooperation movement. He was arrested for taking part in banned processions but released since it was his first offense. This was to be the first of many arrests for Lal Bahadur. He worked during the evenings in a khadi shop and studied while studying for the degree of Shastri (Bachelor) in Philosophy. Lal Bahadur graduated at the head of his class.

He then went on to do social work among the Harijans, working to make their lives better. Two years later he married Lalita Devi. Lal Bahadur and Lalita moved to Allahabad where Lal Bahadur served as secretary of the District Congress Committee. He attended the 1929 Lahore session of the Congress, and upon his return to Allahabad actively spoke out against the British Raj and for "Purna Swaraj". As protests continued more and more people were arrested for participating in the struggle. When Lalita Devi mentioned to Lal Bahadur that the jails were full, he replied in his characteristic fashion, "Yes, but there is still room for me."

He was arrested a few days later. During his stay in jail his wife gave birth to their first child Kusum. He had two other children, Hari and Suman.

His total commitment to Gandhiji and the non-cooperation movement resulted in many jail terms. Since the Congress party was banned by the British Government, Lal Bahadur and his associates spent their time travelling around India spreading Gandhiji's message. He was soon arrested for these activities, and jailed for seven months at an unknown location. Eighteen months later Lalita Devi was granted permission to meet her husband

Lal Bahadur was finally released from prison in 1946. On August 15, 1947 India gained independence. Lal Bahadur was appointed Minister of Police in Nehru's cabinet. In 1951 Jawaharlal Nehru was re-elected Prime Minister for a second term, and Lal Bahadur was appointed General Secretary of the Lok Sabha. While in Nehru's cabinet, Lal Bahadur was entrusted with portfolios for Minister of Railways, Minister of Communications and later Home Minister. He served as Nehru's right hand. On May 27, 1964 Pandit Jawaharlal Nehru died. May of that year Lal Bahadur Shastri became India's second Prime Minister. His term is best known for introducing measures to make India self-sufficient in food production.

In 1965 Pakistan attacked India on the Kashmiri front and Lal Bahadur Shastri responded in kind by punching toward Lahore. In 1966 a cease-fire was issued as a result of international pressure. Lal Bahadur Shastri went to Tashkent to hold talks with Ayub Khan and an agreement was soon signed.

Lal Bahadur passed away in Tashkent before returning home. He was posthumously conferred with the Bharat Ratna Award.

5

Freedom Struggle and Lal Bahadur Shastri

BIOGRAPHY OF LAL BAHADUR SHASTRI

Lal Bahadur Shastri was born at 2nd October in 1904 at Mughalsarai (seven miles away from Kashi), Uttar Pradesh in a simple family and died on 10th January in 1966. His father name was Mr. Sharada Prasad and mother name was Mrs. Ramdulari Devi. His father died when he was only a year old. He was Srivastava but he never added it as his surname because he did not want to point out his caste. His father was a school teacher followed by a clerk in the Revenue Office of Allahabad.

His mother lost him when he was just three months old. She went to bathe in the Ganga with him and in the crowed she lost her child as he slipped away from her arms into the cowherd's basket. She was very sorrow and made a complaint with the police. Finally, police traced the child. Cowherd wept resentfully in returning the child.

One of another incident of his childhood (when he was six years old) taught him an important lesson of his life. Once upon a time he was returning with friends from his school and went to an orchard which was on the way to home. His friends climbed on a mango tree in order to get mangos and he was stand below the tree. In the meantime, the gardener reached there and started to beat him by mistake. He begged too much to gardener in order to get free from him and told that he was an orphan. Gardener said to Lal Bahadur Shastri that as you are an orphan, it is most important for you that you have to learn much better manners." That event impressed him deeply and he decided to behave better in his future.

He got his education from the East Central Railway Inter College in the Mughalsarai, Varanasi. He had completed his graduation from the Kashi

Vidyapeeth, Varanasi in the year 1926 and awarded with the title of Shastri ("Scholar"). He was much influenced by the great Indian leaders such as the Mahatma Gandhi and Bal Gangadhar Tilak. He became the father of six children including Hari Krishna Shastri, Anil Shastri, Sunil Shastri who became politician in the Congress party and Ashok Shastri who became a BJP politician.

He joined the Servants of the People Society as a life member (working for the development of the Harijans) and became the Society President.

HIS CAREER

Marriage

He got married to the Lalitha Devi of Mirzapur on 16th of May in 1928 and took a charkha and few yards of Khadi as a marriage gift.

Non-cooperation movement

Till the age ten he stayed at his grandfather's home and had passed the 6th standard. He has completed his higher education from Varanasi. He had joined the non-cooperation movement against British Government in 1921 by Mahatma Gandhi when he was only seventeen years old. Even he was arrested during that movement but he was firm in his decision. He took part in that movement even after advice from his mother and relatives to not to do so.

The servants of the people society

He joined the Kashi Vidya Peeth after his release and completed his philosophy study. He got the degree of Shastri in 1926 and after leaving Kashi Vidya Peeth he had joined the "The Servants of the People Society" started by Lala Lajpat Rai in 1921. The aim of the "The Servants of the People Society" was to aware youths about their responsibilities towards country.

Civil Disobedience Movement

In 1930, he joined the Civil Disobedience Movement as there was call to him from Gandhi Ji. He was called to join that movement in order to encourage people to oppose to pay land profits and taxes to the government. He had to go in jail for two and half years. He got familiar with all the works of western philosophers, revolutionaries as well as social reformers in the jail.

Individual Satyagraha

Individual Satyagraha was launched by the Congress in 1940 in order to demand freedom just after the Second World War in 1939. He got arrested for one year during that Individual Satyagraha as well. He again got a call from Gandhi Ji on August 8, 1942 for Quit India Movement. He took part very actively and got arrested for long. He met with the Pandit Govind Vallabh Pant and got good comments for his hard work throughout the 1946 provincial elections. He was appointed as the Parliamentary Secretary of Pandit Govind Vallabh Pant (when Pandit Govind Vallabh Pant became the Chief Minister of UP). He became the Police and Transport Minister in Pant's Cabinet in 1947.

He became the Congress Party's General Secretary as soon as India became Republic. He again appointed as the Minister of Railways and Transport in the Central Cabinet in 1952 by Jawahar Lal Nehru. His contribution for travelers in third class compartments is unforgettable because he had deducted the huge difference between the Railways first class and third class. He resigned from Railways in 1956 after a railway accident.

Again, when Congress came into the power, he became the Transport and Communications Minister and later Commerce and Industry Minister. In 1961, after the death of the Govind Vallabh Pant, he became the Home Minister. He had well maintained the internal security of the country in the India-China war in 1962.

He was respected the Bal Gangadhar Tilak too much and used to see him for long as well as hear his speech. Once Bal Gangadhar Tilak visited Varanasi and Lal Bahadur Shastri was fifty miles away from Varanasi in a village. He took some money from his friend and traveled in a train to see and hear the speech of Tilak. Tilak's speech ringed in his ears always and had great effect on his life. The greatest effect on his life was that of Mahatma Gandhi and he devoted his life to the country.

POLITICAL CAREER OF LAL BAHADUR SHASTRI

As a State Minister

After the independence of India, he was selected as the Parliamentary Secretary in his own state, Uttar Pradesh. On 15th of August in the year 1947, he allotted as the Minister of Police and Transport under the Chief Ministership of the Govind Ballabh Pant. He was the first Transport Minister who employed women conductors and Minister of Police who ordered to use jets of water in place of lathis to the police to scatter the public crowds.

As a Cabinet Minister

He was selected as the General Secretary of All-India Congress Committee in the year 1951 when Jawaharlal Nehru was the Prime Minister. As a General

Secretary, he was in charge for the candidates selection and all the activities related to the election. On 3rd of April in 1952, he was nominated to the Rajya Sabha from UP and appointed as the Railways and Transport Minister in the Central Cabinet from 13th of May, 1952 to 7th of December, 1956. After a railways accident at Mahbubnagar in the month of September in 1956, he resigned from the Railways and Transport Ministership which was rejected by the Nehru. After a second railway accident at Ariyalur in the Tamil Nadu, he again resigned from the Railways and Transport Ministership.

He returned to the Cabinet in the year 1957 as a Minister for Transport and Communications and then Minister of Commerce and Industry. He also became the Union Home Minister in the year 1961 and worked on the Prevention of Corruption in the India.

As a Prime Minister of India

In 1964, after the death of the Jawaharlal Nehru, he became the second Prime Minister of India and led India to get success in the war from the Pakistan in 1965. That was very difficult time for the country and everyone were facing huge challenges. Country was facing food shortage and Pakistan had attacked India. He was a man of great valor and will and he has given a slogan "Jai Jawan Jai Kisan" in order to assemble the support of country throughout the war. His leadership was admired all across the world. He lived his life with the immense simplicity and truthfulness and was a great source of motivation to all the Indians.

During his Prime Ministership lots of good and bad events have occurred including Indo-Pak war and his mysterious death. Details of some of the events are mentioned below:

His Contribution in the Domestic Policies through solving the Madras anti-Hindi agitation

When he was assigned as a Prime Minister of the India after the death of the former Prime Minister, Jawaharlal Nehru on 27th of May in 1964, he retained various earlier members from the Council of Jawaharlal Nehru such as Yashwantrao Chavan as a Defence Minister of India, Swaran Singh as an External Affairs Minister, Indira Gandhi as a Minister of Information and Broadcasting, Gulzarilal Nanda as a Minister of Home Affairs of India, T. T. Krishnamachari as a Finance Minister of India and etc.

He also has involved in solving the Madras anti-Hindi agitation in the year 1965. As Indian mother tongue (sole national language) is Hindi, it was opposed by some of the Indian states talking non-Hindi language like English.

In order to handle that situation, he decided in his meeting with Indira Gandhi to continue the English as an official language by the non-Hindi speaking states of the India. After his positive assurance the riots was settled to calm.

His Contribution in the Economic Policies through his White Revolution and Green Revolution Campaign

During his Prime Ministership, he had involved in maintaining as well as enhancing the Indian economy through his great policies. He made his own policies for enhancing the Indian economy as well as continued the socialist economic policies of the former prime minister. He had promoted the most famous national campaign of increasing the supply and production of milk called White Revolution through supporting various dairy companies like Amul milk co-operative of Anand of Gujarat and setting up the National Dairy Development Board.

His great involvement to the management of chronic food shortage all over the India can never be forgotten. He had requested to the Indian people to give up their one meal of the day on their own will in order to save some food for the people living in the affected area of food shortage. He had promoted the Green Revolution campaign (by creating his slogan "Jai Jawan Jai Kisan") all over the India in order to boost up the food production all across the India during the food shortage during 22 days long Indo-Pak war of 1965.

His Contribution to the Country through his Slogan "Jai Jawan Jai Kisan"

He was a great Prime Minister of India as he had given his outstanding supports and efforts in making the country a developed country. He is remembered all over the country by the people at his birthday anniversary and death anniversary each year. Even after being an ordinary Indian person he worked so great like an extraordinary man to lead his country.

He became a successful Prime Minister of the India as he led the India during its most disastrous conditions like Indo-Pak war, food shortage and tec. He had created his own slogan of Jai Jawan Jai Kisan to solve the problem of food shortage all over the India during the Indo-Pak war of 1965.

His Contribution in the Foreign Policies

He had paid great involvement in the foreign policies to enhance the country defense budget by increasing the closer relationship with the Soviet Union after the disastrous condition of the country of Sino-Indian War in 1962. He had decided to increase the defense budget of armed forces of the country after the military ties of Chinese People's Republic and Pakistan. He also had signed the agreement of Srimavo-Shastri Pact (Bandaranaike-Shastri pact) in 1964 with the Prime minister of Sri Lanka (Sirimavo Bandaranaike) considering the Indian Tamils status in the then Ceylon. During this agreement sign up a big settlement was done between India and Sri Lanka, around 600,000 Indian Tamils were freed up and around 375,000 were granted citizenship of Sri Lanka. However, on 31st of October in 1981, this settlement was lapsed by India due to the death of the Lal Bahadur Shastri and only 300,000 Indian Tamils were repatriated and only 185,000 were granted citizenship by the Sri Lanka.

Indo-Pak War

He was a great warrior who led the India to get victory in the Indo-Pak War in the year 1965. He had said in his statement that during the economic development of the country, we would favor to be alive in the poverty for long time according to the necessity but we never let our freedom to be threatened. The purpose of Pakistan was Kashmir during the Indo-Pak War, however, Lal Bahadur Shashtri made them clear that force would be answered only with force. After a long period of time, the Indo-Pak war finished on 23rd of September in the year 1965 with the involvement of United Nation to ceasefire peaceful coexistence.

After the end of war between India and Pakistan, Lal Bahadur Shastri and Pakistani President Muhammad Ayub Khan went for a meeting in the Tashkent where both of them had signed the Tashkent Declaration on 10th of January in the year 1966.

LAL BAHADUR SHASTRI DEATH MYSTERY

He endured a fatal heart attack some hours after signing a treaty on 10th of January in 1966, in which India and Pakistan have the same opinion to not to interfere in each other internal affairs as well as never force or settle disputes between them by the peaceful means. He died on 11th of January in the year 1966.

Great achievements:

He played a great and leading role for the freedom of India. He became the Pandit Govind Vallabh Pant's Parliamentary Secretary followed by the chief minister of UP. In the Pant's Cabinet he became the Minister of Police as well as Transport and allotted as the Minister of the Railways and Transport in the Central Cabinet. He also apprehended the assortments of Commerce and Industry, Transport and Communications, as well as the Home Ministry in the Central cabinet.

Bharat Ratna

He was a dazzling star of an Indian history. The President of India bestowed him the award of "Bharat Ratna" after his death.

Lal Bahadur Shashtri Quotes

- "True democracy or the swaraj of the masses can never come through untruthful and violent means, for the simple reason that the natural corollary to their use would be to remove all opposition through the suppression or extermination of the antagonists".
- "That loyalty to the country comes ahead of all other loyalties. And this is an absolute loyalty, since one cannot weight it in terms of what one receives".
- "Those who govern must see how the people react to administration. Ultimately, the people are the final arbiters."
- "Success in science and scientific work come not through the provision of unlimited or big resources, but in the wise and careful selection of problems and objectives. Above all, what is required is hard sustained work and dedication".
- "We believe in peace and peaceful development, not only for ourselves but for people all over the world. Our main preoccupation is with economic and social development at home and peace and friendship abroad".
- "The emphasis on religion as a basis of defining majorities and minorities in a secular state is quite misplaced and contradiction in terms. You all understand, I am sure, that religion does not aim at dividing. On the other hand, all true religions have a basic unity".
- "In this vast country of ours, people profess different religions, speak different languages, dress differently and observe different customs; but we are one nation; the history of our struggle for independence and our faith in our future development are our common bonds".
- "Sampling out corruption is a very tough job, but I say so in all seriousness that we would be failing in our duty if we do not tackle this problem seriously and with determination".
- "India will have to hang down her head in shame if even one person is left who is said in any way to be untouchable".
- "If Pakistan has any ideas of annexing any part of our territories by

force, she should think afresh. I want to state categorically that force will be met with force and aggression against us will never be allowed to succeed."

Monuments of Lal Bahadur Shastri in India

Lal Bahadur Shastri is a famous person all over the India for his great Prime Ministership and outstanding efforts towards the country. For his big achievements and great job he has been honored with the honorable Indian award called Bharat Ratna. There are various memorials has been made all over the country by the government of India behind him in order to commemorate him and his outstanding supports for the country. Some of the memorials made behind him are listed below:

- Vijay Ghat in Delhi.
- Lal Bahadur Shastri National Academy of Administration in Mussorie, Uttarakhand
- Shastri Indo-Canadian Institute.
- It has been declared by the government of India in 2011to make a biographical museum at this ancestral house in Ramnagar, Varanasi.
- Lal Bahadur Shastri International Airport, Babatpur, Varanasi (Varanasi International Airport).
- Lal Bahadur Shastri National Memorial Trust at 10 Janpath, Motilal Nehru Place, New Delhi.
- A Street in the Tashkent, Uzbekistan is named after him.
- Lal Bahadur Shastri Sagar (Almatti Dam), Northern Karnataka.
- A Cargo Ship is named as MV Lal Bahadur Shastri.
- Five rupee coins, having image of Lal Bahadur Shastri and written his name as "LALBAHADUR SHASTRI BIRTH CENTENARY", were released by the RBI at his 100th birth anniversary in 2004.

Lal Bahadur Shastri Timeline

1904: Born on 2nd of October in Mughalsarai, India.

1926: Completed Graduation in 1st class honor from the Kashi Vidyapeeth and awarded with the title of Shastri ("Scholar").

1921: He had joined Indian Independence Movement.

1928: Got married to the Lalita Devi from Mirzapur on 16th of May.

1930: Started participating in the Salt Satyagraha of Mahatma Gandhi.

1937: Chosen as organizing secretary of the Parliamentary Board of U.P.

1940: went to the jail for one year because of his active participation to the Indian freedom movement.

1942: Went to the jail for years till 1946 for his active participation in the Quit-India Movement.

1947: He was selected as the Parliamentary Secretary in Uttar Pradesh and on 15th of August he became Home Minister of the Uttar Pradesh state.

1951: He was selected as the General Secretary of All-India Congress Committee in the Prime Ministership of Pt. Jawaharlal Nehru.

1952: He entered to Rajya Sabha after getting elected from U.P. and became Railway and Transport minister.

1956: In the month of September he resigned from the post of Railway ministry after a big accident which was unaccepted by the Pt. Nehru.

1956: In the month of December he again resigned from the same post after another railway accident in the Tamil Nadu however that was accepted.

1957: He entered again into the Cabinet.

1961: He again elected as the Home Minister.

1964: On 9th of June, he became the most honorable Prime Minister of India.

1964: on 11th of June, he had given his first speech as a Prime Minister of India.

1964: He signed an agreement with the Prime minister of Sri Lanka (Sirimavo Bandaranaike) regarding the status of Indian Tamils.

1965: He solved the Madras anti-Hindi agitation by assuring people about the continuation of English language as an official language.

1965: He had supported the Amul and White Revolution in order to create a National Dairy Development Board in India as well as requested people to skip at least one meal a day to deal with the food shortage in country.

1965: In the month of August and September, he courageously faced the War with Pakistan and encouraged Indian people by giving the slogan of "Jai Jawan – Jai Kisan".

1965: On 23rd of September, the war with Pakistan was ended in his Prime Ministership with the ceasefire mandated by UN.

1966: On 10th of January, He signed the Tashkent Declaration with the Ayub Khan of Pakistan.

1966: On 11th of January, He died in Tashkent because of the Heart Attack

1966: He became the first person of India to be awarded with the Bharat Ratna.

1966: In the honor of him, the National Academy of Administration of India was renamed as "Lal Bahadur Shastri National Academy of Administration".

THE YOUNG SATYAGRAHI

In 1921, Mahatma Gandhi launched the non-cooperation movement against British Government and declared that the country would not cooperate with the Government in its unjust rule. Lal Bahadur was then only seventeen years.

When Mahatma Gandhi gave a call to the youth to come out of Government schools and colleges, offices and courts and to sacrifice everything for the sake of freedom, Lal Bahadur came out of his school.

His mother and other relatives advised him not to give up his studies. But Lal Bahadur was firm in his decision-Lai Bahadur joined the procession, which disobeyed the prohibitory order. The police arrested him. But as he was too young, he was let off.

Lal Bahadur did not go back to his school. He became a student of Kashi Vidya Peeth. During his four years' stay there, he made excellent progress. Dr. Bhagawandas's lectures on philosophy went straight to his heart. In later life Lal Bahadur displayed surprising poise in the midst of conflict and confusion. This he learnt from his teacher, Bhagawandas.

'The Servants of the People Society'

It was in 1926 that Lal Bahadur got the degree of 'Shastri' and left the Kashi Vidya Peeth. The whole country became the arena of his activity. He became the life-member of The Servants of the People Society, which Lala Lajpat Rai had started in 1921. The aim of the Society was to train youths that were prepared to dedicate their lives to the service of the country.

One of the rules of the Society required the members to take an oath to serve the Society at least for twenty years and to lead a simple and honest life till the end. Lal Bahadur earned the love and affection of Lajpat Rai by his earnestness and hard work. Later he became the President of the Society.

Shastriji married in 1927. Lalitha Devi, his bride, came from Mirzalyur. The wedding was celebrated in the simplest way. All that the bridegroom took as a gift from father-in-law was a charaka and a few yards of Khadi

FREEDOM'S SOLDIER

The struggle for freedom was intensified all over the country in 1930. Mahatma Gandhi started the 'Salt Satyagraha'. Lal Bahadur took a leading role in it.

At the age of seventeen Lal Bahadur had participated in a procession against the British Government. The government had arrested him and then freed him. But this time it did not let him off easily. He had been calling on people not to pay land revenue and taxes to the government and the government had been keeping a wary eye on him. Now he was sent to prison for two and a half years.

From this time onwards prison became his second home. He was sent to prison seven times and was forced to spend nine long years in various prisons on different occasions.

His going to prison was a blessing in disguise. He had time to read a number of good books. He became familiar with the works of western philosophers, revolutionaries and social reformers. He translated the autobiography of Madam Curie (a French scientist who discovered radium) into Hindi.

Lal Bahadur's virtues shone even in the prison. He was a ideal prisoner. 'He was a model to others in discipline and restraint. Many political prisoners used to quarrel among themselves for small things. They used to cringe for small favours before the officials of the prison. But Lal Bahadur used to give up his comforts for others.

Sense of Honour

The greatness of Lal Bahadur was that he maintained his self-respect 'even in prison. Once when he was in prison, one of his daughters fell seriously ill. The officers agreed to let him out for a short time but on condition that he should agree in writing not to take part in the freedom 'movement during this period. Lal Bahadur did not wish to participate in the freedom movement during his temporary release from prison; but he said that he would not give it in writing. He thought that it was against his self-respect to give it in writing. The officers knew that he was truthful. Therefore they did not insist. Lal Bahadur was released for fifteen days.

But his daughter died before he, reached home. After performing the obsequies he returned to his prison even before the expiry of the period.

A year passed. His son was laid up with influenza this time. Lal Bahadur was permitted unconditionally to go home for a week. But the fever did not come down in a week. Lal Bahadur got ready to go back to prison. The boy pleaded dumbly with his tearful eyes.

In a weak voice he urged his father to stay.

For a moment the father's mind was shaken. Tears rolled down from his eyes.

But the next moment his decision was made. He bade good bye to all and left his home for prison. His son survived.

Two qualities, which the leader of any nation must have, are devotion and efficiency. Lal Bahadur had both the qualities in a large measure. He would not swerve from his aim, come what may. When the people of India. Were fighting for freedom he brushed aside all thought of personal happiness and plunged into the freedom struggle. His daughter's death, his son's illness, poverty-none of these made him swerve from his selection path. Even when he became a minister and, later, the Prime Minister he was never attracted to a life of luxury and comfort.

In Prison Again

When the Second World War broke out in 1939, the leaders of our country were in a dilemma. When the people of India were slaves how could they support the cause of Britain?

In the end they decided to launch a 'Satyagraha' against the British Government for the freedom of the country (1940). Satyagraha means opposition based on Truth. Lal Bahadur was one of those who offered individual Satyagraha. He was sent to prison for one year for this.

The freedom struggle became more widespread and intense. The prisons were bursting with political prisoners.

On 8th August 1942, the Indian National Congress which led the fight for freedom decided at its historic meeting in Bombay to sound the trumpet for the final struggle against the British in India. It called on the British to 'Quit India'. The people were determined to 'do or die'.

The government reacted sharply to these calls and arrested many leaders. Prisons became over-crowded. The government used all cruel methods of suppression to nip the movement in the bud.

Lal Bahadur, who had just then come out after a year in prison, travelled from Bombay to Allahabad by train. He got off at a station, unknown to the police. For a whole week he used to send instructions to the freedom fighters from Anand Bhavan, Jawaharlal Nehru's home in Allahabad.

Vijayalakshmi Pandit, the sister of Nehru, lived in Anand Bhavan at the time. The police came there to arrest her and to take possession of the house. Lal Bahadur destroyed all-important documents. Luckily, the police arrested only Vijayalakshmi Pandit and went away.

A few days later Lal Bahadur who was underground came out and shouted slogans against the government. The police arrested him then.

A New Arena

India got freedom in 1947. Lal Bahadur's administrative ability and skill in organization came to light in the days following India's freedom. He was an expert in the art of bringing together people and winning their hearts. Pandit Govind Vallabh Pant, the leader of Uttar Pradesh, was the first to recognize this talent of Shastriji and to encourage him. He earned the love of Pant by his hard work during the elections of 1946 in the provinces. The Congress Office had become Shastriji's home during that period. The Congress won a resounding victory in the elections.

When Govind Vallabh Pant became the Chief Minister of Uttar Pradesh, he wished to train able young men to run the government. But it was not easy to please him. Lal Bahadur did not want any office; yet he was appointed as Parliamentary Secretary to Pant. Pant praised him as 'likable, hard-working, devoted, trustworthy and non-controversial'.

THE RESPONSIBILITY OF FREEDOM

Later, in 1947, Lal Bahadur became the Minister of Police and Transport in Pant's Ministry. He took many steps to bring discipline into the administration. As Transport Minister he subjected government buses to discipline. He was the first to appoint women conductors. Usually the minister in charge of the Police Department will not remain popular for long. But Lal Bahadur Shastri never allowed the police to resort to lathi charge and firing. He ordered that using jets of water instead of lathis should disperse unruly crowds. Though there were many strikes in Uttar Pradesh when he was in office, there was not a single occasion when people shouted slogans against him.

Lal Bahadur was a lover of cricket. Once he was watching a match at Kanpur. Trouble broke out among the spectators. The Police and young men came to blows. Since Shastriji was on the spot the situation did not go out of control. The young men demanded that the red turbans' (the police) should not be found on the cricket ground and Lal Bahadur agreed. But the police were there the next day. The young men became angry with Shastriji and protested. Lal Bahadur laughed and said, "I fulfilled my promise to you faithfully. You did not want red turbans to be here. You see the police are now wearing khaki turbans." The spectators laughed and dropped the matter.

THE MIGHT OF PEACE*

"There come a time in the life of every nation when it stands at the cross-roads of history and must choose which way to go. But for us there need be no difficulty or hesitation, no looking to right or left. Our way is straight and clear – the building up of a socialist democracy at home with freedom and prosperity for all, and the maintenance of world peace and friendship with all nations".

Lal Bahadur Shastri in his first broadcast as Prime Minister-June 11, 1964.

Son of a humble school-master and orphaned at a tender age, he (Lal Bahadur Shastri) knew what poverty meant and understood the people's wants and suffering...

Lal Bahadur was a tireless worker. The only rest he got was in jail where he spent various terms of imprisonment during the national struggle. In all, he was in jail for nine years.

Ideal Successor

The unusual combination of qualities in Lal Bahadur – his high sense of purpose, his zeal, his gentleness and humility, his moderation in speech and decisiveness in action, his homespun wisdom, his humour and unwavering common sense – these and his ability to master intricate matters and find amicable solutions made him an ideal successor to Jawaharlal Nehru. On June 2, 1964, six days after the death of Nehru this unusual person who had risen gently to the top of Indian politics without making a single enemy was unanimously chosen by the Congress party to be its Parliamentary leader and in that capacity to serve as Prime Minister of India.

Primary Task

He regarded it as one of his primary tasks to find a way in which India and Pakistan could live amicably. Indo-Pakistan relations were to occupy so much of his attention during his brief but memorable 19 months in office that it is worth remembering what he said at the very outset of his onerous stewardship. "India and Pakistan", he declared in his first broadcast as Prime Minister, "are two great countries linked together by common, history and tradition. It is their natural destiny to be friends with each other and to enter into close co-operation between these two countries will not only be of immense benefit to them but will make a great contribution to peace and prosperity in Asia. For too long have India and Pakistan been at odds with each other... We must reverse the tide. This will require determination and good sense on the part of the governments and people of both India and Pakistan".

But before the tide was reversed – that was to be Lal Bahadur's crowning achievement at Tashkent – much was to happen. Early in 1965 Pakistan sent its troops, equipped with heavy armour, across the border in Kutch to enforce its claim to territory in that region. The terrain and timing of this action gave the advantage to Pakistan. But Lal Bahadur acted with decision and courage...

Confrontation in Kutch

In his report to the Lok Sabha on the confrontation in Kutch the Prime Minister said : "Ever since the attainment of Independence, India has stood for peace, international amity and goodwill. India has a living and vital stake in peace because we want to concentrate attention on improving the living standards of millions of our people. In the utilization of our limited resources, we have always given primacy to plans and projects for economic development. It would, therefore, be obvious for anyone who is prepared to look at things objectively that India can have no possible interest in provoking border incidents or in building up an atmosphere of strife.... In these circumstances, the duty of Government is quite clear and this duty will be discharged fully and effectively ... We would prefer to live in poverty for as long as necessary but we shall not allow our freedom to be subverted".

Infiltration in Jammu & Kashmir

While he was till explaining to the people the importance of settling issues through discussions rather than through military action, armed infiltrators from Pakistan began entering the State of Jammu and Kashmir on August 5, 1965. Greatly distressed at this turn of events, the Prime Minister made it clear to Pakistan that force would be met with force.

The fighting between Pakistan and India came to a halt on September 23, 1965, under the terms of a resolution of the U.N. Security Council. As Lal Bahadur had earlier declared, what was important was not to live from cease-fire to cease-fire but to achieve a viable peace. In a broadcast to the nation on the day the cease-fire came into force he also outlined how this viable peace could be brought about. Said the Prime Minister: "While the conflict between the armed forces of the two countries has come to an end, the more important thing for the United Nations and all those who stand for peace is to bring to an end the deeper conflict.... How can this be brought about? In our view, the only answer lies in peaceful coexistence. India has stood for the principle of coexistence and championed it all over the world. Peaceful coexistence is possible among nations no matter how deep the differences between them, how far apart they are in their political and economic systems, no matter how intense the issues that divide them".

Victory for Peace

An opportunity to make a start in this direction was provided by the Chairman of the Council of Ministers of the U.S.S.R., Mr. A. N. Kosygin, who invited the Prime Minister of India and the President of Pakistan to meet in Tashkent to discuss peace. The two statesmen accepted the invitation.

After six days of discussions, the President of Pakistan came to appreciate the Indian viewpoint that a firm declaration ruling out recourse to force would create the right kind of climate for settling Indo-Pakistan differences. So an agreement was reached at Tashkent, an agreement which was rightly hailed as a victory for peace rather than for either India or Pakistan. (PIB Features)

HIS ROLE IN THE FREEDOM STRUGGLE

At the age of 17, he was very impressed with Gandhiji's call for freedom through non-violence and so took part in the Non-co-operation Movement of 1921. He courted arrest but was let off because of his age. But he was not so lucky when he followed Gandhiji in the Satyagraha Movement and spent approximately 8 years in jail over a period of time. Even though he was made to undergo tremendous hardships, he survived with the help of his prayers and physical exercises. He spent this time reading different authors like Hegel, Kant, Marx, Russell and Lenin. He also did some translations and wrote about the Quit India Movement.

Post Independence

He served the Congress in various positions before becoming Prime Minister. He was First General Secretary, and then Home-Minister. In U.P. he made some progressive reforms in the police department, and in 1962, Pandit Nehru invited him to join the Union cabinet as a Minister for railways. A post from which he resigned after taking responsibility for a railway mishap, that happened during his tenure.

Lal Bahadur Shastri showed remarkable abilities of oratorship and courage during the Indo-Pakistan War. He inspired his people through his leadership and offered them a slogan that has been passed down the ages-'Jai Jawan Jai Kisan'. The Indo-Pak war would have continued, but fortunately, the Russian Government intervened and both India and Pakistan were forced to sign the 'Tashkent Agreement' on January 11, 1966. A day that saw the passing away of this great leader, just a few hours after signing this historic agreement.

He was awarded the 'Bharat Ratna' posthumously, in light of the services rendered to the country. His memorial 'Vijayghat' in Delhi is a constant reminder of a great administrator and a fantastic human being.

Lal Bahadur Shastri was a well-known freedom fighter. After Jawaharlal Nehru's death, he became the second Prime Minister of India. He believed in high thinking and simple living.

In 1965, when Pakistan attacked India, Shastri proved to be a man of steel. The Indian troops were victorious, but being essentially a man of peace, Shastri agreed to a peace treaty (The Tashkent agreement), which was fair to Pakistan.

The following speech (abridged) was given by Lal Bahadur Shastri at the convocation of the Aligarh Muslim University.

THE RESPONSIBILITY OF YOUNG MEN

Whatever your station in future life, each one of you should first of all think of yourselves as citizens of the country. This confers on you certain rights, which are guaranteed by the Constitution, but it also subjects you to certain responsibilities, which also have to be clearly understood.

Ours is a democracy, which enjoins freedom to the individual, but this freedom has to be subjected to a number of voluntary restraints in the interests of organized society. And these voluntary restraints have to be exercised and demonstrated in everyday life.

A good citizen is one who obeys the law, whether there is a policeman around or not, and who takes delight in performing his civic duties. In the olden days sense of self-restraint and discipline was inculcated by the combined effort of the family and the teacher. The economic stresses of present-day life unfortunately do not leave enough time to the parents to look after the children.

In the educational institutions the numbers have grown so large as to take away the benefits, which used to accrue formerly by personal contact between the teacher and the taught. Inevitably, our young students are often left much to their own resources. Often this creates problems, which we all know about. This is an important aspect, which needs thorough examination. The responsibility of our young citizens is great. In my view every station in life is important in itself. Work has its own dignity and there is great satisfaction in doing one's own job to the best of one's ability. Whatever the duties, we should apply ourselves with sincerity and devotion. Such an approach, apart from being good in itself, also has the added advantage of opening avenues for further advancement. We have to see whether we have done our own job well before thinking of criticizing anybody else. All too often, we succumb to the temptation of decrying others without bothering to look to ourselves.

Never forget that loyalty to the country comes ahead of all other loyalties. And this is an absolute loyalty, since one cannot weigh it in terms of what one receives. It is essential to remember that the entire country is one and that any one who fosters or promotes separatism or fissiparous tendencies is not our true friend. What I have said stems from a desire to see that the youth of our country prepares itself in a disciplined and determined manner for the responsibilities of tomorrow. A democratic country is sustained not by the greatness of a few but by the co-operative effort of the many. The future of the country is in your hands and as the older generations complete their task the new ones come along to take their place. If they are well equipped as individuals and as citizens, the country's future will be bright indeed. At a time when you are at the threshold of a new period in your life I would urge you to play your role with confidence and dignity.

Our position with regard to secularism is known so well that it hardly needs any reiteration. It is embodied in our Constitution, which ensures equal respect for all religions and equal opportunities for all citizens, irrespective of their caste and creed and the faith which they profess. In spite of a seeming diversity, there is a fundamental unity in India, which we all cherish and it has to be our constant endeavour to maintain and strengthen this unity. The country can progress only if it does away completely with fissiparous tendencies and emerges as an integrated whole. And it is in the field of education that the seed of secularism has to be sown at the earliest stages, so that the plant can be carefully nurtured as it grows.

The world is at the moment passing through very difficult times. In fact, it would not be wrong to say that never before in the recent past had mankind to grapple with problems of as complex a nature as are confronting it today. It is imperative that satisfactory and, as far as possible, lasting solutions should be found to these problems without undue delay, otherwise there is a danger of the situation getting out of hand. Mutual suspicions, hatred and ill-will between nations and groups of persons have to be removed at all costs and sincere and determined efforts have to be made to ensure that differences and outstanding problems are resolved by mutual discussion in a spirit of understanding, and not by the use of force. Wars and conflicts, as we know to our cost, always create more problems than they succeed in solving. The great advances made by science and technology, particularly in the field of nuclear and thermonuclear energy, have placed an almost unlimited power at the disposal of mankind. This power can be used either for constructive or for destructive purposes and it is up to us to try to derive the fullest possible benefit from it.

We, in India, have our own special problems. No one can deny that some of them are of a serious nature and must be tackled with vigour and determination. Our national objective has been defined clearly and unambiguously. We aim that every citizen should be provided with the basic necessities of life and should have complete freedom to lead the life of his or her own choice. We aim at a democratic society, strong and free, in which every citizen, irrespective of his religious belief, will occupy an equal and honoured place, and will be given full and equal opportunities for growth and service. We aim at the removal of untouchability and the doing away of the prevailing serious inequalities in status and wealth. We are opposed to the concentration of wealth in a few hands. Our rich cultural heritage extending over countless centuries is not the culture of this community or that but the synthesis of the cultures of the great peoples who lived here at various times in the past. The objectives I have mentioned are by no means easy of achievement in their entirety. I know that we have met with only a limited degree of success so far, but we have to persevere until the goal is achieved.

It must be remembered that the vast majority of Indians are extremely poor and it is only a small minority that live in relative comfort and have the benefit of university education and other worthwhile things. It is when we look at the Indian scene in such a perspective that Hindus, Muslims, Christians, Parsecs and others, instead of feeling that they are different, will together begin to put forth a tremendous effort to fight poverty, to eradicate disease and banish illiteracy.

THE FORGOTTEN PRIME MINISTER

Lal Bahadur Shastri was a man of considerable achievement and also, being a politician, of the odd failure as well.

DEBATES may rage on who was India's best Prime Minister, but there can be no question of who has been its most unjustly forgotten Prime Minister: Lal Bahadur Shastri. This remains so even in this, the centenary year of his birth. His memory was briefly exhumed on his hundredth birthday, October 2, 2004, when, at a desultory function in Delhi, he was described by a Union Minister as a "devoted disciple of Mahatma Gandhi and a legendary loyalist of Jawaharlal Nehru". And that, it appears, was the end of the commemoration for the year — and — perhaps for all time to come.

Commitment to Nationalism

Shastri was both a disciple of Gandhi and an admirer of Nehru, but he was also his own man. Born in Mughalsarai, in a Kayasth family of modest means, he studied first with a *maulvi* and later at the Kashi Vidyapeeth. His commitment to the nationalist cause came early, and remained steadfast. He spent some nine years in Jail (in seven stints) while working his way up the Congress ladder. After Independence, he played a key role in organising his party's campaign in the first General Elections of 1952. He then served for several years as Union Railway Minister, before resigning after a serious train accident for which he felt he must own moral responsibility.

Underestimated

Because of his small size — he was barely five feet tall — and his self-effacing nature, Shastri was consistently underestimated by all those around him — whether journalists, officials, or fellow Ministers. But one who properly appreciated his qualities of head and heart was Jawarhalal Nehru. In 1961 Nehru brought Shastri back into the Cabinet. For the next three years he was (as one contemporary put it) "India's premier compromiser, conciliator and co-ordinator" — the "most popular man in the Congress party and the main channel of communication between Nehru and the party organisations". Among the crises he solved at the Prime Minister's behest were those caused by language riots in Assam and by the theft of a holy relic in Srinagar's Hazratbal mosque.

In and out of office, Lal Bahadur Shastri acquired a reputation for probity of character, unusual even in those generally honest times. When he was asked to demit office under the Kamaraj Plan in 1963, Shastri wrote to an associate of how, without a Minister's salary, his family had decided now to eat one less vegetable every meal and to wash their clothes themselves.

When Nehru died, Shastri was chosen by the Congress to succeed him. These were difficult years, with the country's morale affected by defeat in the war with China, continuing tensions in the borderlands, and serious scarcities of food. Shastri met these challenges with resolve and fortitude. He called for the planners to lay a greater focus on agriculture, and himself supervised the re-organisation of the Indian Council of Agricultural Research. On the industrial front, he rejected the prevailing "export pessimism", arguing that India had both the capital and the expertise to begin exporting chemical and engineering products as well as traditional agricultural commodities such as tea and rubber. (As it since has).

LAL BAHADUR SHASTRI 1904-1966

In a world where political leaders and moral values stand miles apart, Indian history was blessed with a man who always stood for things which were right and was ready to go to any extent for preserving the same.

The man who was short in stature, stood tall and his name will always glitter in gold letters in the annals of Indian history.

Today when leaders have to be reminded of their moral responsibility time and again, our former Prime Minister Lal Bahadur Shastri stood tall because of his principles. Power and berth in the Cabinet held no importance for this great man.

While serving as the Minister of Railways and Transport at the Centre, in 1956, he offered his resignation after a railway accident at Mahbubnagar led to 112 deaths accepting moral responsibility for the mishap.

However, the then prime minister Jawaharlal Nehru did not accept his resignation. Three months later, he resigned accepting moral and constitutional responsibility for a railway accident at Ariyalur in Tamil Nadu that resulted in 144 deaths.

While speaking in the Parliament on the incident, the Nehru, stated that he was accepting the resignation because it would set an example in constitutional propriety and not because Shastri was in any way responsible for the accident. Shastri was an exemplary figure, despite of his short stature and insignificant personality.

Brief Life History

Lal Bahadur was born in the year 1904 in Ramnagar, as Lal Bahadur Srivastava to Sharada Prasad, a poor school teacher. His father later became a clerk in the Revenue Office at Allahabad.

However, destiny had hardships in store for this man and Lal Bahadur's father died when he was only a year and a half old. His mother Ramdulari

Devi took him and his two sisters to her father's house and settled down there. His schooling could not be done at the native village as there were no schools which offered education after Class X. He later went to Varanasi for further schooling where he stayed with his maternal uncle and joined the Harischandra High School.

The turning point in his life came when he heard the speech of Mahatma Gandhi at Varanasi in 1915. Lal Bahadur, unaware of his potential as a future leader, dedicated his life to the service of the country. He also dropped his surname, as it indicated his caste and he was against the caste system.

In 1930, he threw himself into the freedom struggle during Mahatma Gandhi's Salt Satyagraha. Following India's independence, Shastri was appointed Parliamentary Secretary in his home state, Uttar Pradesh. He became the Minister of Police and Transport under Govind Ballabh Pant's Chief Ministership.

He was the first one to appoint women conductors during his term as the Transport Minister. As the minister in charge of the Police Department, he ordered that Police use jets of water instead of lathis to disperse unruly crowds.

In 1951, Nehru nominated him to the Rajya Sabha and he served as the Minister of Railways and Transport in the Central Cabinet from 1951 to 1956. In 1961, he became Minister for Home. As Union Home Minister he was instrumental in appointing the Committee on Prevention of Corruption under the Chairmanship of K. Santhanam.

In a major blow to India, Jawaharlal Nehru died in office on May 27, 1964 after which began the search for a man who would fill the vaccume left by Nehru. The major figures of the Congress Party were unable to find enough support and finally Shastri was elected as the compromise candidate. He took charge of the office of the Prime Minister on June 9, 1964. Shastri, though mild-mannered and soft-spoken, was a Nehruvian socialist. "There comes a time in the life of every nation when it stands at the cross-roads of history and must choose which way to go. But for us there need be no difficulty or hesitation, no looking to right or left. Our way is straight and clear – the building up of a socialist democracy at home with freedom and prosperity for all, and the maintenance of world peace and friendship with all nations," he said in his first speech after taking over as the prime minister.

Apart from emphasizing the Green Revolution, he was instrumental in promoting the White Revolution. The Indo-Pakistan War of 1965 was the chief problem for Shastri's administration. The war ended on September 23, 1965 with a United Nations-mandated ceasefire. After the declaration of ceasefire, Shastri and Pakistani President Muhammad Ayub Khan attended a summit in Tashkent (former USSR, now in modern Uzbekistan), organised by Kosygin.

On January 10, 1966, Shastri and Khan signed the Tashkent Declaration which is considenred as one of the milestones in the history of the two neighbouring nations.

The next day Shastri, who had suffered two heart attacks earlier, died of a heart attack. He is the only Indian Prime Minister, and indeed probably one of the few heads of government, to have died in office overseas. Some conspiracy theories allege his death to be of unnatural causes.

Shastri was known for honesty and humility. He was the first person to be posthumously awarded the Bharat Ratna, and a memorial "Vijay Ghat" was built for him in Delhi.

A NEWSEXTRAXT FROM 1956

Thirty Congress MPs have, in a signed appeal, requested Prime Minister Nehru to reverse his decision to advise the President to accept Mr. Lal Bahadur Shastri's resignation. They said they were shocked at the tragic news of the railway disaster at Ariyalur, but "we are equally shocked by your decision to accept the resignation of the Railway Minister." They added, "It was quite noble of him (Mr. Lal Bahadur) to have offered to resign for the disaster but we feel that in a technical Ministry like the Railways, it is the Railway Board which is directly responsible for the administration of the Railways and not the Railway Minister. The recurring train disasters have brought to light the necessity of efficient Railway administration and we, as well as the country, have faith in the efficiency of the Railway Minister."

6

Shastri and Pakistan

How much the Nation Owes to Shastri. That was the time when massive Pakistan military infiltration had taken place in Jammu and Kashmir and war clouds were hovering over the country.

Referring to Chinese protests, "The Chinese are claiming that we have made bunkers in their territory", he told the nation. "Well, if it is their territory they are welcome to destroy them", he added to a thunderous applause. That was Lal Bahadur Shastri, our Prime Minister. No logic could be more simple; no message more direct. A physically small man who stood much taller in his boldness to take political decisions. On the anniversary of our 1965 war, it would be appropriate to recall his contribution to the nation.

Both India and Pakistan have followed divergent paths since Independence. While India chose to become a democratic, secular and welfare state wanting to be left alone, Pakistan chose to foster an obsessive hatred of India and to prevent India from going forward by any means, fair or foul.

Historically, peace between the two has been possible only when Pakistan had a fear of military retaliation from India, mainly from 1971 till 1989. On becoming nuclear, and assuming to be immune to attack from India, it stoked a jihad in Kashmir. Another such period of fear on part of Pakistan was prior to 1962 when Ayub Khan had a very high opinion of the fighting prowess of the Indian Army and had stated in a public meeting that he did not want to lose Pakistan for the sake of Kashmir.

All that changed in 1962, when the famed India Army was humbled and humiliated in a totally one-sided conflict with China. Ayub seems to have concluded that the India Army was no more the same feared fighting machine that it used to be. Death of Indian Prime Minister Jawaharlal Nehru and his succession by a diminutive, seemingly unimpressive Lal Bahadur Shastri seemed to have further emboldened Pakistan. The result was the Indo-Pak war of 1965.

Kashmir has always been a handy pretext for Pakistan to justify its obsessive hostility towards India. Of course, there can be any number of such pretexts between two countries sharing such a long border. One such chosen by Pakistan in April 1965 was the Rann of Kutch.

Pakistan planners decided to test Shastri and also to draw out Indian Army far way from Kashmir, where they planned to fight their real battle. The Rann of Kutch gave Pakistan every tactical advantage. India had hardly any troops in Gujarat; the nearest unit was in Jam Nagar and they were under Bombay area, a peace formation not geared for fighting a war. The only rail communication was a metre gauge railway incapable of transporting tanks and artillery.

Pakistan, on the other hand, had better rail and road communications right up to the chosen battlefield. The entire Rann became a sea during monsoon and India would be obliged to withdraw troops before the rains started. The only problem was the fact that Pakistani Air Force bases were far away in Punjab, while Indian bases were in Gujarat and Rajasthan.

To overcome this problem, the Pakistan Air Force C-in-C Ashghar Khan tried the usual dirty trick and called up his old senior from pre-Partition days ACM Arjun Singh Chief of Indian Air Staff to suggest that the two air forces stay out of the conflict. As subsequent events proved, the latter was just too shrewd and too thorough a professional to get taken in by such a ruse. Pakistan created a border dispute in Rann totally out of the blue and sent a Brigade group supported by heavy artillery and Patton tanks under Brigadier Tikka Khan who was later to become notorious as Butcher of Bangladesh.

The Indian High Command, having sensed a trap, refused to bite the bait and the then Chief of Army Staff General J.N. Chowdhary was categorical that we would fight at the place of our choosing and not the one chosen by Pakistan. Though we lost some territory and considerable prestige in the world by refusing to fight and accepting a face saving formula that left our territory in Pakistani hands, it saved the day for us later when the real action started. Emboldened that Indian leadership was shy of a war, Pakistan launched its Operation Gibraltar by sending thousands of infiltrators into the Kashmir valley. The major route was through Haji Pir. Our Para battalion under Ranjit Dayal captured it and not only blocked further infiltration but also cut off the supplies etc. for those that were already in Jammu and Kashmir.

Pakistan unleashed its previously planned Operation Grand Slam on September 1, 1965 aimed to capture Akhnur bridge over Chenab cutting off Punch and Rajauri and then capture Jammu along with a pincer from Sialkot, bottling up all Indian troops in Jammu and Kashmir. On Sept 3, Ayub Khan sent his favourite General Yahya Khan (who though a Shia was instrumental in bringing Ayub Khan to power in the October 1958 coup as a senior operational staff officer in GHQ then at Karachi), to command this battle and get all the honours.

As the situation in Akhnur sector was getting critical and untenable, India opened a second front across the international border to relieve the pressure there and a full scale war was on. A war on a wide front favours a country with more resources in manpower and material and slowly as we started getting an upper hand, the ceasefire came about on Sept 23, 1965.

Two events during the war stand out not only for their boldness but also for the impact on the outcome of the war. Both were political decisions taken under the leadership of Lal Bahadur Shastri, who had earlier set an example of moral courage by resigning as the Railway Minister following a train accident.

First was the decision to use the Air Force on the evening of Sept 1 when the Army's situation had become untenable and Akhnur was in imminent danger of falling to the enemy. That far-reaching and bold decision he took within minutes of being apprised of the critical situation by the Army and Air Chiefs.

The second decision was to open another front across the international border. An attacker chooses the time and place of his attack and is the strongest in the chosen sector. Militarily, it makes more sense for a defender to launch a counter-stroke elsewhere to force the attacker to divert his resources into defending his own territory and thus weakening his attack. In the 1948-49 Kashmir operations, the fighting had remained confined to the ceasefire line and did not spill over to the international border. Pakistan, obviously, expected a repeat of the scenario and had prepared accordingly.

When India opened up the Punjab front, they were surprised and Ayub's dreams of glory and consummation of the "ideology of Pakistan" ended in the plains of Punjab, thanks primarily to a diminutive man but with the heart of a lion. The nation owes this lion an everlasting gratitude. Without his bold leadership, the outcome of that war could and would have been different and the political map of the subcontinent of India would have been very different today.

The Indian Railway Centenary Day celebrations were held on April 16 in the Railway Exhibition grounds at New Delhi. Mr. Lal Bahadur Shastri, Minister for Transport & Railways; Mr. 0. V. Alaggesan, Deputy Minister; Mr.

Shah Nawaz, Parliamentary Secretary; Members of the Railway Board and senior railway officials received Dr. S. Radhakrishnan, the Vice-President, at the New Delhi ceremonial platform. Dr. Radhakrishnan deputised for Dr. Rajendra Prasad, the President, who was indisposed. After inspecting the guard of honour provided by the Northern Railway, he was conducted to the special train arranged to take the party to the exhibition grounds, where a large audience including Cabinet Ministers, diplomats, and senior officials awaited.

Mr. S. S. Vasist, Member for Transportation, Railway Board, said that today the Indian railway system was the largest in Asia and the fourth largest in the world. The capital outlay, Rs.38 lakhs in 1853, was Rs.862 crores in 1951-52. It was to be hoped that before long the railways would not only be meeting the current requirements of trade and industry but also developing facilities and services to get ahead of the nation's expanding industrialisation. Mr. Vasist then introduced to the audience Mr. Durga Manoo, the oldest serving railwayman in India, who was appointed on the Indian Midland Railway in 1900.

The Minister for Transport & Railways recalled that railways appeared in India at a time when there were scarcely any internal communications worth the name and nothing could have been more welcome to the country than the changes which they brought about. The second world war and the partition of the country which followed profoundly affected the Indian railways. Nevertheless in six years their progress had been such as to satisfy the severest critic. The railways had been regrouped successfully into six zonal systems, an organisational change of far-reaching importance. Dismantled lines had been restored and new lines opened. Chittaranjan works was now producing locomotives and a large coach building works at Perambur was being built.

Dr. Radhakrishnan, to whom the Minister for Transport & Railways presented a commemorative volume on Indian railways, looked forward to a lessening of international tension which would release more money for constructive purposes and therefore enable them to allot more funds to the railways. He congratulated the Railway Minister, the members of the Railway Board and every railwayman on the success which they had achieved.

A documentary film entitled 'A Century of Progress' was then shown, with a running commentary on the developments during the period. In the evening there was a centenary dinner in the exhibition grounds.

The day was observed as a holiday on all railways, and celebrations also were held at other places. That at the Victoria Terminus in Bombay had a special significance as the first train in India ran from Bombay (Borce-Bunder) to Thana. At the meeting held in the afternoon of April 16, attended by Mr. F. C. Badhwar.

Chairman of the Railway Board, Mr. Gida Shanker Bajpai, Governor of Bombay, presided. Mr. H. P. Hira, General Manager, Central Railway, who welcomed the guests, traced the development of the system to its present mileage and organisation. Mr. Badhwar compared the function to a birthday party, and added that as presents were usual on such occasions the public might offer one in the form of consideration and understanding of their problems. Mr. Bajpai praised the efficient work of the railwaymen. There was an exhibition of old and new rolling stock, and models.

At a meeting of the officers and staff of the Western Railway at Bombay, held on the lawns adjoining the Churchgate Building, Mr. K. P. Mushran, General Manager, spoke on the importance of the occasion. At Calcutta there was a celebration at the Garden Reach office of the Eastern Railway, presided over by Dr. H. C. Mukerjee, Governor of Bengal. Mr. K. B. Mathur, General Manager of the Eastern Railway, reviewed in a speech the history and progress of the system. The Governor's speech referred appreciatively to the contributions made by railways to the economic progress of the country. Dr. B. C. Rey, the Chief Minister of West Bengal, emphasised the importance of the railways to the economy of Eastern India. A the headquarters of the North Eastern Railway at Goraklipur, Mr. G. Pande, General Manager, addressed the officers and staff.

Headquarters offices, workshops and important stations were illuminated on all railways. The illuminations at Victoria and Churchgate, Bombay, were elaborate and attracted thousands of sightseers. At Delhi, the main station and the headquarters offices at Baroda House and at Calcutta the Fairlie Place offices, and Howrah and Sealdah stations were illuminated. Undeterred by an electricity cut, the Southern Railway brought out wick and oil lamps to illuminate the frontage of Egmore Station, Madras, in a manner reminiscent of the Deepavali, or Festival of Lights.

LAL BAHADUR SHASTRI

The 27th of May 1964 is an unforgettable day in the history of India.

On that day the citizens of Delhi woke and attended to their routine work.

During the day came shocking news from Teen Moorti Bhavan. The first Prime Minister of free India, Jawaharlal Nehru, lived in Teen Moorti Bhavan; the citizens learnt that he had a heart attack.

'After Nehru, Who?'

A few months before Nehru had suffered a mild heart attack. But he had recovered from it quickly. He was certain that he would live for some more years.

But he passed away on May 27, 1964.

Nehru was no more. It was unbelievable but true. One question echoed from Kashmir to Kanyakumari: 'After Nehru, who?'

The leaders of the ruling party, the Congress Party, thought deeply over the question. They counted a few suitable names on their fingers. Which of them was the best choice? Who could be the Prime Minister?

'Bharat Ratna'

Lal Bahadur was a star of great brightness in the history of India, After his death the President of India conferred on him, on behalf of the nation, the award of ' Bharat Ratna'; it was a most fitting.

A small bodies but mighty man-so runs a kannada proverb. It applies to several great men. Shivaji was not tall. But like a magnet he attracted people, and organized and built a great empire. Napoleon was short. But he shook the whole world. Lal Bahadur Shastri was not taller than those two; but he was not second to them in greatness. Firmness, love of adventure, patience and skill in administration cannot be acquired in a day or a year. Only when we study his growth from childhood can we understand how he acquired all these qualities.

The Fatherless Child

Lal Bahadur was born on October 2nd, 1904 at Mughalsarai, seven miles from Kashi. His parents were Sharada Prasad and Ramdulari Devi. They were agriculturists. Srivastava was part of Lal Bahadur's name. He dropped that part indicating his caste when he grew up. He did not like such indications of caste.

Lal Bahadurs father was a poor teacher at first. Then he became a clerk in the Revenue Office at Allahabad. Here, too, he earned very little. But, even though he was poor, he never accepted bribes. He lived a life of honesty and integrity.

Sharada Prasad died when Lal Bahadur was only a year old. Ramdulari Devi felt as though the skies had come down on her.

Her father gave shelter to her and her three children, a boy and two girls.

The Loving Grandfather

Lal Bahadur's grandfather Hazari Lai's family was very large. His brothers, their wives and children, besides his own children and grand children, lived under the same roof. It was a small world in itself and Hazari Lai was the fountain of love and affection to all of them. He looked after every one in the family with love. He was especially fond of little Lal Bahadur. He always affectionately called him 'Nanhe' which means 'tiny'.

An interesting incident took place when Lal Bahadur was only three months old. The mother went to bathe in the holy Ganga with her child. In the milling crowd at the bathing ghat she lost her child. The child had slipped from his mother's arms into a cowherd's basket.

The cowherd had no children, So he took the child as a gift from God and celebrated the event with great joy. The mother was lost in grief. A complaint was lodged with the police. They traced the child. The foster parents wept bitterly to give back the child. Lal Bahadur, who was destined to govern the country, narrowly missed the 'good fortune' of becoming a cowherd.

Lal Bahadur stayed at his grandfather's house till he was ten. By that time he had passed the sixth standard examination. There was no high school in that place. They sent him to Kashi for further education

Strong and Self-respecting

Courage and self-respect were two virtues, which took deep root in him from his childhood. While in Kashi, he went with his friends to see a fair on the other bank of the Ganga. On the way back he had no money for the boat fare. His self-respect did not allow him to ask his friends for money. He slipped from their company without their knowledge. His friends forgot him in their talk and boarded the boat. When the boat had moved away, Lal Bahadur jumped into the river; as his friends watched breathlessly he swam to the other bank safely.

Though Lal Bahadur was, a man of small build, he was unusually strong. His moral strength was even greater. As in water so in life he swam quite successfully. Twice he was about to be drowned but was saved. It is said that when he was saved the second time, he had his teacher's three-year-old baby on his shoulders.

Lal Bahadur acquired virtues like boldness, love of adventure, patience, self-control, courtesy and selflessness in his childhood.

Even as a boy he loved to read books. He read whatever books he came across, whether he understood them or not. He was fond of Guru Nanak's verses.

He used to repeat the following lines often:

"O Nanak! Be tiny like grass,
For other plants will whither away, but grass will remain ever green."

The Lesson

An incident, which took place when he was six years old, seems to have left a deep mark on his mind. Once he went to an orchard with his friends. He was standing below while his friends climbed the trees. He plucked a flower from a bush.

The gardener came in the meantime and saw Lal Bahadur. The boys on the trees climbed down and ran away. The gardener caught Lal Bahadur. He beat him severely.

Lal Bahadur wept and said, "I am orphan. Do not beat me."

The gardener smiled with pity and said, "Because you are an orphan, you must learn better behaviour, my boy."

The words of the gardener had a great effect on him. He swore to him, "I shall behave better in future. Because I am an orphan I must learn good behaviour."

Though short he was not timid at school. All boys were friendly with him. Like the grass he always looked fresh and smiling. Not only during his school days but also in his later life he did not hate anyone. It seems he used to act in plays at school. He played the role of Kripacharya in the play 'Mahabharatha'. Kripacharya was in the court of Duryodhana and yet was loved by the Pandavas. Lal Bahadur Shastri had acquired the same worth.

Tilak and Gandhi

Even when Lal Bahadur was a student of Harischandra. High School at Varanasi a whirlwind had disturbed India.

Everywhere there was the cry of 'Freedom'! "Swaraj is our birth right"- Bala Gangadhara Tilak had declared. This had become the nation's battlecry.

Lal Bahadur reverenced Tilak. He longed to see him and hear his speech. Once Tilak visited Varanasi. Lal Bahadur was away in a village fifty miles from Varanasi. He borrowed money and travelled in a train to see and hear Tilak. He saw him and heard his speech. It reverberated in his ears like Krishna's conch, the Panchajanya. Like Bharata, carrying Rama's sandals on his head, Lal Bahadur carried Tilak's message in his heart. This message guided him all through his life. The greatest influence on Lal Bahadur was that of Mahatma Gandhi. Lal Bahadur was electrified when he heard a speech of Gandhi at Varanasi in 1915. Then and there he dedicated his life to the service of the country

1965 CRISIS

After the war Soviet Premier, Kosygin, decided to play the role of a peace maker. He invited both Prime Minister Shastari and President Ayub to meet at Tashkant for peace settlement. Both accepted his invitation. Indian delegation including Foreign Minister Swaran Singh, Defense Minister Y. B. Chawan and Indian Ambassador at Moscow, T. N. Kaul. Pakistan delegation included its Foreign Minister, Z. A. Bhutto. The meeting began on January 4th, with an opening address by Kosygin in the course of which he said "India and Pakistan are our southern neighbors. We always came out not only for the strengthening of friendly relations between Soviet Union and India and Pakistan but also for the reign of peace and friendship between these countries themselves." He did not utter a word which could be considered as sympathetic to India which had been subjected to unprovoked aggression. Deliberations continued till January 10, when Tashkent Declaration was adopted and initiated by Lal Bahadur Shastri and Ayub Khan on behalf of India and Pakistan.

Tashkent Declaration was a collection of platitudes. Its only concrete and operative part was clause-II which said "The Prime Minister of India and President of Pakistan have agreed that all armed personnel of the two countries shall be withdrawn not later than 15 February, 1966 to the positions they held prior to August 5th and both sides will observe the ceasefire terms on the ceasefire line."

This was a clear rebuff to India. It not only put the aggressor and the aggressed on par but also committed India to withdraw from Haji Pir and Kargil Heights which belonged to India, had been illegally occupied by Pakistan and had been liberated by Indian armed forces at a heavy cost. It virtually gave legal validity to Pak occupation of the territory it had occupied in 1947-48 without prejudice to its claim on the rest of the state which was still with India.

Lal Bahadur had assured the people and armed forces before his departure for Tashkent that he would not accept any suggestion for the return to Pakistan of Haji Pir pass and Kargil Heights. He stood firm on his word to the nation till the last day. But his aides, Swaran Singh, Y. B. Chawan and T. N. Kaul, pressurred him to accept the Pak demand for withdrawal of troops from there for fear of alienation of USSR. It implied that it was the presure of the Soviet Union which forced India to accept a patently unjust settlement. Had India not put all her eggs in Soviet basket and had it maintained dialogue with USA also before and after going to Tashkent, it might have been saved from the predicament in which Shastri had to sign the Tashkent Declaration against his better judgement.

Prime Minister Shastri was found dead in his room at Tashkent on the morning of January 11, 1966. It was given out that he died of heart failure. But suspicion that he was poisoned to death lingers on. No detailed inquiry into his death was made. Indian physician Dr. Chugh, who had accompanied him to Tashkent was mysteriously liquidated sometime later.

Death of Shri Shastri Shastri was the greater loss suffered by India at Tashkent. Had he returned to India alive, he might have given new orientation to India's foreign policy and ended her total dependence on Soviet Union which had proved not only undependable but also dubious.

Soviet leaders were more concerned with global interests and global strategy of Soviet Union than with national interests of India. Independence of character and commitment to national interest above everything else that Lal Bahadur Shastri had displayed during his short tenure was not to the liking of Soviet Union and its supporters in India. They wanted a more pliable person committed to Nehruvian foreign policy to toeing the Soviet line even at the cost of vital national interest of India. That explained the interest Kosygin, who overstayed in Delhi for 4 days after the funeral of Lal Bahadur Shastri, showed in the election of Mrs. Gandhi as Leader of Congress Parliamentary Party to fill the place of Lal Bahadur Shastri.

Pakistan was not sincere about Tashkent Declaration. This became clear from the statement made by Altaf Gauhar, Press Secretary of President Ayub, soon after the signing of this Declaration. He was reported to have said that nothing but withdrawal of troops to August 5, position which suited Pakistan had been agreed upon and that Pakistan reserved the right to continue its efforts to secure Kashmir by force. President Ayub confirmed this in his statement made at Hamburg in November, 1966. He said, "It (Tashkent Declaration) settled nothing. All it did was to enable the two countries to disengage their armies from each other." From the Indian point of view, the futile Pak attempt to grab Kashmir by force had some positive results. In the first place even those parties in India like the Swatantra Party which had been advocating settlement with Pakistan about Kashmir in terms of UN resolutions conceded that Pakistan had forfeited its claim on Kashmir by taking resort to arms. Mrs. Indira Gandhi, the new Prirne Minister, also declared at New York on March 31, 1966, "It is now too late to talk of plebiscite. The second invasion of Kashmir by Pakistan last autumn has destroyed whatever marginal or academic value the old UN resolutions might have had. Kashmir is now also vital to defense of Laddakh against China. Any plebiscite today would by definition amount to questioning the integrity of India. It will rouse the demand for accessation against which is fought a civil war. We cannot and will not tolerate a second partition of India on religious ground. It will destroy the very basis of the Indian states.".

Secondly, it had a salutary effect on the minds of those Kashmiris who had been wistfully looking to Pakistan.

Had the government of India taken advantage of this situation to fully integrate Kashmir with the rest of India and had it extended Indian Constitution to that State and enabled Indians from other parts of the country to settle there, the Pak design on Kashmir might have been effectively scotched for ever.

But that was not to be. Mrs. Gandhi had the same weakness for Sh. Abdullah and his concept of Kashmiri nationalism which had prevented her father to adopt a realistic and nationalistic approach to Kashmir issue. Her policies soon destroyed the wholesome effect of 1965 war on Kashmiri mind.

The net result of Second Indo-Pak war on Kashmir went in favour of Pakistan, as in the case of First War of 1947-48. Pakistan had gained 30,000 sq. miles of Indian territory by the war of 1947-4B. It regained some of this territory which had been taken back by Indian army in the war of 1965. It also established its right on the territory illegally occupied by it since the ceasefire of 1949. It was also able to push out lakhs of Hindus from both wings of Pakistan as refugees into India. Furthermore, it confiscated Indian properties and assets in Pakistan worth hundred of crores of rupees. Thus, in spite of its failure to grab Kashmir by force it was able to strengthen its position against India both internally and externally.

ROLE OF THE PRIME MINISTER

Nehru set the pattern for the formation of Indian foreign policy: a strong personal role for the prime minister but a weak institutional structure. Nehru served concurrently as prime minister and minister of external affairs; he made all major foreign policy decisions himself after consulting with his advisers and then entrusted the conduct of international affairs to senior members of the Indian Foreign Service. His successors continued to exercise considerable control over India's international dealings, although they generally appointed separate ministers of external affairs.

India's second Prime Minister, Lal Bahadur Shastri (1964-66), expanded the Office of Prime Minister (sometimes called the Prime Minister's Secretariat) and enlarged its powers (see The Executive, ch. 8). By the 1970s, the Office of the Prime Minister had become the de facto coordinator and supraministry of the Indian government. The enhanced role of the office strengthened the prime minister's control over foreign policy making at the expense of the Ministry of External Affairs. Advisers in the office provided channels of information and policy recommendations in addition to those offered by the Ministry of External Affairs. A subordinate part of the office—the Research and Analysis Wing—functioned in ways that significantly expanded the information available to the prime minister and his advisers. The Research and Analysis Wing gathered intelligence, provided intelligence analysis to the Office of the Prime Minister, and conducted covert operations abroad.

The prime minister's control and reliance on personal advisers in the Office of the Prime Minister was particularly strong under the tenures of Indira Gandhi (1966-77 and 1980-84) and her son, Rajiv (1984-89), who succeeded her, and weaker during the periods of coalition governments under Morarji Desai (1977-79), Viswanath Pratap (V.P.) Singh (1989-90), Chandra Shekhar (1990-91), and P.V. Narasimha Rao (starting in June 1991). Although observers find it difficult to determine whether the locus of decision-making authority on any particular issue lies with the Ministry of External Affairs, the Council of Ministers, the Office of the Prime Minister, or the prime minister himself, nevertheless in the 1990s India's prime ministers retain their dominance in the conduct of foreign relations.

Giving an overall assessment of the achievement of Lal Bahadur Shastri's steely leadership ordering the Indian Army to launch a counter-attack on Pakistan and march towards Lahore and Sialkot during the September 1965 Indo-Pakistan War, Lt. Gen. Harbaksh Singh, the then GoC of the Western Command, writes in his War Despatches, Indo-Pakistan Conflict 1965 (Lancers, New Delhi 1991): "The illusion that Pakistan could steamroll into India with the help of gifted American equipment had been replaced by a hearty respect for the Indian jawan who forced the opponent to the knees in a straight contest. Our slow, simple and ponderous tanks, nicknamed 'Ancient Hulls' challenged and vanquished the ultra-modern Pattons to rub in the lesson that in the ultimate test of battle it is the man behind the gun that counts. The Pak Army was, in short, cut to size.

Shastri Retrieved India's Prestige

"And there is yet another achievement that overshadows all.

The humiliation heaped upon the Indian Army at home and abroad, consequent upon the NEFA debacle in 1962 had always ramkled deep in our minds and made us bend our heads in shame. This slur had been wiped out. In the eyes of the nation, the army ensured a prestige rarely equalled before. To the world at large it has re-established its traditional fame. Within the army itself our faith has been restored. These are mighty gains, far greater than any stretch of enemy territory or the destruction of her military potential." In fact, as admitted by Gen. Ayub Khan's then Information Secretary Altaf Gauhar in his memoirs, after the utter rout of Pakistan's Ist Armoured Division in the Khem Karan offensive, costing it destruction or loss of 97 Patton tanks, war was practically over for Pakistan on September 11, 1965, though the ceasefire came 12 days later. In contrast, what was the situation after the NEFA debacle in October-November 1962, under Prime Minister Nehru from which Shastri redeemed the nation? There was demoralisation from top to bottom.

Nehru himself had suffered such deep shock that not only his health deteriorated rapidly, he lost even "the will to live", as even his sister Vijay Lakshmi Pandit lamented. A friend of veteran journalist Frank Morales remarked to him, "Nehru really died two years before his actual death. He died on the day the Chinese crossed our borders." As the Chinese mounted attack, "Gone was non-alignment. Now military aid was welcome from any quarter." In this context, two eminent writers have painted the 'picture of pity' that Jawaharlal Nehru had become in his last days. One is that given by Gen. S.S.P. Thorat who was superseded for the post of Army Chief after retirement of Gen. Thimayya in 1961. As Corps Commander of NEFA, Thorat had prepared a plan to meet the Chinese challenge but was bypassed and retired to favour the mediocre, Gen. P.N. Thapar. In fact, so headstrong Krishna Menon and Nehru's favourite 'political general' B.M. Kaul had become that they were on a look out for a pretext to shunt out even Manekshaw (then a Brigadier).

He was 'A Picture of Pity' after the Chinese Attack

However, when after the debacle, Thorat sought time and went to meet Nehru, he was filled with pity to see him so haggard and woe-begone. Nehru sat aimlessly for sometime in his chair cutting a cigarette into small pieces with scissors. After long silence, he asked Thorat, What went wrong? As once reported by Manohar Malgonkar in the Statesman, Thorat replied he really couldn't say as he was forced to quit a year before the Chinese attack. But, says Thorat in his memoirs, the contrast between present and past Nehru shook him to the bones. Another graphic picture of Nehru's last days is drawn by former Indian diplomat Budruddin Tyabji (in his Memoirs of An Egoist), as he called on him in his last year after he had delegated all his authority to Lal Bahadur Shastri in January 1964. As Tyabji sat waiting in his first floor sitting room, Nehru came walking very slowly almost dragging, his feet into the room. How ill and discoloured he looked! He gave a pale smile with a swollen face. He sat there, saying nothing and silence became unbearable in that large room". At last Tyabji said, now that he had delegated many responsibilities he must have enough time to concentrate on large issues. But Nehru raplied, now he had more time than he knew what to do with it. At last, Tyabji took leave, haunted by the memory of once charismatic leader now completely played out. A Nation living on Secular Lies Kennedy's counter-sermon to Nehru after the NEFA debacle.

THE DAY A COLOSSUS PASSED AWAY

May 27, 1964 was just like any other summer day in New Delhi. The scorching heat had slowed down the pace of life and nothing much was likely to happen till the rains which were still weeks away. But by the afternoon of that day Jawarhalal Nehru, India's first Prime Minister, had passed away. An era had ended. The architect of India's foreign policy, the founder of the non-aligned movement, the motivating spirit behind the process of planned economic development, the chain of national laboratories and a thousand other things was no more.

I was then an Information Officer in the Public Relations Directorate of the Ministry of Defence. Our Director, G G Mirchandani, held a meeting of officers, the first thing in the morning. We were taken aback when he told us that the Prime Minister had been taken seriously ill, an emergency surgical operation was under way and the worst was feared. Our Director asked us to stop all routine work and to get busy if the worst happened.

The signs of an approaching end were there for anyone to see but the Indian people who looked upon Nehru as their idol refused to recognise that there might be a day when he was not there. The Chinese aggression in October-November, 1962 had come as a rude shock to him. A fond dream had been shattered. A severe blow had been inflicted on his reputation as a statesman of international repute. He survived the attacks against his leadership at home but just about. Questions were asked openly about his stewardship of foreign affairs. Many like me had gone to Parliament House to hear Nehru speak on the resolution on the Chinese attack, hoping to hear a speech on the lines of Winston Churchill's famous 'tears, blood and sweat' speech. What we got was a rambling speech with little fight in it. The Chinese aggression had suddenly accelerated the ageing process. The eyes had a glassy look and the reply to greetings was now just a mechanical gesture. The smile, which once captivated the people, young and old, was no longer there. The man who took two steps at a time while climbing stairs had, after he suffered a stroke, difficulty in walking. And yet he continued to work 16 hours a day attending to myriad problems. He had returned from a short holiday in the hills, just a few days before and had confidently said that he would be around for quite some time.

All these thoughts crossed my mind as I busied myself with the share of work allotted to me. The major responsibility of arranging a state funeral fell on the Army and the machinery had started moving. But there was one difficulty. It was 16 years earlier, in 1948 that there had been a state funeral – of Mahatma Gandhi in New Delhi. Most of those associated with it at a senior level had long since retired from service. Old records were therefore searched and people still in service consulted about the modalities. The troops in New Delhi were not enough. The Army Chief, Gen. J. N. Chaudhuri, informed the Defence Ministry that he was calling troops from Meerut. But the sudden movement of troops gave rise to misgivings. Why were these troops coming to Delhi in such large numbers? The misgivings were soon removed but were symbolic of the large question mark and the void created by Nehru's sudden death.

Parliament was in session but the heart and the mind of the members were not in the legislative business. Attendance was thin and the members had gathered in the lobbies and the Central Hall sitting in clusters, hoping for the best and yet fearing for the worst. Indian writers had generally been reticent in discussing an India without Jawaharlal Nehru. Western writers had no such inhibitions. Earlier, the question asked was 'After Nehru, Who'? Ten likely names were mentioned and discussed in a book of that title. Then the question asked was 'After Nehru, What?', implying that after Jawaharlal Nehru there was likelihood of total anarchy in India. It is quite another matter that these prophets of doom were proved wrong. The transition to Lal Bahadur Shastri and a year later from Shastri to Indira Gandhi was brought about in an orderly manner. By mid-day, the fact that Nehru was seriously ill was known all over the country and 'What Next"? was the question in the mind of everyone.

A little after 2.30 p.m. Parliament was informed by C. Subramaniam that Jawaharlal Nehru had passed away. I was asked to rush to Teen Murti House. I had no specific duty to perform but was only to watch and see for any unforeseen developments. A pall of gloom had descended on Teen Murti House. Soon after I reached there, Ministers and Members of Parliament began arriving. It was a varied lot. There were Ministers, former Ministers and Members of Parliament from all political parties. It was as representative a political gathering as it could be. Some who were close to the family were allowed to go to the bedroom on the first floor where the body lay. Others remained on the lawn below.

Shock, grief and loss was written large on everyone's face. But I have a vivid impression of the agony on the face of two persons. One of them was Acharya Kripalani. He had been a colleague of Nehru for nearly 30 years but had now parted company. As he walked with his head covered by a small *dupatta,* one could see that political differences apart he was feeling the loss of someone who had been a comrade in arms during the freedom struggle. The other person was V K Krishna Menon. He had come under severe criticism for India's failure to meet the Chinese attack in 1962. Nehru had tried to defend him for a time but had ultimately to give in before the storm of public anger. It must be said to the credit of Menon that neither then nor at any time later did he try to pass on the blame to Nehru as many others did.

Even in the atmosphere of gloom, permutations and combinations of a future political line-up were being discussed by politicians in small groups. One Minister known for his belief in astrology was going round telling all those who would listen that he had long ago been told by a leading astrologer of Delhi that Nehru would not see the end of May. Meanwhile, arrangements were being finalised to bring Nehru's body to the foyer so that people could have a glimpse of the departed leader. Nearby in the South Block, the machinery had started moving for a State funeral. It was also known that leaders from other countries would be coming to New Delhi in large number to bid good bye to Jawaharlal Nehru.

When I left Teen Murti House, the crowds had gathered outside and the gates were closed. People could get in only with difficulty. If the politicians inside were discussing the political fallout, the people outside were in a state of shock almost bordering on personal loss.

Lakhs turned out in the scorching May sun to say good bye to Nehru as his body was taken for the last rites. He had been a darling of the masses for more than 30 years and his picture as he rode a white charger to preside over the Lahore session of the Indian National Congress in 1929 adorned many drawing rooms. Even his opponents in political life held Nehru in esteem. The most moving tribute to him in Parliament after his death was by Mr Atal Bihari Vajpayee, then a member of the Jana Sangh opposition party.

It is easy to find fault with a political personality and to say that he could have done more. This is particularly so when he is no more. There are many who hold that Mahatma Gandhi was wrong when he nominated Nehru and not Sardar Vallabhbhai Patel as his political successor. A visitor asked this question of Morarji Desai when he was Prime Minister. Desai's reply surprised me because like many others, I had thought that he would say that Patel would have made a better Prime Minster. Desai said that Patel was a great leader and a great administrator but was not known outside India. When India became free it was not strong economically or militarily. Nehru, who was known abroad, managed to win respect for India at the international level, which would have been difficult for Patel. But this thought did not enter the minds of the lakhs who turned out to have a last glimpse of Nehru. What Nehru meant to them was brought home to me a few days later. A house owner abused the woman who swept the street. The woman burst out in tears and said, "*Ab Panditji nahi hain is liye aap gali de rahe ho*". Nehru would certainly have not come to save the woman but her reply was symbolic of the image of Jawaharlal Nehru as the protector of the downtrodden.

TRIBUTE TO A "GENTLE LEADER"

A world-renowned figure who is affectionately remembered as India's "gentle leader." He was a leader of great compassion. He was, at the same time, unrelenting in his commitment to building peace and prosperity. His all-too-brief stewardship as Prime Minister of India (June 1964-January 1966) created the groundwork for a transformed society; indeed, a transformed region.

Domestically, India's continuing efforts to promote policies and programs for people-centred growth are in keeping with the orientation of his beliefs. His selection of Mr. C. Subramanian as Minister of Agriculture was a stroke of genius. Mr. Subramanian's international task force, which included two CGIAR figures-M.S. Swaminathan and Ralph Cummings Sr.-mapped out India's agricultural transformation. Externally, the five-point doctrine, based on mutual trust and respect among sovereign nations, which currently governs India's foreign policy is based on the principles Mr. Shastri pressed on his contemporaries repeatedly, including at Tashkent in 1966. Truly, his legacy is a continuing influence and inspiration.

Like so many of this country's leaders, Mr. Shastri received his earliest training through political imprisonment in the heyday of India's freedom struggle and went on, after independence, to serve his country both in a provincial setting, and in the central government.

He faced a range of challenges with patience, skill, and loyalty to a set of defining principles:

- domestic strength as a pre-requisite for external, mainly regional, stability,
- a powerful nationwide campaign against hunger and poverty, as the foundation of domestic strength, and
- adherence to consensual politics, in order to promote the widest possible acceptance of the policies and programs he proposed.

The consensus-building process he championed is arduous and time consuming. I can testify to this from my experience as Chairman of the CGIAR where all decisions are reached by consensus, not by head-counting. I am sometimes surprised and of course, gratified, that decisions are reached at all through such a hectic exchange of views among women and men of great intellectual capacity and strongly-held positions.

So, too, must it be in India, where contention and disputation have been celebrated in prose and verse. But experience tells us that decisions reached through discourse and persuasion are usually long-lasting.

Whether Mr. Shastri was grappling with the prickly issues of regional peace and stability; moving toward promising, new vistas of bilateral engagement; responding to the sensitivities of provincial concerns in the domestic polity; or encountering the heartbreak of food crises; his emphasis was on constructing principles and undertaking programs that would endure.

The long-last lasting impact of his policies is evident even today. We salute his wisdom and applaud the way he used it on behalf of the weak and the vulnerable.

In that spirit, let me briefly touch on India's achievements in an area that was so dear to Mr. Shastri's heart: modernizing agriculture so as to build food security and change forever the fortunes of the rural poor. Let me then, while drawing important lessons from the past, look to the future, not only in India, but in a global context of complex food security challenges.

ELEMENTS OF SUCCESS

"To the hungry," Gandhi once said, "God is bread". That sage assessment reminds us that the hungry are both physically and spiritually malnourished. The possible repercussions of this condition were vividly, if starkly, described in the sixties by Nobel laureate and CGIAR scientist Norman Borlaug who visited a group of Indian farmers in their fields and said to them: "If there is no more food, a volcano will erupt under the political leaders of this land."

Mr. Borlaug spoke at a time of growing concern in many circles that a Malthusian nightmare threatened much of the developing world, and particularly South Asia. For some, concern fuelled a pessimism that soon turned to a certainty of doom. Paul Ehrlich's often quoted comment summed up their viewpoint. He said:

> *"Some time between 1970 and 1985 the world will undergo vast famines — hundreds of millions of people are going to starve to death. That is, they will starve to death unless plague, thermonuclear war, or some other agent kills them first. The United States should announce that it will no longer ship food to countries such as India where dispassionate analysis indicates that the unbalance between food and population is hopeless."*

Today, some thirty years later, I am proud to share with you the triumph of knowing that reality proved Mr. Ehrlich hopelessly wrong. India, through a concerted effort that represents an exemplary turnaround of national fortunes, overcame the crises that caused such predictions.

By 1985, the closing year of Mr. Ehrlich's prediction, famine, a wracking feature of the past, was just a part of history. And in November last year, Prime Minister Deve Gowda, reflecting the growing confidence of India's agricultural sector, told the World Food Summit:

> *"There have been periodical predictions of shortfalls in the world's food production and, often, major disasters are predicted by agricultural pundits. I am a grassroots farmer and may I assure you that as a grower of food grains on my own land, I do not believe the prophets of doom."*

The agricultural sector supports about 65 percent of the labour force, contributes almost 30 percent of GDP, and contributes substantially as well to the total value of the country's exports. During the post-green revolution period, i.e. after 1967-68, the growth rate of agricultural production has consistently been around 2.8 percent annually.

An institutional assessment from the World Bank is optimistic about India's agriculture. A recent examination of agricultural performance says that "between 1980 and 1996, agricultural growth has accelerated and spread to the eastern regions and rainfed areas, and real rural wages have improved. Together, this has contributed to an unprecedented decline in rural poverty, except during droughts and economic recession."

Consider these facts:

- Cereals output in India has risen from 80 mill t (1966) to 221 mill t (1996)-an increase of 176 percent increase or 5.8 percent per year,
- Cereal yields increased from 0.86 t/ha (1966) to 2.2 t (1996)-156% increase or 5.2 percent per year,

- India is the world's second largest producer of rice, after China,
- Paddy production rose from 46 mill t (1966) to 125 mill t (1996)-an increase of 172 percent or 5.7 percent annually,
- Rice yields increased from 1.3 t/ha (1966) to 3 t (1996)-a 170 percent increase or 5.7 percent per year,
- India is now the world's second largest wheat producer, behind China but ahead of the US,
- Wheat output rose from 10 mill to (1966) to 64 mill t (1996)-a 540 percent increase or 18 percent per year,
- Wheat yields increased from 0.83 t/ha (1966) to 2.5 t (1996)-a 167 percent increase or 5.6 percent per year,
- The output of pulses rose from 9.8 mill t (1966) to 15.4 mill t (1996)-a 57 percent increase or 1.9 percent per year,
- Potato production rose from 4 mill t (1966) to 18 mill t (1996) — yields rose from 8.5 t/ha (1966) to 16.5 t (1996)-a 94 per cent increase or 3.1 percent per year,
- Agricultural land under irrigation increased from 25.9 million ha (1964) to 48.0 million ha (1994) or 85.3 percent,
- Forest land increased from 61 mill ha (1964) to 68.5 mill ha (1994), or 12.4 percent over a period of 30 years,
- Fuelwood and charcoal production doubled over the same period, and industrial roundwood production tripled.

These achievements do not imply that agricultural development has reached its zenith in India, thereby eradicating poverty. Much has been done. Much remains to be done by way of revamping trade policy, reviewing subsidies, and targeting poverty reducing measures. What they do mean is that India has crossed the boundary from despair to hope-and beyond.

Confidence in India's agriculture was not always so strong, as we know, and it is useful to remember that the seeds of achievement were actually sown at a time of seeming distress; the sixties. How was that possible? How did a situation close to despair change into one of promise? The nature of the problems encountered were a catalyst in themselves. They were so severe, so deeply entrenched, and so debilitating that they required responses which were both creative and far reaching. Anything less would have fulfilled the predictions of doom.

India's leaders defined a set of goals and reached out to them single-mindedly. Five crops were chosen for improvement-rice, wheat, maize, sorghum, and pearl millet. Price supports were provided for rice and wheat.

Specific targets were set up for the production and distribution of inputs. Administrative machinery was mobilized to give agricultural programs coherence and vigour. Floor prices were announced before sowing commenced, and mechanisms were established for implementing government policies including prices and the distribution of inputs. The private sector was fully engaged. So were external partners, for this was a time when development cooperation was considered a civilized responsibility not an odious burden.

In addition to political will, sound decision-making, effective policy implementation, and unity among many elements, a strong contribution was made by scientific research which created what are now widely known as "green revolution technologies." India's scientists and their colleagues in the international agricultural research centers produced new technologies that were used to increase the productivity of the five crops selected for a special effort. The new technologies have their detractors and their concerns must be respected as the world moves into the next phase of agricultural development. The undeniable fact, however, is that application of the new technologies saved millions from starvation or death. For this, the credit goes to scientists *and* farmers.

India's farmers have always been a powerful force. In 1932, for instance, the colonial administration placed a ban on the activities of *Kisan Sabhas* (peasant organizations) because their involvement in the freedom struggle was formidable. In the sixties and beyond, farmers applied those same creative energies to agricultural transformation. As former Minister of Agriculture C. Subramanian, the father of modern agriculture in India, puts it: "Indian scientists responded to the challenges in a magnificent way. More than that, the farmers were prepared to take risks, they were prepared to use new varieties. That is how the green revolution became a reality."

Farmers were the first scientists. They carried out the first experiments, asked themselves numerous questions and, through their answers, served as creative providers. So, however high we set our sights, we should never forget that in the distilled experience of farm women, men, and children reside wisdom that has to be integrated within the new science. If we fail to do so we will have to ask ourselves, as the British poet T.S. Eliot did:

Where is the wisdom we have lost in Knowledge"? And where is the knowledge we have lost in information:

Facing New Challenges

The "new" agriculture was not restricted to India. At the global level, one of the greatest achievements of this century has been the phenomenal increase of agricultural productivity through the application of science-based technologies. In Asia, the data is nothing short of stunning. Over the thirty years ending in 1991, rice production increased by 123 percent, largely through an increase in yields of some 88 percent. Wheat production rose by 338 percent in the same period, with yields increasing by 204 percent. Consumers gained over time from lower prices of basic foodstuffs made possible by increased supply. The poor benefited greatly because they spend a higher proportion of their resources on foodstuffs than no others.

In a report prepared for the World Food Summit, the World Bank pointed out that real progress was achieved in the past twenty five years in improving the condition of the world's poor. For instance:

- the proportion of the world's population living in poverty has dropped,
- average incomes per person have doubled,
- real food prices have fallen by more than 50 percent,
- average calorie supplies per person have risen by some 30 percent,
- infant mortality has been reduced by half, and
- average life expectancy has increased by ten years.

And yet, the sights and sounds of poverty are all around us. The paradox of our times is that both in the North and the South poverty and plenty co-exist. Women and men of goodwill in the North grapple continuously with the demeaning effects of homelessness, societal collapse, and the frustrations of an almost permanent underclass. The South faces problems so challenging as to frighten the faint-hearted.

As we move towards the new millennium and beyond, when the world's population will be about 8.5 billion, 7 billion in developing countries, the world's very poor will number one and a half billion. Some 70 percent of them will be women. At the dawn of the 21st century, India's population will be some 1 billion. Within the next 30 years no less than 80 countries, 43 of them in Africa, will double their populations.

During the same period, urbanization and increased income in developing countries are likely to change dietary habits, with the demand for livestock and high value agricultural products increasing. This, in turn, will increase the demand for cereals and coarse grains to be used as animal feed, not only as food for people.

Simultaneously, current trends suggest that the world will continue to face serious environmental concerns such as soil degradation (water and wind erosion, loss of soil nutrients, salinization, and water logging), tropical deforestation, and loss of biodiversity unless corrective measures are taken.

India itself, despite its impressive advances on so many fronts, faces numerous problems as well.

- Every minute — 48 children are born,
- Every minute — the population increases by 42 people,
- Total population rose from 495 million (1965) to 936 million (1995) and is projected to increase to 1.32 billion in 2020,
- The rural population rose from 402 million (1965) to 685 million (1995) of which 78 comprises the agricultural population,
- Some 300 million live below poverty line; and India has the largest concentration of poor people,
- Silent hunger is a menace, with child undernutrition still as high as 63 percent,
- Infant mortality high stands at 70 per 1000 births,
- About half the population lacks access to safe water,
- Only 16 percent of the population has access to sanitation,
- Over 141 million hectares are subject to water and wind erosion,
- Over a million hectares are damaged as a result of shifting cultivation annually,
- Some 40 million hectares are flood prone.

Such realities in India and across the world could very easily be interpreted as constituting, once again, a catastrophe scenario. Last year's temporary increase of the price of wheat, and fears that yield increases of major cereals have reached a plateau, adds to the concerns. Indeed, catastrophe is an ever-present danger, if circumstances are not scientifically assessed and, as necessary, countered. Agriculture is at the heart of any effective solution to this nexus of problems encompassing population growth, environmental destruction, poverty reduction, and food security. Over 70 percent of the world's land and water are used for agriculture. Over 75 percent of employment in the poorest countries is based on agriculture. If we do not transform agriculture to be more productive, we will curtail food abundance, which is the basis of food security. If we do not transform agriculture to be sustainable, we will destroy natural resources, the foundation of productivity and human sustenance. If we do not transform it to benefit the poorest and focus especially on women, we will help to perpetuate the very inequities that should be destroyed.

The Changing Paradigm of Science

As we look to the future, therefore, we know that action on a broad front is required to meet the objectives of poverty reduction, food security, and natural resources management. In the short-run, reducing hunger must focus at the household level with enabling actions by nations. Globally, only adequate supplies and food aid can help. In the medium-term, the emphasis must be more at the national and international levels, focusing on reducing poverty and generating sustained economic development for all. Central to that vision are concerted national and international efforts to generate appropriate agricultural technology to improve the productivity and profitability of millions of farmers in developing countries. In the long-term, global food supplies must increase in sustainable production systems to feed more than 8 billion people, and a fair trading system is vital.

India's outstanding experience in the green revolution shows us that in the past, government policies compiled with good science and an effective extension service which took the results of science to the farmers were adequate to meet the challenges of the time-provided that the technology package was appropriate.

Today's problems are more complex. Science can help us to meet them, but the mobilization of science has to be reshaped, as science itself changes. Science must be used in three crucial areas:

- Defining the problem,
- Identifying partnerships and the new role of all partners in the global agricultural research system, and
- Making decisions on how science is practiced-bringing together all members of the "science family" together in a single constructive enterprise.

Getting the Facts Right

The world has seen a science explosion. The wonders of science and their potential for further improving the condition of the human family are all around us. We must put that potential to the best possible use, beginning with a concerted effort to define our problems accurately; to get the facts right.

So much of the debate among policymakers, advocacy groups, and in the media is based on partial figures and incomplete or inaccurate information. Sensible discussion and appropriate policies are thereby made elusive. What virtue is there in carrying out an impassioned debate on food production in China when the protagonists use vastly divergent figures of the acreage of Chinese land under cultivation on which the yield figures depend?

India was a pioneer in matching the requirements of agricultural development and information technology through its Satellite Instructional Television Experiment (SITE). Now is the time to be bold again, and to ensure that new breakthroughs in Geographic Information Systems (GIS) and computing will make it possible for more accurate figures to be obtained on the kinds of questions that determine policy. More importantly, such developments will enable the ecological site-specific data and the socioeconomic data to be mapped at the local to the supranational levels, offering for the first time the possibility of substantial relational databases being developed with all the advantages for analysis that such developments entail. Maintaining and making available proper databases thus becomes another major contribution that scientists can make to the better understanding of the issues and the monitoring and evaluation of trends by countless researchers and groups. Beyond using GIS/computing, databases, and scientific interpretation, the international scientific community can state problems accurately, define areas of uncertainty and risk, identify new technologies, and help set the boundaries of debate.

The debate will be wide ranging and through it will emerge an agenda for today and tomorrow. Let me review some of the issues that will have to be confronted.

- Favoured or less-favored areas. This is not an either/or choice. The real question is how much of each receives priority attention by researchers in a period of finite resources. How does one weight poverty reduction for poor subsistence farmers against low food prices for the rural landless and the urban poor? How does one focus on the particular target groups we want to help—the poorest, women, and those who cultivate fragile environments?
- Traditional versus exotic crops. How can we improve the productivity and the income potential of poor farmers in the semi-arid tropics and arid zones? Should we invest in improving the yields of indigenous crops—millet and sorghum—or should we try to improve the stress resistance of higher yielding nontraditional maize? Should we invest in developing "tropical" wheat or potatoes or improve yams, sweet potatoes, and cassava?
- Time horizon choices. What should be the time frame of expected impact? Often, improved agronomic practices such as spacing, seeding time, weed control, and planting depth can have short-term yield impacts, whereas genetic improvement, particularly involving complex characteristics, takes much longer but has higher long-run yield potential. How much should the international system invest in small, incremental improvements (including removing impediments to application of known technologies); how much on the development

of radical new technologies such as transgenic techniques for apomixis and plant resistance?

- Environmental improvement versus yield maximization. Frequently this is posed as a major trade-off in priority choices, but it cannot persist as such. Clearly a major challenge to agricultural science is to turn this apparent win-lose situation into a win-win guarantee.
- The integration of traditional knowledge and new science. The documentation of traditional knowledge, including identification of wild races, should be undertaken as a matter of urgency before it is lost. It must be integrated in a two-way commerce of ideas with modern science, and the poor farmers who are the custodians of this knowledge should benefit from these efforts. Taxonomies will show us different ways of approaching these problems.
- The search for integrated farming practices that reflect local specificity's versus the search for new technologies with very broad applications. Such farming practices would reduce the vulnerability of the smallholder farmer and/or increase her or his income. These require international reach but local adaptation, such as the introduction of multipurpose leguminous trees e.g., sesbania or calliandra, or the introduction of fish ponds for super tilapia, which help with on-farm water management in addition to producing fish. How much attention should be given these types of activities versus the use of cutting-edge technologies such as transgenic biotechnology to attack the problems of the developing world?
- Preserving biodiversity. This is a crucial aspect of the agricultural research process, an area in which many groups need to work together to ensure that we can increase our use of this biodiversity and that our common heritage is protected and preserved for the future.
- Greater use of biotechnology. This could be the most exciting contribution that science can make to food security in the next century. Radical and rapid changes in our understanding of molecular biology have spawned a potential biotechnology revolution. The application of biotechnology was pioneered in the medical sciences, but agricultural science has been catching up. There has undoubtedly been concern that the application of biotechnology in agriculture is occurring more slowly than its enthusiasts predicted. Yet today, some fifty plant varieties—from alfalfa to wheat—have been altered through biotechnology since the first success was recorded in gene manipulation in the 1980s. The value of sorrel products from biotechnology in agriculture in the U.S. market alone is US$380 million in sales in 1996,

with predicted growth in the market of 20 percent per annum over the next decade.

The opportunities for producing transgenic varieties are endless. Plants and animals that use water more efficiently, grow in highly adverse conditions, resist pests and diseases, and use fewer inputs have enormous potential to contribute to the sustainability of agricultural production systems and are representative of the range of possibilities which may develop through biotechnology. Biotechnology also has great potential in livestock and fish production, and in the modification of biological control agents.

Genetically altered varieties, especially those that are sensitively responsive to the specifics of complex smallholder farming systems, can be introduced to less-favored areas offering undreamed of opportunities to the poor. However, the research agenda must also address areas of concern with biotechnology. The correct balance has to be established on weighing the benefits against the risks of biotechnology. Not everything that is technically feasible is ethically desirable. The technology potential involves science and economics. The ethical issue has many complexities. We cannot accept hunger and poverty as the permanent legacy of the disadvantaged. We cannot accept the notion that deprivation should forever be imprinted on the genes of the poor and destitute-that misery is their inevitable or even karmic destiny-because of fears about the use of biotechnology. Both sets of issues need to be boldly confronted.

Getting the Roles Right

Science has created the basis of a new interconnectedness. And yet there is potential for dangerous divisions. Aspects of the application of intellectual property rights could lead to limitations on the free flow of germplasm, thus drastically curtailing agricultural development. The collaborative nature of science and its application run the risk of being transformed into a competitive race — not by scientific or communications obstacles but by legal requirements.

Indeed, research today is subjected to dual pressure. On the one hand, it must take account of the diversity of natural and human environments and therefore come to terms with location-specific realities. It is equally influenced by globalization factors: the awakening of a planetary conscience against common challenges, the revolution of basic sciences, particularly in biology; the interconnection of communications networks; economic liberalization, and so on. The emergence of a "global system" is manifest.

However, in this area, as in others we must ensure that this "globalization" of research does not translate into a few powers dominating a world where the vast majority are relegated to facing the specter of environmental loss, and seeing the impact of continuing inequities on the poor, there can be no room for divisiveness in the agricultural research effort. "Public assets" and "private assets" each have their own logic. These must be clearly understood, and their differences as well as their complementarities respected. We need a new paradigm of research. The real challenge is to ensure that all usable assets are deployed for the production of public goods. This principle applies to the protection of intellectual property and in the field of biological research. We need an overall system that promotes interaction to help each actor contribute to the best of its comparative advantages so that the whole is much more than the sum of the parts. When such a system is in place, the synergies in agricultural research will acquire their own momentum, providing more productive links among public and private actors, national and international agencies, rich and poor countries, and formal and informal sector institutions of the civil society.

Getting Partnerships Moving

To address all these issues, what should be the distribution of responsibilities among local, national, regional and international research? Should every country have a full-blown research system? What role should multinational firms play in the global research systems? What are truly public research goods—nationally and internationally? What level of public investment is required for the production of public goods? How can the strengths of the private sector be integrated with public endeavour?

These are difficult issues, but nobody said that development would be simple. Think of the Finance Minister of any small country in the South who, three weeks before Budget Day, has to choose between allocating money for an emergency program to clean out small irrigation reservoirs or an emergency program to build a network of rural dispensaries. The choices of development are rarely easy. But, just as the crises of the fifties and sixties in India brought forth effective responses, I am convinced that today's challenges are also today's opportunities. They are opportunities for building partnerships, creating and implementing effective policies, for acting in areas both directly and indirectly connected with food security issues, for reaching out to the weakest among us and helping them to begin their ascent from poverty.

We all recognize that the challenges of tomorrow will require the mobilization of the talents, resources and abilities of all the actors, from the public and the private sectors, local, national and international agencies, the private sector and the civil society. How does one bring them together? How does one find a non-bureaucratic forum to enable them to share ideas and help shape the agenda? To define new partnerships and work out new forms of collaboration? Indeed, steps to do just that have already been taken. A Global Forum, which took place in Washington last October, was the start of this dream of a common commitment by one and all for the better future of humanity and of our planet.

Clearly, the voice of the NARS and their regional fora must be central in helping shape the future programs of this new Global Forum. The single most important challenge facing this Global Forum is that of devising both the priorities of and the modalities for action. But such action must be guided by principles designed to create a truly participatory and inclusive system. Based on this, the emerging global system can have a shared vision in which the programs of each benefit from the successful work of the others. This will give substance to real research partnerships in the battles against poverty, hunger, environmental degradation, and inequity.

The CGIAR sees itself as an active participant in the further development of the global agricultural system, as CGIAR centers continue with the mission of carrying out cutting-edge research. Beyond the content of their work and the manner in which they design and carry out research programs with their partners, these centers of scientific excellence must act as dynamic catalysts, as platforms for the exchange of information and the development of true networks of scientists between the South and the North.

In preparation for its deepening involvement in a partnership mode within global agricultural systems, the CGIAR undertook an 18-month program of renewal-which was launched in this city in May 1994. The program was completed on schedule in October of 1995.

As a result the CGIAR is today a fully South-North enterprise, its participatory mechanisms have been greatly improved and the mode of operations of some centers have changed or are changing. ICRISAT, headquartered near Hyderabad, is one such centre.

It is reducing the size of its staff, orienting itself much more than before to operating through partnership, and is sharply refocusing its research agenda. Utmost care is being taken to cushion the personal impact of the changes underway.

Periods of change are hard, nevertheless, and I share the concerns of those who are personally affected. Commiseration is easier than hardship. Many hundred staff are affected; national and international. The CGIAR is profoundly concerned about the personal difficulties that are being experienced. I, personally, have appealed for more resources to prevent current developments, and wish that other courses could have been followed. Those affected will be cared for, to the fullest extent possible. Our thoughts are with them, and we hope that the adjustment process will soon be completed. The plus side of an otherwise negative situation is that programmatic and administrative changes now in progress at several CGIAR centers will enable them to be even more effective partners of national scientists than before. The NARS will have to undergo their own transformation, taking on new responsibilities, and working out effective distributions of tasks among themselves and other components of the global agricultural research system. Let us all do our bit to ensure that the changes will not only be made, but will be part of the new science paradigm.

INTO THE FUTURE

Inspired and strengthened by past achievements we must face the future with hope, determination, and confidence-but not over-confidence which could be as damaging as complacency. We must be willing to acknowledge how formidable the challenges of today and tomorrow might be. And we must be ready to mobilize science and scientists to meet those challenges.

The effectiveness of science is no longer dependent only on the quality of scientific breakthroughs, but by the speed at which nations can embrace the change and incorporate the new.

Klaus Schwab, head of the World Economic Forum, has said that "we are moving from a world in which the big eat the small to one in which the fast eat the slow." None of us wants to be destroyed because we are unable to absorb and use new science speedily. To hold our own, we must all transform ourselves into learning nations, leaving none behind in the process. The most skilled scientists and the poorest farmers must all be involved in this common enterprise. We need to transform society from the inside out, something like turning out a sock.

These are formidable challenges. They can be overcome if all of us who share the same concerns and strive for the same goals work in partnership and unity.... if we pool resources and combine forces to create a just future for today's marginalized. We must be driven by a sense of moral outrage against the continuance of poverty and hunger. And we must mobilize a scientific dynamism that cares for the neglected, reaches out to the unreached, feeds the hungry, and empowers the weak.

What can India do? Very much. One out of every six persons on earth is Indian. India is a leader of the South, with the capacity to blaze trails that others will follow. Your success is the key to global success. The Indian agricultural research community is the pride and envy of the whole world. Indian scientists, supported by policymakers, can carefully select problems for solution in terms of their potential for impact. This will have to be done in such a way that a balance is created among basic, strategic, adaptive and applied research.

Sixty years ago, Jawaharlal Nehru said of India: "The promised land may be far from us, and we may have to march wearily through the deserts, but who will dare to crush the spirit of India which has found rebirth again and again after so many crucifixions." So it is with us today. Who will dare crush our spirit or thwart our purpose, if we are determined to persevere until success is ours?

SASTRI'S VIEW ON NUCLEAR TEST

India tried three approaches to resolve its nuclear dilemma. One, it sought security guarantees from the United States, Soviet Union and Britain to cope with a hostile nuclear China on her borders. India was rebuffed by all three. Two, it attempted to develop a multilateral solution by calling for a non-proliferation treaty under which the nuclear powers would give up nuclear weapons and others would not acquire them.

The NPT that came out of the multilateral negotiations turned out to be entirely different. Three, Prime Minister Lal Bahadur Shastri decided in 1965 to go ahead with a sub-terranean nuclear explosion project (SNEP). But both Shastri and Bhabha died in January 1966. And given the large political and economic crisis that India went through in that period, SNEP was postponed. In May 1964, Prime Minister Nehru died. He was succeeded by Mr Lal Bahadur Shastri. Pakistan intensified its anti India campaign and decided that 1965 was the right year to force a settlement of the Kashmir issue that had eluded them in 1947-48.

During 1964, delegations headed by Defence Minister Chavan held discussions with America, Russia and Britain regarding assistance for India's Defence Plan 1964-69. America could not offer what India wanted. Russia offered the Army and Navy what they sought.

The Army contracted for light tanks and artillery. The Navy did not want to strain its connections with the British Navy and waited for the outcome of discussions with Britain.

The Defence Minister's delegation visited Britian in end 1964. It found that Britain's decision to reduce the size of its Navy precluded it from meeting the Navy's immediate requirements of ships and submarines. However, negotiations were concluded for British collaboration in the construction in Bombay of the British Navy's latest design of Leander class frigates.

In end 1964, Britain's economy was under serious strain. A major review of defence and foreign policy had concluded that Britain could neither afford its overseas defence commitments nor the size of its Navy. It was mutually agreed that the burden of Cold War naval deployment in the Indian Ocean should be borne by America.

In due course, the British withdrew from Gan in Addu Atoll and America established its presence in Diego Garcia. Likewise, the American Navy gradually replaced the British Navy's presence in Bahrein in the Persian Gulf. By 1965, there were sharp differences in Britain about Indian Ocean policy. In one view, Britain's economic difficulties and the conclusions of the strategic defence review carried out in 1964 required that Britain withdraw from the Indian Ocean and concentrate on Europe.

The opposite view was that in view of China's nuclear explosion in 1964, Indonesia's confrontation with Malaysia in the east and Egypt's 'subversion' of Aden and the Persian Gulf in the west, Britain should not withdraw from the Indian Ocean, because it would leave friends and allies in the lurch. Even though Indonesia and Egypt were not overtly communist, the British viewed their actions as serving communist objectives. In their view, the security of the Indian sub-continent was central to Indian Ocean Policy and it would not avail to stand fast on the Himalaya, if the western and eastern flanks of the area were turned. (Note: Letter to the London Times 29 Apr 65 by Sir Olaf Caroe and others).

In May 1965, Pakistan intruded into the Rann of Kutch. At the same time, there was a marked increase in intrusions in the Nicobar Islands. The Navy recommended an immediate increase in naval presence in the Bay of Bengal. This precipitated the decision to accept the ships and submarines which Russia had offered to the Defence Minister's delegation in 1964 and to base them in Visakhapatnam.

Within a brief period of four years between 1961 and 1965, the geopolitical and economic compulsions of America and Britain had led India's Air Force, Army and Navy to accept Russia's generous offers of its latest conventional defence systems on extremely favourable financial terms. The 1956 Rupee-Ruble Trade Agreement was extended also to defence sales from 1965 onwards.

During the 1965 war, Indonesia's stance was markedly pro-Pakistan. There was an increase in the sightings of unidentified submarines and aircraft in the Andaman and Nicobar islands. In response to Pakistan's request for assistance, the Indonesian Navy sent two submarines and two missile boats to Karachi. The Indonesian Naval Chief even volunteered to distract India by making moves to take over islands in the Nicobars (For details see "The First Round" by Air Marshal Asghar Khan, Page 45). It was this vulnerability in August 1965 that impelled Naval Headquarters to keep the Indian Fleet in the Bay of Bengal for as long as possible, so as to deter adventurist Indonesian naval moves.

After the 1965 Indo Pakistan War, Russia's mediation at Tashkent helped to negotiate the postwar settlement. From 1966 onwards, Russia tried to wean Pakistan away from American and Chinese influence by offering defence assistance and economic aid. By 1969, it was clear that this had not succeeded.

In the same year, discussions started on what in August 1971 was to become the Indo Soviet Treaty of Peace, Friendship and Cooperation (Note: for details see "War and Secession" by Sisson and Rose, Page 197). Russia offered to sign a similar treaty with Pakistan provided they got out of CENTO, SEATO and the American Military Assistance Programme. Pakistan rejected the offer.

In the 1960's, America's naval policy in the Indian Ocean had many ingredients. The foremost was to deter Russia from interrupting the flow of oil from the Persian Gulf countries to America and Europe. Politically, this entailed American support of Iran to counter Russian influence in Iraq. It entailed maintaining a naval presence in the Persian Gulf, and wherever possible, in the countries on the rim of the Indian Ocean, not only to secure the sea lines of communication which criss-crossed the Indian Ocean but also to inject military force from seaward when required. By 1968, the American Navy had effected the necessary adjustments in its global naval deployments. In 1968, Britain announced its intention to withdraw from East of Suez by 1971 and generated debate on "the Vacuum in the Indian Ocean". Russia's naval presence in the Indian Ocean increased to keep pace with the American naval presence.

America felt that Russia was articulating anxiety to forestall American naval deployment. The Russians on the other hand, felt that the establishing of communication facilities in Diego Garcia and in Northwest Cape in Australia could be interpreted clearly as reflecting an intention to deploy submarines in the Indian Ocean whose ballistic missiles were targeted on Russia. Fears of a naval vacuum in the Indian Ocean were soon overtaken by fears of the militarisation of the Indian Ocean. America neither denied nor acknowledged the deployment of submarine launched ballistic missiles. The Russian Navy started showing its flag in the Indian Ocean, partly to fill the naval vacuum, partly to counter the American Navy and partly to demonstrate to the littoral states that the Russian Navy was a force to contend with. Since Russia lacked naval bases in the Indian Ocean, an anchorage was developed off Socotra near the Gulf of Aden. Overall, there was a steady increase in the presence of American and Russian naval ships.

In 1969, American President Nixon's "Twin Pillar" strategy entrusted the security of the Persian Gulf region to the monarchies in Iran and Saudi Arabia. America started heavily arming both countries under the Nixon Doctrine. In 1970, the Russians became active in the Dhofar rebellion in Oman, which was a Persian Gulf choke-point. These moves towards militarisation of the Indian Ocean triggered countermoves to make the Indian Ocean a Zone of Peace. And both these moves and countermoves had to take into account the overall American hyper-sensitivity regarding West Asian oil supplies.

In 1971, the Indo Soviet Friendship Treaty and Russia's veto in the Security Council during the Indo Pakistan war helped India to liberate Bangladesh so that ten million refugees could return to their homes. America made its gesture of support to Pakistan by sending the ENTERPRISE carrier group into the Bay of Bengal. The Russian Navy, in an equally reassuring gesture of support to India, shadowed the American Navy's task force into the Indian Ocean. After the 1971 war, the Russian Navy worked alongside the Indian Navy to clear the mines laid by the Pakistan Navy in the approaches to Chittagong harbour.

In 1971 also, the concept of the Indian Ocean as a Zone of Peace crystallised in the UN. The original idea of the Non Aligned Movement was that the Great Powers should not enhance their military presence in the Indian Ocean area. The UN's 1971 resolution for an Indian Ocean Peace Zone was very specific about the scope of the Zone. The Indian Ocean covered not only the ocean, but also its natural extensions like the Red Sea, the Persian Gulf etc. It did not include the adjacent land mass. The main thrust of the resolution was directed against Great Power rivalry in the Indian Ocean. It did not try to find a solution to the politics of the littoral. Nor did it make the acceptance of the Zone of Peace by the Great Powers conditional upon reciprocal obligation by the littoral and hinterland states. However, since this did not suit the Cold War interests of the two super powers, the UN's Adhoc Committee attempted to reverse the priorities. The Great Powers were able to divert attention from their own obligations by demanding that the regional powers should themselves accept de-nuclearisation first. And, as usual, they were able to manipulate regional dissensions and rivalries to stall the convening of a Zone of Peace Conference.

In 1972, Iraq nationalised her oil companies. The Iraqi Navy established a naval base and positioned Russian supplied missile boats at Umm Qasr at the head of the Persian Gulf in the Shatt-el-Arab, not far from the Iranian oil fields of Abadan. America commenced the construction of naval facilities on Diego Gracia to support a carrier task force for 30 days. Three submarine pens were to be constructed for the attack submarines which accompany a carrier battle group. The runways were to be lengthened to operate B 52 strategic bombers. America indicated that it did not intend to employ nuclear weapons on these B-52's nor deploy submarine launched ballistic missiles from Diego Garcia.

In 1973, the Arab Israeli war persuaded the OPEC states to use oil pricing as a weapon against the West to offset the continued economic, political and military arms support for Israel. They raised the price of oil. The results were many and diverse. The nations of the West reacted with hysteria to start with, but soon turned it to advantage. There was a massive increase in wealth for the OPEC states, who then significantly increased their military expenditures and arms purchases. The Western banks, faced with mounting deposits of petro dollars, increased their lending to non OPEC Third World countries. This credit boom offered an excellent opportunity to upgrade defence equipment, particularly as Western suppliers were increasingly keen to export state of the art weapons and equipment to offset domestic economic decline and balance of payment difficulties, both of which were being aggravated by rising oil prices. Concurrently, extensive plans were initiated for oil substitutes and diversification of oil supplies. The number of new producers increased. Soon supply exceeded demand, prices fell and the crisis shifted from the consumers to the producers.

In 1973 also, America decided to create a Quick Reaction Force to deal with crises in the Persian Gulf. The Russian Navy symbolised its presence when it helped to clear mines in the Red Sea. In 1974, Russian influence started building up in Somalia and the Russian Navy helped in clearing the Suez Canal of mines.

Pakistan's naval relationship with China started in September 1970 when the C-in-C Navy first visited there. By this time, unrest was brewing in East Pakistan and China agreed to strengthen the Navy in East Pakistan by supplying small shallow craft for riverine patrols. The patrol craft could not be delivered until after the establishment of Bangladesh, when the contract was amended. In subsequent years, China supplied the Pakistan Navy with hydrofoil torpedo boats, gunboats, missile boats and large patrol craft. (Story of the Pakistan Navy Page 302).

In the years after the 1971 war, the Pakistan Navy acquired one more Daphne class submarine, two Agosta class submarines and Atlantic maritime patrol aircraft from France, frigates and anti submarine Seaking helicopters from Britain and destroyers on loan from America.

Prime Minister Lal Bahadur Shastri with President Mohammad Ayub Khan of Pakistan and Soviet Prime Minister Alexei Kosygin in Tashkent on January 10, 1966. Shastri died in Tashkent the next day.

The result is that even solution of contentious issues becomes easier because sentiments change. If 20 years ago somebody had asked us to have CBMs with China, many in India would have reacted with a great deal of emotion. The same situation prevails with Pakistan. I had personally suggested that we put the issue of Kashmir on the backburner. We did not mean that they should forget about it.

Two years ago, in a Track Two meeting in Pakistan, I suggested to the then Prime Minister, Benazir Bhutto, that there is a Sino-Indian border agreement and that she should look at it. She was not responsive. Ultimately when a contentious issue which has so much historical and emotional baggage has to be solved, this model is a very relevant one.

THE BANK AND 1966 FOREX CRISIS

Due to heavy dependence on external aid, imports and the growing burden of outward remittance of profits of foreign companies, the next great foreign exchange crisis came. This crisis coincided with the succession crisis caused by Nehru's death. At this time, the World Bank became more critical of the direction of Indian economic policy. A World Bank mission headed by Bernard Bell visited India in 1964 and issued a report calling for the devaluation of the rupee and abolition of many of the foreign trade controls then in effect. It said "There is no particular evidence that the licensing system has in fact served any positive economic purposes.

It has, like the Import control system, protected and preserved inefficiency by, in effect, allocating market shares and restraining the growth of more efficient enterprises." India's first answer to Bell's recommendation was defiance. T.T. Krishnamachari, who had sparred with Eugene Black in 1956, was again the Minister of Finance who picked up the gauntlet thrown down by the Bank by insisting that devaluation was not the answer. However, the Indo-Pakistan war in 1965 led to an abrupt suspension of American aid to India. In early 1965 Nehru's successor, Lal Bahadur Shastri died abruptly in Tashkent, USSR.

The Bank and Devaluation

Mrs. Indira Gandhi was chosen the new Prime Minister of India. The new government immediately softened the hard-line towards the Bank and its western creditors. Mr Krishnamachari was removed from the Finance Ministry for his opposition to the Bank's insistence on devaluation.

The Planning Minister, Ashok Mehta, with some socialist leanings, paradoxically, became an active supporter of the Bank. The following year, the Prime Minister, Planning Minister and the new Finance Minister visited Washington. When Mrs. Gandhi went to Washington she was informed that resumption of Aid—which was cut off as a result of war with Pakistan—was dependent on India coming to terms with the World Bank. The United States made the bank its intermediary and arbiter with respect to aid to both India and Pakistan. From its past role as fund raising organizer and chairman of AIC, the Bank moved into a more active role in evaluating Indian and Pakistani economic plans and advocating, economic reforms *a al* the United States.

The Bank's recommendations, echoing the Bell Mission report, were for a devaluation of the rupee accompanied by dismantling of the plethora of import controls and export subsidies. The government announced devaluation of rupee by 37.5% (from Rs4.75 to Rs 7.50 to a dollar) and the associated import liberalization measures in June 1966.

When the Finance Minister was asked why the government had not waited another six months to see whether a good monsoon might make the devaluation unnecessary. He replied, *"If we had waited another six months, we would have had absence of imports in India"*. The implication was that aid was made conditional on the devaluation. According to him *"action could not be postponed because all further aid negotiation hinged on it."*

However, the devaluation package did not yield results. The expected boost to exports did not materialize, instead they declined. The reasons were obvious. The previous structure of import tariffs and export subsidies had amounted to a de facto devaluation by raising the prices of imports and lowering the prices of exports. A Post-mortem declining exports decline confirmed suspicion that exports suffered due to abolition of subsidies and gained little from the devaluation.

Two days after the devaluation was announced, the World Bank called an urgent meeting of the AIC in order to raise $900 million in non-project aid which was promised. But failed, as the consortium members failed to pledge the necessary amounts. Even five months after devaluation, India had received only $465 million of the promised amount.

The project and non-project aid fell from $1.6 billion in 1966-67 to $0.64 billion in 1967-68 and $0.76 billion in 1968-69, as against $1.7 billion per year promised by the World Bank. This led to sharp criticism of Government's policies by many political groups in India. *"You sold the country and have not even got the price"* a parliamentarian accused the government.

Thus, the devaluation became very unpopular in India. The unpopularity of the devaluation was believed to be a reason of defeat of the Congress Party in 1967 general election. In response to public criticism and on aid disappointment, Mrs Gandhi took a sharp swing to the left by abolishing privy purse and nationalization of banking and insurance sectors. She also signed Indo-USSR treaty to show her displeasure with the western world. This created a very popular image of Mrs Gandhi.

Subsequently, she fought and won a battle for control of the Indian National Congress in 1969 and opted for hard-line against the World Bank and US pressures. The slogan of self-reliance, almost forgotten in the decade—1956-66 had become a favourite phrase once again.

The Post-1966 Period

India's dependence on the Bank and other creditors reached a high in 1966 when the Fourth Five Year Plan, supposed to begin in 1966, had to be postponed for 3 years for obvious reasons. The plan was dependent on uncertain external aid to allow the execution. As a result of this dependency, the Bank sent a second Bell Mission in 1967.

Its recommendations were supportive of the Green Revolution which was already underway in India. This strategy aimed at the creation of a stratum of prosperous capitalist farmers and use of expensive commercial inputs such as chemical fertilizers. The Bank exerted direct pressure during the 1966 exchange crisis for obtaining favourable conditions for foreign investment in India's fertilizer industry.

With the nationalization of coal and oil industry in the 1970s, this option for private foreign capital was foreclosed. But this move did not affect the area of influence of foreign capital. In the post-independence period, foreign companies were moving away from their traditional sectors of investment, i.e., extractive and trading activities.

The manufacturing sector gained prominence during this period and adopted priorities set by developed countries. Thus foreign private capital was taken as inescapable by the policy makers.

The table on page 18 shows that over the last 45 years, certain sectors have been the focus of the Bank's abiding concern. Progressively over the years, it has therefore been pumping aid into these sectors which are power, mining and exploration, irrigation, agriculture and, to some extent, telecommunications and railways. The table not only shows a secular increase in World Bank funding to these sectors, but also during 1980s—the beginning of India's *"dance to freedom"*.

ALL THE BANK'S MEN

In the recent years, most of the key positions in the economic policy establishment in India has passed into the hands of ex-World Bank officials. The list includes the present Finance Secretary, Mr. Montek Singh Auliwalia; Economic Advisor to the Finance Ministry, Mr. Percy Mistry; Chief Economic Advisory Council to Prime Minister, Dr. Bimal Jalan who loined as India's Executive Director in the World Bank; Economic Advisor in Ministry of Industry, Mr. Rakesh Mohan; and Economic Advisor, Ministry of Commerce, Mr. Jayanto Roy.

It is evident that the increase of Bank loans is phenomenal by any count ranging from 200% to over 2500%. More so in the case of agriculture, irrigation and power where even the preceding period shows a phenomenal increase.

In Irrigation and Agriculture, a closer look at the desegregated project list shows minimal Bank loans till 1960s, with the solitary exception of one IBRD loan of $10 million in 1949 towards agricultural machinery.

It is not too far fetched to see the post-1980 period of the Bank's loans and aid was one of preparation for the grand and royal entry of foreign capital. By building up infrastructure—power generation, mining and exploration of new reserves, proper roads and rail facilities, trained technical manpower, etc. In fact, the Bank and the IMF inspired policies have facilitated a new phase of the operation of foreign capital in India. This phase of economic liberalization began in 1980 with the SDR 5 billion loan from the IMF. It weakened the real economy, created the preconditions for export orientation and facilitated the recomposition of the industrial sector in subordination to world capital. This was followed up by another wave of liberalization which included devaluation, lifting of trade barriers and greater impetus to foreign capital and market forces in India.

7

Shastri, Kashmir and the 1965 War

Operation Gibraltar is a major event in the history of Pakistan and Kashmir. Whatever its intent and purpose, it had a far reaching affect on the history of India, Pakistan and Kashmir. It changed the course of history in the Sub-Continent. To majority of the Pakistani and Kashmiri people it was a daring military expedition to 'liberate' the Indian held Kashmir; but the reality appears to be somewhat different. Some writers and retired army men claim that it was a 'conspiracy'. If it is true, then the question is conspiracy by who and against who.

It is very controversial area which requires considerable but careful research and analysis. No researcher can ever claim to uncover the whole truth in a research of this nature. I don't claim that I have discovered the whole truth, but I can certainly present the alternative view with solid arguments and prove that the planners of the 'Operation Gibraltar' had more than one target in their minds and the 'liberation of Kashmir' was not their first priority. Had it been their priority then they must have given attention to the following:

1. Very careful planning with clear objectives.
2. Proper training and resources to achieve those objectives.
3. Close co-ordination with the bodies or organizations who could have helped to achieve those objectives, in this case the Azad Kashmir Government which was set up to liberate Kashmir; or those political organizations which believe in the liberation of Kashmir.
4. Broad-based consultation with the local people and win their confidence whose independence was to be achieved. Without their active support and participation this 'Operation' could not even survive in hostile place never mind of its success.

5. Above all dedicated and sincere leadership which believed in the plan, and had the ability to implement it.

Let us now examine these on the available evidence and see what was in the minds of the planners of this 'Operation', and how successful they were in achieving their target or targets.

Background Situation

Pandit Jawhar Lal Nehru's successor Lal Bahadur Shastri, rushed through a series of "Constitutional amendments, (Articles 356 and 357 of the Indian Constitution) despite strong opposition." The aim was to bring the State of Jammu and Kashmir in line with other States of the Indian Union. The head of the State under new law was not to be elected by the State Legislature, rather the Delhi government had a right to nominate anyone. Also under the new law four seats were allocated in the Indian Parliament, Lok Sabha, to the State of Jammu and Kashmir. And for the first time the Kashmiri people would contest for seats in the Indian Parliament. This really meant a gradual erosion of the Article 370 which gave special status to Kashmir. There was a strong reaction to this in the Valley. Sheikh Abdullah declared on May 7 1964, that 'no solution will be lasting unless it has the approval of all the parties concerned, namely India, Pakistan and the people of Kashmir'.

It is believed by some people that Nehru towards the end of his life felt that despite his best endeavours India had failed to win the hearts and souls of the Kashmiri people; and that he needed to find a more realistic solution to the dispute. There were some influential people like Jayaparkash Narayan who also felt that the Kashmiri people should be given a chance to decide their future. In an article published in the Hindustan Times on 20 April 1964, he said, I might be lacking in patriotism, but it is difficult for me to believe that the people of Kashmir had already voted to live with India on the basis of the 1957 and 1962 elections which are highly controversial and are alleged to have been rigged. Why not give the Kashmiris a real chance to decide about their future. If we are sure that they want to live with us then what fear is there.

So it was with this kind of thinking Nehru released Sheikh Abdullah who was in prison since 1953, and allowed him to fly to Pakistan. It is believed that the aim was to sell to Ayub Khan a proposal of confederation between India, Pakistan and Kashmir. It is claimed that Sheikh Abdullah discussed the idea with Ayub Khan but due to untimely demise of Nehru on 27th May 1964, Abdullah flew back to Delhi and with it this plan aborted. 1 Many commentators think that the scheme was to partition the State on more 'realistic' and 'practical grounds', and by granting some kind of 'independence' to a part of the State with joint supervision of both countries.

Later Sheikh Abdullah and Afzal Beg toured Europe, West Asia and Makkah. Abdullah's meeting with the Chinese Prime Minister Chou-in Lai in Algiers was disliked by India; and on their return to Delhi, both leaders were arrested. This further aggravated the already tensed situation.

The Pakistani government was clearly very perturbed by all this and believed that India was paving the way for the 'merger' of the State of Jammu and Kashmir. So alarm bells were sounded in government circles that some thing had to be done, but It was not clear what. It was not possible for any Pakistani government to remain quiet and let India, arch enemy, get away with all this. It was more of a political requirement then any commitment to the Kashmiri people or any ideology.

Leaders and Planners

Apart from that the people of the Indian held Kashmir were angry and agitated with the disappearance of a relic of the Prophet Mohammed (peace be upon him), which was kept at Hazrat Bal, in Srinager. All these events put together provided an attractive opportunity to some 'ambitious high ups' in the Pakistan government who thought it was right time to intervene in Kashmir. President Ayub was induced to launch "Operation Gibraltar" to free Kashmir. The White Paper on Kashmir published in 1976, stated that, at the time of Sino-India war some one close to President Ayub Khan suggested to him that it was the right time to attack India and free Kashmir. The President who fully understood the horrors of a modern war, reported to have said that he was thinking of either sending him to mental hospital or shoot dead for suggesting this kind of dangerous thing.

This clearly explains what the President Ayub thought of war with India. War, understandably, is not a joke and must be taken very seriously, and every effort must be made to avoid it. Then the question is why Pakistan started the war of 1965. It is no longer true to say that it was India who started the 1965 war. Only last month September 1997, in a statement in newspapers, also published in Daily Jang London, the then Air Chief Marshal, Noor Khan said that it was Pakistan who started the war.

A part of the answer to this question as to why Pakistan started the war is provided by a very senior freedom fighter and renowned journalist Mir Abdul Aziz. According to him a very senior retired officer told him that Ayub Khan was very upset about anti-Ayub demonstrations, even though he was at that time an 'elected' president. He was advised that:

'This was the chance to strike in Kashmir and he would become the darling and hero of the Pakistani and Kashmiri people. On this Ayub Khan was convinced and the Operation Giberaltor was put into practice."

Apart from that it must be noted that it was the same leadership in Pakistan which endeavored to negotiate the division of Kashmir in 1963. At that time Ayub Khan was the President, and Z.A. Bhutto was the Foreign Minister of Pakistan. It is inconceivable that the leadership which was prepared to accept the partition of Kashmir, and settle for whatever piece of land they had, was all of sudden overcome by 'patriotism' and 'love' for the Kashmiri people, and risked a war with India, hence lives of thousands of innocent people.

After the sino-India war, under the pressure of the Western powers, especially the United States of America, India and Pakistan had a series of bilateral talks in 1962/3, in which Bhutto represented Pakistan and Sardar Sawarn Singh represented India. The division of the State of Jammu and Kashmir was discussed and no agreement was reached mainly because India refused to accept the Pakistani proposal for the division of Kashmir.

These negotiations started on 27 December 1962 and finished on 16 May 1963. The Indian delegation presented its plan for the division of Kashmir and called it 'Political Settlement'. Pakistan by continued talking on the division plan, in principle, accepted that Kashmir can be divided provided the right price was paid to Pakistan. Moreover in the Calcutta meeting, Pakistani delegation headed by Z.A. Bhutto, put forward its own plan for the division of Kashmir. Pakistan demanded the whole districts of Mirpur and Poonch and Riasi, in return Pakistan was prepared to accept the postponement of the decision regarding the future of the Valley; or accept that the Valley may be 'internationalised' for ten years. India refused to accept this plan, and that was the end of this round of bilateral talks.

For more details see India-Pakistan Relations by G.W. Choudhry page 138. This book is written by a known writer who was a Minister in Pakistan Government.

OPERATION GIBRALTAR REJECTED BY THE ARMY CHIEF

Brigadier (R) Farooq who was an officer in the force which was sent to 'liberate Kashmir' claims in his book, 'Operation Gibraltar', that Zulfiqar Ali Bhutto, the then Foreign Minister of Pakistan was one of the brains behind this. 5 According to him, Bhutto set up a ' Liberation Cell ', which included people like:

- Mr Aziz Ahmed
- Mr Nazir Ahmed
- Mr Ayub Buksh Awan
- Mr NA Farooqi
- Mr Ahmed
- Mr Altaf Goher

(although the later did not attend any of the meetings)

General Musa, Commander in Chief of the Pakistan Army at that time, confirms the existence of this 'Cell', which was set up in August of 1964. 6 The majority of the members of this 'Cell' were from the 'Qadiani sect'. This 'Cell' had the support of some senior army officers, including Major General Akhtar Malik, who was also known to be a 'Qadiani'.

When this ambitious plan was first sent to the GHQ, General Musa opposed it and wrote the following points to the President Ayub Khan:

A. Guerrilla war in Kashmir can only be successful if the people of Kashmir take part in it, and in my opinion we need more time to prepare people for this.

B. During the guerrilla war if India realized that it is losing the war in Kashmir, she will attack Pakistan.

C. As long as Pakistan is not in a position to defeat India militarily, we should not venture such operation in Kashmir.

D. In order to defeat India we need more army, better arms and better training.

(General Musa asked for money to set up two more army divisions to face the challenge. General Ayub in principle agreed with this idea, but the Finance Minister Mr Shoaib persuaded him against this by saying that the Pakistan economy cannot afford it. And this idea was dropped. It is ironic that no such army was raised before the start of the 'Operation Gibraltar' or during its operations, but after the war, in the same month, two divisions were set up).

It is amazing to note that Air Marshal Asghar Khan, who retired from his position on 23 July 1965 was not consulted on this important issue. It was quite obvious that with an ' Operation ' of that nature there would be some serious response from India, which could lead to a full scale war, and for that the assistance of the air force was must. The planners, for what ever reason, assumed that like 1947 India would limit the war to the State of Jammu and Kashmir. Pakistan had pay heavily for this wrong, rather foolish assumption.

Despite this opposition from the senior army men, including the Commander in Chief, the go ahead was given to this 'Operation'. In Brigadier (R) Farooq's view, Mr Bhutto played the leading role in persuading Ayub Khan. According to him, Bhutto must have said to Ayub Khan that:

1. You missed an opportunity of liberating Kashmir in 1963, while India was engaged in a war with China.
2. You are just as great and important as Mao-se-Tang of China, General Charles De Gaul of France, and Marshall Tito of Yugoslavia. You have made Pakistan a strong and viable country. Pakistan needs you, and his (Bhutto's) wish is that Ayub Khan remains president for life. This can only be done if some how Kashmir is liberated and joined with Pakistan. If this can happen then it will establish him in the history as a great leader and conqueror, and there will be no parallel to his greatness.
3. Furthermore Bhutto is what he (Ayub Khan) has made him, and it is his desire to serve him as the Foreign Secretary to pay his due.

Another writer, Arshad Ahmed, in an article on the 1965 war said: Zulfiqar Ali Bhutto wanted to deprive Ayub Khan of his power, and this was not possible until the strength, ego and pride of the army was not smashed.

This view was supported by Marxist leader Tariq Ali, who was close to the Peoples Party which Bhutto formed after disagreements with the Ayub Khan Government, said in an interview in America that, he had asked Bhutto about the 1965 war, and Bhutto told him: Until these generals are not defeated it is not possible to get in power in Pakistan.

According to the writer this view is also supported by prominent people like Major General Rao Farman Ali, Lt. General Atiq Ul Reman, Major General Ahesan Ul Haq, Col. Ghafar and Altaf Goher.

Brigadier Arshad who was the Director Military Intelligence also opposed this 'Operation', but later agreed to go along with the tide, perhaps he had realized the trend and did not want to oppose this and jeopardies his promotion prospects. He later retired as a Lt. General. According to Brigadier (R) Farooq General Musa was a simple man.

He gave his opinion about the 'Operation' and then did not make it a matter of pride and remained quiet if he and General Sher Bahdar who also opposed the idea, had resigned then there would have been no 'Operation Gibraltar'

A top level meeting was held at the Headquarters of the 12th Division in May 1965. Once again, General Musa opposed the plan, and to this President

Ayub Khan: 'Musa I have been assured by the Foreign Office that India would not be involved in a full scale war' When both General Musa and General Sher Bahadar said that if we are to start a guerrilla war at that level, it is very likely that India would react and attack Pakistan. President Ayub Khan reacted by saying: 'We will have to take heart sometime'

Apart from the assurance to which President Ayub Khan made reference that India would not attack Pakistan, Pakistani planners of this 'Operation' were led to believe that India is not in a position to launch attack against Pakistan until 1966 or 1967.

It was emphasized that we do not waste any more time, and start our action as soon as possible.

During this time the plan was discussed with Col. Syed Ghafar Mehdi, the Commander of the Special Services Group, whose officers were also to take part in this Operation. After reading it he said:

> *'The whole concept of this Operation is wrong, and the planning is wrong too. The planners have not used their common sense and intelligence. This is a product of a bankrupt mind, and it is possible that this may prove to be "Bay of Pigs" for Pakistan.'*

Objectives of the Operation

We have looked at the planners and the leaders of the 'Operation', now let us examine at its objectives. According to Brigadier (R) Farooq it was assumed that as the result of this guerrilla war the Kashmir problem would be settled within weeks; if this did not happen, at least, it would force the United Nations to intervene and have a cease fire.

India had started calling Kashmir as its 'integral part', this was contrary to the UN resolutions and India's pledges regarding Kashmir. The aim of the 'Operation' was:

- To expose the Indian claim on Kashmir by the guerrilla war-present it as the Kashmiri peoples struggle against the Indian rule in Kashmir.
- Force India to take some kind of military or political action which will prove to the world that there is still some trouble in Kashmir; and that the Kashmir dispute has not been resolved as claimed by India.
- To persuade the local people to fight against India. It was assumed that the support for this was already there and all they had to do was to give them a call, and people would be ready to fight and defeat world's fourth biggest and well trained army. Perhaps this was also assumed that the Kashmiri people do not need any kind of training to achieve this gigantic task.

Preparation for a Guerrilla War

Mao Se Tang, who successfully waged a guerrilla war in China, said, in order for the guerrilla war to succeed there must be a:

- Strong public support.
- Excellent organization and administration.
- Strong fighting force with sufficient arms supplies.
- Territory suitable for commando actions.
- Economic stability/ self sufficiency.

If we look at Mao's rules for the guerrilla war, the first priority is given to the public support, whatever it takes to get that support. Without the mass support of the local people there is absolutely no chance of winning this kind of war. If the purpose was to wage a successful guerrilla war against India and liberate Kashmir, then the Kashmiri people must have been taken into confidence. The local people must have been trained for this purpose, the people of Azad Kashmir could have been there to provide extra help and support. The people who were sent to fight a guerrilla war were not familiar with the territory.

Commenting on this point, General Musa, who was Commander in Chief of Pakistan Army at the time of war, in his book, 'My Version' said that the Kashmiris of the Valley were not taken into confidence about the 'Operation' that was to be started to liberate them. He wrote:

We had not even consulted the public leaders across the cease fire line about our aims and intentions, let alone associating them with our planning for the clandestine war.....

Any one with any sense can see and understand that the people of the area to be 'liberated' must have be taken into confidence, if the people organizing this gigantic task really meant business. Without the help of the local people outside army cannot win a war or even survive. Not only the people of Kashmir living on the other side of the cease fire line were not taken into confidence, also the people of Azad Kashmir, even the Azad Kashmir Government was not taken into confidence. When the 'Operation' was put into practice then the planners realized that they need to have some Kashmiri support for this.

They already had set up a Liberation Council, and compelled by circumstances they announced that Choudhry Ghullam Abbass was leading this Liberation Council. They did not have the courtesy, even at that time, to speak to the top Kashmiri leader on this side of the border before making this announcement. Choudhry Ghulam Abbass was already very annoyed with all this, he immediately rejected that in a news statement in the Nawa E Waqat the following day: that he had nothing to do with all this, and that he did not know anything about the 'Operation'.

General Musa also confirms the above position, he said:

> *Because of the haste with which the 'Operation' was launched, even Azad Kashmir leaders were not taken into confidence by the advocates of Guerrilla raids. Helplessly they remained in the background. Their co-operation was also very necessary and would have been very helpful. They could have assisted the mujahideen in various ways by themselves and in conjunction with the Kashmiris of the Valley.*

It must be noted here that the total number of commandos who were sent to 'liberate' Kashmir were 3000, with 4000 volunteers (mujahids) and they were from Azad Kashmir Regular Forces. According to Brigadier (R) Isahaq and Brigadier (R) Salah Udin 98% of the mujahids were forcibly included in the force, and these were those people who had no means to pay bribe to the local police.

I have interviewed a number of local people of Mirpur and Bhimber who testified that the local people were forcibly included to fight a guerrilla war. Even people from my own village, including some of my relatives, were rounded up and taken to the training camps. Majority of them had never held a rifle in their hands before, and it was expected that these men would drive out highly trained Indian army from Kashmir.

Training

As discussed earlier for a task like this to be successful, there has to be perfect planning, first class leadership to CO-ordinate and implement the planning; and of course high quality training. When we analyse the whole plan nothing was in order.

According to experts, guerrilla war fare has a number of stages which must be completed before embarking on the venture:

- Agreement by the leadership on practical and achievable objectives.
- Selection of a capable commander who firmly believes in those objectives.
- organizational set up and distribution of duties.
- Recruitment and training of those who are to take part, this includes the training of the officers.
- Intelligence network to support and advise the leadership.

- Supply Line to provide the guerrillas all what they require to accomplish the task.
- Distribution of task and areas that different groups can function independently but can help and co-ordinate in case of difficulty.
- Last but not least the resources.

There are a number of stages and procedures within all of the above which requires further break down and careful analyses of each one, but this will be divergence from the main point, and I don't want to make this a chapter on the working of the guerrilla war.

Generally speaking other countries spend many months, and some times more than a year, preparing before the first bullet is shot. The planning is made in such a way that the struggle can be maintained for years, as exampled by the guerrilla struggle in Vietnam, China, Algeria, Ireland etc. For example, in Vietnam initial training was for nine months followed by ideological training for four months. Whereas the 'Operation Gibraltar' was 'pushed through' all the stages in a record six weeks, and the planning was to fight for a short period. On 16 May 1965 a meeting was held in Murree to discuss the mechanisms of the 'Operation' and on the next day General Akhtar Hussain Malik put forward 19 pages plan. Some people claim that it was prepared by LT. Col. Waqee Ul Zaman who was also a Qadiyani.

According to Brigadier (R) Farooq the Plan was prepared by amateurs that is why no attention was given to many important things. No one thought of impact of this venture on the situation inside the country, or on the international community. No missions were sent out to persuade the international community or to explain what was the situation in Kashmir. No consideration was given to economy of the country. Can we sustain this kind of 'Operation' for a period of time; and what if India crossed the international border, is our economy and military ready to take up this challenge. Or was it enough that the Foreign Office had assured us through a third party that India would not cross the international border.

He further said that everything was rushed through and we missed out on many stages of the preparation, and even the officers had no practical experience of fighting a guerrilla war. Some of them must have read books written on the subject and that was about it. It was assumed that all the officers were also experts in the guerrilla war fare as well. The reality was that some of the officers heard of the guerrilla war tactics during our training. 28 He said, 95% of us did not know anything about the history and geography of Kashmir. Also we had no idea of their social and culture, out of six commanders only one (Salaudin) had some knowledge on Kashmir.

COMMENTS ON THE 'OPERATION GIBRALTAR'

Brigadier Isahaq, who was second in command in the implementation of the Operation Gibraltar, commented on the 'Operation' in 1985:

> *Unfortunately we could not create the situation in the Valley as we expected. We could not win the confidence of the local people. Despite that they helped us and looked after our needs; and above all they did not inform the authorities about us.*

Aslam, was one of the Officer who led the force in Kashmir in 1965 commented:

> *The purpose of this was good but when we look at the planning and its implementation, it appears that a third rate and useless army has done a quick job. But I want to emphasis that we are not third rate army. All those who had planned this and took part in this are known to be professional soldiers, to them if this Operation was not practical then they should have resigned rather than flattering.*

Another Commentator, known as HJN said: without any hesitation I can say that no matter how important is the expedition, it can only be completed if there is sincerity and dedication. It is unfortunate to note that both of these were not present in this. Our planning and actions lacked vision and consistency. In reality the planning and actions has made us a third rated army, which we are not.... Our officers were professionals I wonder they accepted to complete this in such a short time...... Integrity in an officer demands that he should speak his mind about operations and actions.....

> *...... Kashmir is very suitable for these kinds of small operations, but they must have the support of the local people. These small groups could not control an area for a long time, they must be helped by a regular army. I have not read in history that an area was liberated by these small groups without the support of a regular army. Therefore when the regular army could not reach there it was impossible for you (guerrillas) to remain there. Under these conditions it was wrong to expect that you (guerrillas) would be able to liberate Kashmir....*

....It is amazing what was planned by the planners, and how and why people in the high power circles approved this. Despite the passage of long time (more than two decades), it is difficult to understand if it was a conspiracy, why no heads were rolled. Was it a conspiracy or simple incompetence and insincerity. Or shall I say treason. In my opinion those people who planned it, and those who agreed to implement it without suggesting any improvements and criticising it, have committed treason. It is difficult to find another words for this.

Some commentators say that the Kashmiri support for Pakistan was taken for granted. But this may not be the case. The evidence shows that the plan lacked proper planning. Perhaps one could add that the planners lacked sincerity as well; and the purpose of this war may not have been the liberation of Kashmir.

One may ask, how could a government, which only two years ago were engaged in bilateral talks with India (S Sing-Z A Bhutto Talks 1963) to divide Kashmir; and which at one time offered India 'Joint Defence', be so sincere to wage a war to liberate Kashmir. According to Qudrat Ullah Shoahb, he spoke to Nawab of Kala Bagh, Governor of West Pakistan, about the 1965 War, who said:

> *'This was not Pakistan's war. In fact this war was imposed by Major General Akhtar Malik, M. M. Ahmed, Z A Bhutto, Aziz Ahmed and Nazir Ahmed. The aim was to control Ayub Khan and increase their power and influence, and in doing so if it hurts Pakistan they damn care.'*

Qudrat Ullah Shoahb had been a Minister of Information, Secretary to the President, and an Ambassador in Holland, and he was very informed and well connected person. He further said that:

> *At a time when Major Akhtar Hussain Malik was to take over Akhanoor to pave the way to take Srinager, the capital of Kashmir, he was wrongly removed from the command, and General Yayya Khan was put in his position. Perhaps the aim was to deprive Pakistan success in Akhnoor, Yayya Khan accomplished this task very well.'*

Air Marshal Noor Khan, who was the Air Chief during the war of 1965, said in a statement that ' the thing which is worth noting about the 1965 war is that there was no planning of it at all.'

The question is if there was any planning for the war, which there must have been, then the Air Chief of the Army must have been involved in it; and if there was no planning for the war then one wonders what was the planning for? Was it a conspiracy of some kind, as pointed out by Lt. General (R) Atiq Ul Rehman and Col. (R) Ghafar Mehdi:

> *'India and Pakistan war of 1965 was not won or lost, but it laid down the foundations for the disintegration of Pakistan. This question is still unsolved that the war was over zealous ambition of a few people or a conspiracy of more than one country'*

A well known Kashmiri writer and journalist Mir Abdul Aziz commented:

> *Poor Kashmiris were made the scape-goats. They were never consulted, not even informed that a war of liberation of Kashmir was being started. Those*

who were sent to Kashmir Valley did not even know the Kashmiri language. The whole affair was a wild goose chase.

Dr. Basit, a famous lawyer and writer commented: We want to ask if liberation of Kashmir was your purpose, then why this was kept secret from all the Kashmiri leaders? Was it not necessary for the Kashmiris to take part in their war of freedom?

K. H Khurshid, who was the secretary to Mohammed Ali Jinnah, and also Prime Minister of Azad Kashmir Government commented: I firmly believe that Ayub Khan was not fully aware of the reasons for the war of 1965. Foreign Office, Home Ministry and some senior officers from the Ministry of Kashmir Affairs which included A. B Awan, Nazir Ahmed, Aziz Ahmed and Zulfiqar Ali Bhutto, prevailed on him and assured him that it is only a small programme which would not lead to a war with India. Ayub Khan who offered India 'joint defence' would not have agreed to a full scale war with India.... These men wanted to weaken Ayub's hold on the government, and this is the real reason why he was so angry with them after the war.

Did the Kashmiri People let them Down?

'When the 'Operation' proved to be a disastrous, not only it led to a full scale war with India, it posed serious threat to integrity and stability of Pakistan. Also it did serious damage to the Kashmir cause in the form of the Tashkent Declaration. Apart from that it created some rift between the Kashmiri leadership on both sides of the border and the Pakistani establishment. Kashmiris were angry the way they were treated before, during and after the 'Operation'. The people of Valley, who although were not taken into confidence, went out of their way to support the guerrillas, and when these guerrilla returned back to Pakistan they left helpless people of Kashmir at the mercy of the Indian forces.

The 'Operation' created a number of difficulties for the government of Pakistan, and that time the planners were criticised for their hasty and badly planned action. It is reported by a prominent writer and thinker, Altaf Goher, that in a Cabinet meeting after the war Bhutto and his team were severely criticised for bad planning and misleading the President. At that time Bhutto tried to put forward his case but realizing that he was not cutting any ice, he started crying and said that his political future is ruined.

It was after the failure of the venture when the planners of the 'Operation' turned their propaganda guns against the poor Kashmiris, and claimed that if it was not for the non co-operation of the Kasmiris, the 'Operation' would have been successful. In a systematic manner this misinformation was spread and government resources were used to carry out this propaganda operation. The planners of the 'Operation Gibraltar' were unsuccessful in liberating Kashmir but they were successful in shifting the blame to the Kashmiri people. It is because of this Mir Abdul Aziz, quoted earlier, said, 'poor Kashmiris were made the scape goats'.

Many more quotations of prominent people who were at the helm of affairs in Pakistan, can be given to support that the planners of the war of 1965 had many targets in mind, and Kashmir was very low down on their list of priorities. But it doesn't look necessary to do so. It is, however, important to clarify about the role of the Kashmiri people during the war of 1965. It is alleged that the 'Operation' failed because the people of Kashmir did not co-operate. This is not true. It is however, true that they were not taken into confidence and they were surprised and bewildered when they learnt about the 'liberation' forces.

Already I have quoted General Musa and few other prominent people who confirmed that the people of Kashmir were not consulted about the 'Operation Gibraltar', and despite that they helped the mujahids to the best of their ability. It was bad planning and insincerity by some high ups that the 'Operation' failed; and it is wrong to accuse the Kashmiri people for this failure.

Freedom fighter, writer and well known journalist, Mir Abdul Aziz, in a meeting with this writer said that when Sheikh Abdullah visited Pakistan in 1964, he discussed a possibility of guerrilla war in Kashmir, and Pakistani support for it. He was disappointed with the response of the Pakistani authorities. When he returned back from Haj he was arrested by India and once again put in prison. When Pakistan started the 'Operation Gibraltar' in 1965, he was still in jail, and must have been astonished to hear about 'guerrilla war', if it can be called so.

The first rule about the guerrilla war is that it is fought by the local people-by the son of the soil-people who know the local conditions well. Where people are brought from out side to fight a kind of 'guerrilla war' in an area which is strange to them, then more than likely they will fail in their purpose, as the mujahids failed in 1965. There were many reasons for their failure, one was lack of preparation and consultations with the Kashmiri people. The Mujahideen who were sent to 'liberate' Kashmir, as noted earlier, were from Azad Kashmir and they did not know the Kashmiri language and traditions. They looked different from the people of the Valley and were not aware of the climatic, geographical and social fabrics of the Valley.

The first problem you face when you go to a strange place, especially with hostile intentions, is to hide yourself and get a safe shelter. The language of the people is alien to you, the clothes you wear are different to yours.

The food you eat is also different, in Azad Kashmir people eat 'roti', and in Kashmir Valley people eat rice; and 'roti' is eaten during famine or in extreme poverty and under medical care. It is claimed by Mir Abdul Aziz that some Mujahideen went to shops and asked for 'dho seir ata', meaning two kilo flour, but they asked in weights which were abolished a long time ago. Also the request for 'atta' was enough to expose them that they were not Kashmiris.

One can see from the above that it was not the lack of co-operation of the Kashmiri people which resulted in the failure of the 'Operation Gibraltar'. The Kashmiri people helped them to the best of their ability, even though they were not taken into confidence, and mentally they were not ready to accomplish this gigantic task. According to Col. Mansha Khan, who later became member of the Azad Kashmir Assembly and the Speaker of the Assembly, said that the people of Valley co-operated with them even at times risking their lives. In a detailed interview with Justice Yousaf Saraf, he said that 'they could not have come alive if the Valley people had not risked their lives and honour for the Mujahideen.'

Ayub Khan was assured by his advisors and the Foreign Secretary, Z.A. Bhutto, that India would not cross the international boundary to attack Pakistan. The Indian leaders and ministers were clearly saying that if Pakistan did not stop its adventure in Kashmir, then the conflict could spread to other areas. But Pakistani leaders did not take these threats seriously until the direct Indian attack on the Pakistani cities of Lahore and Sialkot in order to release the pressure on the retreating Indian forces in Kashmir.

It is claimed by some writers, as quoted above, that this operation was 'deliberately mis-planned to topple or weaken Ayub Khan' 44. This topic has become very controversial, but whatever its real motives, it resulted in a full scale war between India and Pakistan. The Security Council arranged a cease fire on 23rd September 1965.

Tashkent Agreement and Kashmir

After the war both India and Pakistan claimed 'victory'. It is open to interpretation what is meant by the word 'victory', and it may be true to some extent that they were both 'victors' because both have in their occupation land which did not belong to them. The only loser in this war game were the

Kashmiri people who were the main suffering party; and who despite huge sacrifices were still divided and oppressed.

Mrs Indira Gandhi was once asked by a foreign journalist that Pakistan claims to have won the 1965 war, and India makes a similar claim; what was her opinion on this. With a smile she said we did not send any one to liberate the area which is under illegal occupation of Pakistan. It was Pakistan which sent the "intruders" in order to get Kashmir from India. Our purpose, at that time, was not to get any more area which is occupied by Pakistan, we simply wanted to drive out the "saboteurs" out of Kashmir. Kashmir is still with us and the "intruders" were successfully pushed out of Kashmir. I want you to be judge and decide who is the 'victor'.

During the war soon it was realized by the both countries that they were not in a position to win the war. India crossed the international border to attack Pakistan in order to release pressure it had faced in Kashmir. Pakistan successfully stopped that offensive, but that was about it. Pakistan was not in a position to take Kashmir from India by force, and India was also incapable of defeating Pakistan militarily. Both countries were not in position to continue war for any longer because of spare parts, supplies and economic impact, so both looked for a cease fire with some kind of honour-without giving this impression to their people that they have lost.

There was international pressure to stop fighting, and the Security Council passed resolutions to this effect. The Indian government agreed to the cease fire conditionally, she wanted Pakistan to withdraw her forces from the State of Jammu and Kashmir. Also she wanted assurance from the United Nations that Pakistan would not commit such acts of 'aggression'. The Pakistani government on the other hand, showed her willingness to accept cease fire if it was to follow an immediate withdrawal of the Indian and the Pakistani forces from the State of Jammu and Kashmir, and replaced by the United Nations forces recruited from Afro-Asian countries. The obvious aim of this was to prepare grounds for a plebiscite in Kashmir to decide if the people of Kashmir wanted to live with India or join Pakistan. India was of course not interested in any kind of plebiscite, as she considered Kashmir to be 'integral' part of India. Anyhow both countries had to accept a cease fire unconditionally on 23 September 1965.

The September War was one of the most important event of President Ayub Khan's rule, and it is amazing that he did not throw any light on it in his book 'Friends Not Masters'. This book was published in 1967, and he was in a position to clarify many aspects of the war and many other important things, which for some reason he did not. According to Qudrat Ullah Shoahab, who had been an Information Minister and Secretary to the President, commented on the war:

When General Akhtar Malik was about to run over Akhnoor (an important town on the Indian side of Kashmir), many generals including General Musa and President Ayub Khan got alarmed that he would emerge as a hero, and this would make him a stronger candidate for the highest post of the Commander in Chief. President Ayub Khan already had a 'suitable' man, General Yayya Khan, for this position. Before General Akhtar Hussain Malik could take over Akhnoor, he was replaced by General Yayya Khan, probably that he could stop Pakistan army to invade Akhnoor, which he did successfully.

Apart from many other damages done to the Kashmir cause by the 1965 war, one serious blow was that for the first time in its long history, Kashmir was taken out of the United Nations to be discussed in Tashkent. This was a serious and delicate matter which required careful consideration, but the Pakistani authorities gave into the pressure and agreed to join discussions in Tashkent. They (Pakistani authorities) were pressurized not to take any action while India was engaged in a war with China, they gave in to the pressure to start the 'Operation Gibraltar', they were pressurized to have a cease fire, then they were pressurized to go to Tashkent for discussions.

On matters of this magnitude and importance there should have been careful consideration and experts, especially in international law and international relations, should have been consulted. Above all the Kashmiri leaders should have been taken into confidence, but there was no such precedent of consulting the Kashmiris. It was assumed that what ever the rulers of Pakistan may decide it would be agreed by them.

Thinking people like Qudrat Ullah Shoahab, who was Ambassador in Holland and happened to be a Kashmiri, warned President Ayub Khan of serious consequences if Pakistan had negotiations with India at Tashkent; and especially it would be bad for the Kashmir dispute. He said that there is a history of bad relationship between the Soviet Russia and Pakistan, especially with regard to foreign policy and the relationship with the West and the Pakistani role in the anti Soviet military alliances. It was as the result of this relationship that the Soviet Russia used its Veto in support of India when resolutions on Kashmir were debated in the UN Security Council. He further said that at Tashkent the whole environment would be against Pakistan and Pakistan would be under pressure to make compromises. And if Pakistan refused to do this and no agreement is made, then this would indicate a

Superpower's inability to act as an influential and may be honest power broker between regional states. This failure would be directly attributed to Pakistan; and this would further deteriorate Soviet-Pakistan relationship.

Apart from that it would not be prudent to discuss Kashmir dispute outside the United Nations. Since the start of the Kashmir crises, its natural and proper forum for discussions has always been United Nations, and whenever we talk about Kashmir dispute its reference is always the UN resolutions. But once we discuss it outside of this international forum, and some kind of agreement is reached there, then from then onwards that would be the new reference on Kashmir not the previous reference of the UN resolutions. If this happened then this would be a serious setback to our stand on Kashmir. It is claimed that President Ayub Khan after reading the telegram sent by Qudrat Ullah Shoaab said, 'There is a lot of sense in what he says'.

But despite that President Ayub Khan ignored this advice and walked into this trap. The Soviet Union wanted to show that it has some role to play in the Asian countries as well. Pakistan had developed friendly relations with China, which became more prominent during the war. This pro-China stance of Pakistan was disliked by Soviet Union and America. It was in the interest of both if the Chinese influence over Pakistan can be reduced or neutralized. So the Soviet Prime Minister Aleksei Kosygin invited Ayub Khan and Lal Bahadur Shastri to Tashkent. The negotiations continued for eight days. India refused to hear about Kashmir, and called it its integral part. Any expectations Pakistan may have had regarding getting some kind of concessions on Kashmir were soon dashed. The failure of the Conference looked apparent and that would have been a serious blow to the image of the Soviet Union, so a lot of arm twisting by Kosigen, the Soviet Prime Minister, resulted in a compromised text which was signed by both India and Pakistan on 10 January 1966. This treaty is known as the Tashkent Declaration, and it only makes a passing reference to the Kashmir dispute.

Whatever edge Pakistan had over India on Kashmir was very 'successfully' lost in Tashkent, and this was a direct result of the 'Operation Gibraltar'. The Indian Prime Minister, Lal Bahdur Shastri, died in Tashkent after signing the Tashkent Pact. It is claimed by many Pakistani commentators that he did not expect any concessions on Kashmir let alone any kind of clear victory, and when he got that 'victory' in the form of the Tashkent Declaration, he was overjoyed and died. Qudrat Ullah Shaoahb, after seeing Ayub Khan carrying the coffin of Lal Bahadur Shastri in Tashkent, commented that with the body of Shastri we wrapped up all the proceedings of the UN on Kashmir as well.

A Pakistani thinker and writer Inayat Ullah commented on the 'Operation Gibraltar';

Our forces (Commandos) prepared the ground for us in Kashmir, the next stage was to launch attack by regular army and capture Akhnoor. If General Akhtar Hussain Malik was not removed then we could have had Akhnoor and 200,000 prisoners of war as well, and Kashmir would have been independent. But our dictator (Ayub Khan) gave Kashmir to India on a tray, and went to Tashkent to get compliment from America and Russia.

On another occasion commenting on the 'Operation Gibraltar' he said: One question which we are ashamed of and which still haunts us is that if our strategy was to please America, Russia and India then why sent our sons to Kashmir to be killed. This question is asked by every commando who went to Kashmir, it is asked by the Pakistan Army and the Azad Kashmir army; it is also asked by the nation and history.

G.W. Choudhry, who was a minister in Ayub Khan and Yayya Khan's governments said: Yet the Indo-Pakistan War of 1965 had disastrous effect both on Ayub's authority and on relations between East and West Pakistan....... many army officers and including some generals, felt that Ayub should have continued the war with Chinese help (which China offered); Indonesia under Sukarno was also willing to help Pakistan. The younger groups of army officers felt that Ayub accepted the cease-fire and the subsequent Tashkent agreement under external pressure and to the detriment of his internal political order...... Ayub's image was tarnished by his alleged surrender of the "national interests" at the Tashkent Conference-a theme on which Bhutto based his major attack against Ayub during the political upheaval of 1969.

Zulfiqar Ali Bhutto Government in 1976 published a White Paper which said: It is a simple political fact that the Tashkent Declaration ended the Kashmir dispute the way India wanted it to end. Pakistan could have ended this kind of speculation by immediately going back to the Security Council.

The "Tashkent Declaration" emphasized that both countries seek a solution to their disputes through peaceful means. The "Tashkent Declaration" was seen as a defeat by the Kashmiri and Pakistani people and there were processions against it. Whatever other achievements of the "Tashkent Declaration," it failed to make any progress on the Kashmir dispute, rather it caused a great disappointment to the Kashmiri people. And as predicted by Qudrat Ullah Shoahab, Kashmir was never to be discussed in the Security Council as a dispute after the Tashkent Declaration. The Tashkent Declaration was followed by another pact (Simla Pact) which Pakistan made with India after the defeat of 1971 war, and now that is the last reference on Kashmir. No matter what Pakistani leaders say, the Kashmir dispute would never be solved according to the UN resolutions on Kashmir, because both governments agreed to solve it bilaterally.

THE TASHKENT DECLARATION 10TH FEBRUARY 1966

The Tashkent Declaration of January 10, 1966 was a peace agreement between India and Pakistan. In September of 1965 before the two had engaged in the short run Indo-Pakistani War of 1965. Peace had been achieved on September 23 by the intervention of the great powers who pushed the two nations to a cease fire for fears the conflict could escalate and draw in other powers.

A meeting was held in Tashkent in the USSR (now in Uzbekistan) beginning on January 4, 1966 to try to create a more permanent settlement. The Soviets, represented by Premier Kosygin moderated between Indian Prime Minister Lal Bahadur Shastri and Pakistani President Muhammad Ayub Khan. The conference was viewed as a great success and the declaration that was released was hoped to be a framework for lasting peace. The declaration stated that

- Indian and Pakistani forces would pull back to their pre-conflict positions
- The nations would not interfere in each other's internal affairs
- Economic and diplomatic relations would be restored
- The two leaders would work towards building good relations between the two countries.

The day after the declaration Indian Prime Minister Shastri died of a sudden heart attack. In Pakistan many civilians felt that they had won the war-though Pakistan had suffered more casualties and territorial losses-and were disappointed at the return to the *status quo ante bellum*. The agreement was criticized in India because it did not contain a no-war pact or any renunciation of guerrilla warfare in Kashmir. The two countries would again be at war in 1971.

The Prime Minister of India and the President of Pakistan, having met at Tashkent and having discussed the existing relations between India and Pakistan hereby declare their firm resolve to restore normal and peaceful relations between their countries and to promote understanding and friendly relations between their peoples. They consider the attainment of these objectives of vital importance for the welfare of the 600 million people of India and Pakistan.

(i) The Prime Minister of India and the President of Pakistan agree that both sides will exert all efforts to create good neighbourly relations between India and Pakistan in accordance with the United Nations Charter. They reaffirm their obligation under the Charter not to have recourse to force and to settle their disputes through peaceful means. They considered that the interests of peace in their region and particularly in the Indo Pakistan subcontinent and, indeed, the interests of the peoples of India and Pakistan were not served by the continuance of tension between the two countries. It was against this background that Jammu and Kashmir was discussed, and each of the sides set forth its respective position.

(ii) The Prime Minister of India and the President of Pakistan have agreed that all armed personnel of the two countries shall be withdrawn not later than 25 February, 1966, to the position they held prior to 5 August, 1965, and both sides shall observe the ceasefire terms on the ceasefire line.

(iii) The Prime Minister of India and the President of Pakistan have agreed that relations between India and Pakistan shall be based on the principle of noninterference in the internal affairs of each other.

(iv) The Prime Minister of India and the President of Pakistan have agreed that both sides will discourage any propaganda directed against the other country and will encourage propaganda which promotes the development of friendly relations between the two countries.

(v) The Prime Minister of India and the President of Pakistan have agreed that the High Commissioner of India to Pakistan and the High Commissioner of Pakistan to India will return to their posts and that the normal functioning of diplomatic missions of both countries will be restored. Both governments shall observe the Vienna Convention of 1961 on diplomatic intercourse.

(vi) The Prime Minister of India and the President of Pakistan have agreed to consider measures towards the restoration of economic and trade relations, communications as well as cultural exchanges between India and Pakistan, and to take measures to implement the existing agreements between India and Pakistan.

(vii) The Prime Minister of India and the President of Pakistan have agreed that they will give instructions to their respective authorities to carry out the repatriation of the prisoners of war.

(viii) The Prime Minister of India and the President of Pakistan have agreed that the two sides will continue the discussion of questions relating to the problems of refugees and evictions/illegal immigrations. They also agreed that both sides will create conditions which will prevent the exodus of people. They further agree to discuss the return of the property and assets taken over by either side in connection with the conflict.

(ix) The Prime Minister of India and the President of Pakistan have agreed that the two sides will continue meetings both at the highest and at other levels of matters of direct concern to both countries. Both sides have recognised the need to set up joint IndianPakistani bodies which will report to their governments in order to decide what further steps should be taken.

The Prime Minister of India and the President of Pakistan record their feelings, deep appreciation and gratitude to the leaders of the Soviet Union, the Soviet Government and personally to the Chairman of the Council of Ministers of the USSR for their constructive, friendly and noble part in bringing about the present meeting which has resulted in mutually satisfactory results. They also express to the government and friendly people of Uzbekistan their sincere thankfulness for their overwhelming reception and generous hospitality.

They invite the Chairman of the Council of Ministers of the USSR to witness this declaration.

INDO-PAKISTANI WAR OF 1965

The Indo-Pakistani War of 1965 was a culmination of skirmishes that took place between April 1965 and September 1965 between Pakistan and India. The conflict began following Pakistan's Operation Gibraltar, which was designed to infiltrate forces into Jammu and Kashmir to precipitate an insurgency against Indian rule. India retaliated by launching a full-scale military attack on West Pakistan.

The seventeen-day war caused thousands of casualties on both sides and witnessed the largest engagement of armored vehicles and the largest tank battle since World War II. Hostilities between the two countries ended after a United Nations mandated ceasefire was declared following diplomatic intervention by the Soviet Union and the United States, and the subsequent issuance of the Tashkent Declaration. Much of the war was fought by the countries' land forces in Kashmir and along the border between India and Pakistan. This war saw the largest amassing of troops in Kashmir since the Partition of British India in 1947, a number that was overshadowed only during the 2001–2002 military standoff between India and Pakistan. Most of the battles were fought by opposing infantry and armoured units, with substantial backing from air forces, and naval operations. The war exposed Pakistan's inadequate standards of military training, its misguided selection of officers, poor command and control arrangements, poor intelligence gathering and bad intelligence procedures. In spite of these shortcomings, the Pakistan Army managed to fight the larger Indian Army. Many details of this war, like those of other Indo-Pakistani Wars, remain unclear.

Despite the cease-fire rendering the conflict militarily inconclusive, both India and Pakistan claimed victory. Most neutral assessments, however, agree that India had the upper hand over Pakistan when the ceasefire was declared. Though officially deemed to be militarily inconclusive, the conflict is widely seen as a strategic and political defeat for Pakistan, as it had neither succeeded in fomenting insurrection in Kashmir nor had it been able to gain meaningful support at an international level.

Internationally, the war was viewed in the context of the greater Cold War, and resulted in a significant geopolitical shift in the subcontinent. Before the war, the United States and the United Kingdom had been major material allies of both India and Pakistan, as their primary suppliers of military hardware and foreign developmental aid. During and after the conflict, both India and Pakistan felt betrayed by the perceived lack of support by the western powers for their respective positions; those feelings of betrayal were increased with the imposition of an American and British embargo on military aid to the opposing sides.

As a consequence, India and Pakistan openly developed closer relationships with the Soviet Union and China, respectively. The perceived negative stance of the western powers during the conflict, and during the 1971 war, has continued to affect relations between the West and the subcontinent. In spite of improved relations with the U.S. and Britain since the end of the Cold War, the conflict generated a deep distrust of both countries within the subcontinent which to an extent lingers to this day.

PRE-WAR ESCALATION

Since the Partition of British India in 1947, Pakistan and India remained in contention over several issues. Although the Kashmir conflict was the predominant issue dividing the nations, other border disputes existed, most notably over the Rann of Kutch, a barren region in the Indian state of Gujarat. The issue first arose in 1956 which ended with India regaining control over the disputed area. Pakistani patrols began patrolling in territory controlled by India in January 1965, which was followed by attacks by both countries on each other's posts on 8 April 1965. Initially involving border police from both nations, the disputed area soon witnessed intermittent skirmishes between the countries' armed forces. In June 1965, British Prime Minister Harold Wilson successfully persuaded both countries to end hostilities and set up a tribunal to resolve the dispute. The verdict, which came later in 1968, saw Pakistan awarded 350 square miles (910 km^2) of the Rann of Kutch, as against its original claim of 3,500 square miles (9,100 km^2).

After its success in the Rann of Kutch, Pakistan, under the leadership of General Ayub Khan, believed the Indian Army would be unable to defend itself against a quick military campaign in the disputed territory of Kashmir as the Indian military had suffered a loss to China in 1962 in the Sino-Indian War. Pakistan believed that the population of Kashmir was generally discontented with Indian rule and that a resistance movement could be ignited by a few infiltrating saboteurs. Pakistan attempted to ignite the resistance movement by means of a covert infiltration, codenamed Operation Gibraltar. The Pakistani infiltrators were soon discovered, however, their presence reported by local Kashmiris, and the operation ended unsuccessfully.

THE WAR

On 5 August 1965 between 26,000 and 33,000 Pakistani soldiers crossed the Line of Control dressed as Kashmiri locals headed for various areas within Kashmir. Indian forces, tipped off by the local populace, crossed the cease fire line on 15 August.

Initially, the Indian Army met with considerable success, capturing three important mountain positions after a prolonged artillery barrage. By the end of August, however, both sides had relative progress; Pakistan had made progress in areas such as Tithwal, Uri and Poonch and India had captured the Haji Pir pass, 8 km into Pakistan-Administered Kashmir.

On 1 September 1965, Pakistan launched a counterattack, called Operation Grand Slam, with the objective to capture the vital town of Akhnoor in Jammu, which would sever communications and cut off supply routes to Indian troops. Ayub Khan calculated that "Hindu morale would not stand more than a couple of hard blows at the right time and place" although by this time Operation Gibraltar had failed and India had captured the Haji Pir Pass. At 3:30 hours, on 1 September 1965, the entire Chhamb area came under massive artillery bombardment. Pakistan had launched operation Grand Slam and India's Army Headquarter was taken by surprise. Attacking with an overwhelming ratio of troops and technically superior tanks, Pakistan made gains against Indian forces, who were caught unprepared and suffered heavy losses. India responded by calling in its air force to blunt the Pakistani attack. The next day, Pakistan retaliated, its air force attacked Indian forces and air bases in both Kashmir and Punjab. India's decision to open up the theatre of attack into Pakistani Punjab forced the Pakistani army to relocate troops engaged in the operation to defend Punjab. Operation Grand Slam therefore failed, as the Pakistan Army was unable to capture Akhnoor; it became one of the turning points in the war when India decided to relieve pressure on its troops in Kashmir by attacking Pakistan further south. In the valley, another area of strategic importance was Kargil. Kargil town was in Indian hands but Pakistan occupied high ground overlooking Kargil and Srinagar-Leh road. However, after the launch of a massive anti-infiltration operation by the Indian army, the Pakistani infiltrators were forced out of that area in the month of August.

India crossed the International Border on the Western front on 6 September, marking an official beginning of the war. On 6 September, the 15th Infantry Division of the Indian Army, under World War II veteran Major General Prasad, battled a massive counterattack by Pakistan near the west bank of the Icchogil Canal (BRB Canal), which was a *de facto* border of India and Pakistan. The General's entourage itself was ambushed and he was forced to flee his vehicle. A second, this time successful, attempt to cross the Ichhogil Canal was made over the bridge in the village of Barki, just east of Lahore. These developments brought the Indian Army within the range of Lahore International Airport. As a result, the United States requested a temporary ceasefire to allow it to evacuate its citizens in Lahore. However, the Pakistani counterattack took Khem Karan from Indian forces which tried to divert the attention of Pakistanis from Khem Karan by an attack on Bedian and the adjacent villages.

The thrust against Lahore consisted of the 1st Infantry Division supported by the three tank regiments of the 2nd Independent Armoured Brigade; they quickly advanced across the border, reaching the Ichhogil (BRB) Canal by 6 September. The Pakistani Army held the bridges over the canal or blew up those it could not hold, effectively stalling any further advance by the Indians on Lahore. One unit of the Indian Jat Regiment, 3 Jat, had also crossed the Icchogil canal and captured the town of Batapore (Jallo Mur to Pakistan) on the west side of the canal. The same day, a counter offensive consisting of an armoured division and infantry division supported by Pakistan Air Force Sabres forced the Indian 15th Division to withdraw to its starting point. Although 3 Jat suffered minimal casualties, the bulk of the damage being taken by ammunition and stores vehicles, the higher commanders had no information of 3 Jat's capture of Batapore and misleading information led to the command to withdraw from Batapore and Dograi to Ghosal-Dial. This move brought extreme disappointment to Lt-Col Desmond Hayde, CO of 3 Jat. Dograi was eventually recaptured by 3 Jat on 21 September, for the second time but after a much harder battle due to Pakistani reinforcements.

On 8 September 1965, a company of 5 Maratha Light Infantry was sent to reinforce a Rajasthan Armed Constabulary (RAC) post at Munabao – a strategic hamlet about 250 kilometres from Jodhpur. Their brief was simple. To hold the post and to keep Pakistan's infantry battalions from overrunning the post at bay. But at Maratha Hill (in Munabao) – as the post has now been christened – the Indian company could barely manage to thwart the intense attack for 24 hours. A company of 3 Guards with 954 heavy mortar battery ordered to reinforce the RAC post at Munabao could never reach. The Pakistani Air Force had strafed the entire area, and also hit a railway train coming from Barmer with reinforcements near Gadra road railway station. On 10 September, Munabao fell into Pakistani hands, and efforts to capture the strategic point did not succeed.

On the days following 9 September, both nations' premiere formations were routed in unequal battles. India's 1st Armoured Division, labeled the "pride of the Indian Army", launched an offensive towards Sialkot. The Division divided itself into two prongs, was forced back by the Pakistani 6th Armoured Division at Chawinda and was forced to withdraw after suffering heavy losses of nearly 100 tanks. The Pakistanis followed up their success by launching Operation Windup, which forced the Indians back farther. Similarly, Pakistan's pride, the 1st Armoured Division, pushed an offensive towards Khem Karan, with the intent to capture Amritsar (a major city in Punjab, India) and the bridge on River Beas to Jalandhar.

The Pakistani 1st Armoured Division never made it past Khem Karan, however, and by the end of 10 September lay disintegrated by the defences of the Indian 4th Mountain Division at what is now known as the Battle of *Asal Uttar* (lit. meaning – "Real Answer", or more appropriate English equivalent – "Fitting Response"). The area became known as 'Patton Nagar' (Patton Town), because of the large number of US-made Pakistani Patton tanks. Approximately 97 Pakistani tanks were destroyed or abandoned, with only 32 Indian tanks destroyed or damaged. The Pakistani 1st Armoured Division less 5th Armoured Brigade was next sent to Sialkot sector behind Pakistani 6th Armoured Division where it didn't see action as 6th Armoured Division was already in process of routing Indian 1st Armoured Division which was superior to it in strength.

The hostilities in the Rajasthan sector commenced on September the 8th. Initially Pakistan Desert Force and the Hur militia (followers of Pir Pagaro) was placed in a defensive role, a role for which they were well suited as it turned out. The Hurs were familiar with the terrain and the local area and possessed many essential desert survival skills which their opponents and their comrades in the Pakistan Army did not.

Fighting as mainly light infantry, the Hur inflicted many casualties on the Indian forces as they entered Sindh. The Hurs were also employed as skirmishers, harassing the Indians LOC, a task they often undertook on camels. As the battle wore on the Hurs and the Desert Force were increasingly used to attack and capture Indian villages inside Rajasthan. It was in this vein that an assault on Kishangarh fort was launched. The attack surprised the Indians and the fort was captured after several days of bitter fighting.

The war was heading for a stalemate, with both nations holding territory of the other. The Indian army suffered 3,000 battlefield deaths, while Pakistan suffered 3,800. The Indian army was in possession of 758.9 miles^2 (1,920 km^2) of Pakistani territory and the Pakistan army held 210 mile^2 (550 km^2) of Indian territory. The territory occupied by India was mainly in the fertile Sialkot, Lahore and Kashmir sectors, while Pakistani land gains were primarily south in deserts opposite to Sindh and in Chumb sector near Kashmir in north. However, some analysts like Lalita Prasada, Manus I. Midlarsky and Col J Francis (Retd) say that the Pakistanis claim that Pakistan held 1600 square miles of Indian territory (1300 of it in the desert).

Aerial warfare

The war saw aircraft of the Indian Air Force (IAF) and the Pakistan Air Force (PAF) engaging in combat for the first time since independence. Though the two forces had previously faced off in the First Kashmir War during the late 1940s, that engagement was very limited in scale compared to the 1965 conflict.

The IAF was flying large numbers of Hawker Hunters, Indian-manufactured Folland Gnats, de Havilland Vampires, EE Canberra bombers and a squadron of MiG-21s. The PAF's fighter force comprised 102 F-86F Sabres and 12 F-104 Starfighters, along with 24 B-57 Canberra bombers. During the conflict, the PAF claimed it was out-numbered by around 5:1.

The PAF's aircraft were largely of American origin, whereas the IAF flew an assortment of British and Soviet aeroplanes. It has been widely reported that the PAF's American aircraft were superior to those of the IAF.

The F-86 was vulnerable to the diminutive Folland Gnat, nicknamed "Sabre Slayer." The Gnat is credited by many independent and Indian sources as having shot down seven Pakistani Canadair Sabres in the 1965 war. while two Gnats were downed by PAF fighters. The PAF's F-104 Starfighter of the PAF was the fastest fighter operating in the subcontinent at that time and was often referred to as "the pride of the PAF".

However, according to Sajjad Haider, the F-104 did not deserve this reputation. Being "a high level interceptor designed to neutralise Soviet strategic bombers in altitudes above 40,000 feet," rather than engage in dogfights with agile fighters at low altitudes, it was "unsuited to the tactical environment of the region."

In combat the Starfighter was not as effective as the IAF's far more agile, albeit much slower, Folland Gnat fighter. Yet it zoomed into an ongoing dogfight between Sabres and Gnats, at supersonic speed, successfully broke off the fight and caused the Gnats to egress. An IAF Gnat, piloted by Squadron Leader Brij Pal Singh Sikand, landed at an abandoned Pakistani airstrip at Pasrur and was captured by the Pakistan Army. The pilot claimed that most of his equipment failed and even if he could get some chance on that, the Starfighters snuffed it. This Gnat is displayed as a war trophy in the Pakistan Air Force Museum, Karachi. Sqn Ldr Saad Hatmi who flew the captured aircraft to Sargodha, and later tested and evaluated its flight performance, was of view that Gnat was no "Sabre Slayer" when it came to dog fighting. The Pakistan Air Force had fought well in countering the much large Indian Air Force and supported the ground forces.

The two countries have made contradictory claims of combat losses during the war and few neutral sources have verified the claims of either country. The PAF claimed it shot down 104 IAF planes and lost 19 of its own, while the IAF claimed it shot down 73 PAF planes and lost 59. According to PAF, It flew 86 F-86 Sabres, 10 F-104 Starfighters and 20 B-57 Canberras in a parade soon after the war was over. Thus disproving the IAF's claim of downing 73 PAF fighters, which at the time constituted nearly the entire Pakistani front-line fighter force.

Indian sources have pointed out that, despite PAF claims of losing only a squadron of combat craft, Pakistan sought to acquire additional aircraft from Indonesia, Iraq, Iran, Turkey and China within 10 days of the beginning war.

The two air forces were rather equal in the conflict, because much of the Indian air force remained farther east to guard against the possibility of China entering the war. According to the independent sources, the PAF lost some 20 aircraft while the Indians lost 60–75. Pakistan ended the war having depleted

17 percent of its front line strength, while India's losses amounted to less than 10 percent. Moreover, the loss rate had begun to even out, and it has been estimated that another three week's fighting would have seen the Pakistani losses rising to 33 percent and India's losses totalling 15 percent. Air superiority was not achieved, and were unable to prevent IAF fighter bombers and reconnaissance Canberras from flying daylight missions over Pakistan. Thus 1965 was a stalemate in terms of the air war with neither side able to achieve complete air superiority. However, according to Kenneth Werrell, the Pakistan Air Force "did well in the conflict and probably had the edge". When hostilities broke out, the Pakistan Air Force with around 100 F-86s faced an enemy with five times as many combat aircraft; the Indians were also equipped with comparatively modern aircraft inventory. Despite this, Werrell credits the PAF as having the advantage of a "decade's experience with the Sabre" and pilots with long flight hours experience. One Pakistani fighter pilot, MM Alam, was credited with the record of downing five Indian aircraft in less than a minute, becoming the first known flying ace since the Korean War. However, his claims were never confirmed by the PAF and is disputed by Indian sources and some PAF officials.

Tank battles

The 1965 war witnessed some of the largest tank battles since World War II. At the beginning of the war, the Pakistani Army had both a numerical advantage in tanks, as well as better equipment overall. Pakistani armour was largely American-made; it consisted mainly of Patton M-47 and M-48 tanks, but also included many M4 Sherman tanks, some M24 Chaffee light tanks and M36 Jackson tank destroyers, equipped with 90 mm guns. The bulk of India's tank fleet were older M4 Sherman tanks; some were up-gunned with the French high velocity CN 75 50 guns and could hold their own, whilst some older models were still equipped with the inferior 75 mm M3 L/40 gun. Besides the M4 tanks, India fielded the British-made Centurion Tank Mk 7, with the 105 mm Royal Ordnance L7 gun, and the AMX-13, PT-76, and M3 Stuart light tanks. Pakistan fielded a greater number and more modern artillery; its guns out-ranged those of the Indian artillery, according to Pakistan's Major General T.H. Malik.

At the outbreak of war in 1965, Pakistan had about 15 armoured cavalry regiments, each with about 45 tanks in three squadrons. Besides the Pattons, there were about 200 M4 Shermans re-armed with 76 mm guns, 150 M24 Chaffee light tank and a few independent squadrons of M36B1 tank destroyers. Most of these regiments served in Pakistan's two armoured divisions, the 1st and 6th Armoured divisions – the latter being in the process of formation. The Indian Army of the time possessed 17 cavalry regiments, and in the 1950s had begun modernizing them by the acquisition of 164 AMX-13 light tanks and 188 Centurions. The remainder of the cavalry units were equipped with M4 Shermans and a small number of M3A3 Stuart light tanks. India had only a single armoured division, the 1st 'Black Elephant' Armoured Division, which consisted of the 17th Horse (The Poona Horse), also called 'Fakhr-i-Hind' ('Pride of India'), the 4th Horse (Hodson's Horse), the 16th Cavalry, the 7th Light Cavalry, the 2nd Lancers, the 18th Cavalry and the 62nd Cavalry, the two first named being equipped with Centurions. There was also the 2nd Independent Armoured Brigade, one of whose three regiments, the 3rd Cavalry, was also equipped with Centurions.

Despite the qualitative and numerical superiority of Pakistani armour, Pakistan was outfought on the battlefield by India, which made progress into the Lahore-Sialkot sector, whilst halting Pakistan's counteroffensive on Amritsar; they were sometimes employed in a faulty manner, such as charging prepared defences during the defeat of Pakistan's 1st Armoured Division at Asal Uttar.

After India breached the Madhupur canal on 11 September, the Khem Karan counter-offensive was halted, affecting Pakistan's strategy substantially. Although India's tank formations experienced some results, India's attack at the Battle of Chawinda, led by its 1st Armoured Division and supporting units, was brought to halt by the newly raised 6th Armoured Division (ex-100th independent brigade group) in the Chawinda sector. Pakistan claimed that Indians lost 120 tanks at Chawinda. compared to 44 of its own But later, Indian official sources confirmed India lost only 29 tanks at Chawinda. Neither the Indian nor Pakistani Army showed any great facility in the use of armoured formations in offensive operations, whether the Pakistani 1st Armoured Division at Asal Uttar or the Indian 1st Armoured Division at Chawinda. In contrast, both proved adept with smaller forces in a defensive role such as India's 2nd Armoured Brigade at Asal Uttar and Pakistan's 25th Cavalry at Chawinda.

The Centurion battle tank, with its 105 mm gun and heavy armour, performed better than the overly complex Pattons.

Naval hostilities

Naval operations did not play a prominent role in the war of 1965. On 7 September, a flotilla of the Pakistan Navy under the command of Commodore S.M. Anwar, carried out a bombardment of the Indian Navy's radar station coastal down of Dwarka, which was 200 miles (320 km) south of the Pakistani port of Karachi. Operation Dwarka, as it is known, is a significant naval operation of the 1965 war contested as a nuisance raid by some. The attack on Dwarka led to questions being asked in India's parliament and subsequent post-war modernization and expansion of the Indian Navy, with an increase in budget from Rs. 35 crores to Rs. 115 crores.

According to some Pakistani sources, one submarine, PNS Ghazi, kept the Indian Navy's aircraft carrier INS Vikrant besieged in Bombay throughout the war. Indian sources claim that it was not their intention to get into a naval conflict with Pakistan, and wished to restrict the war to a land-based conflict. Moreover, they note that the Vikrant was in dry dock in the process of refitting. Some Pakistani defence writers have also discounted claims that the Indian Navy was bottled up in Bombay by a single submarine, instead stating that 75% of the Indian Navy was under maintenance in harbour.

Covert operations

The Pakistan Army launched a number of covert operations to infiltrate and sabotage Indian airbases. On 7 September 1965, the Special Services Group (SSG) commandos were parachuted into enemy territory. According to Chief of Army Staff General Muhammad Musa, about 135 commandos were airdropped at three Indian airfields (Halwara, Pathankot and Adampur). The daring attempt proved to be an "unmitigated disaster". Only 22 commandos returned to Pakistan as planned, 93 were taken prisoner (including one of the Commanders of the operations, Major Khalid Butt), and 20 were killed in encounters with the army, police or civilians. The reason for the failure of the commando mission is attributed to the failure to provide maps, proper briefings and adequate planning or preparation.

Despite failing to sabotage the airfields, Pakistan sources claim that the commando mission affected some planned Indian operations. As the Indian 14th Infantry Division was diverted to hunt for paratroopers, the Pakistan Air Force found the road filled with transport, and destroyed many vehicles.

India responded to the covert activity by announcing rewards for captured Pakistani spies or paratroopers. Meanwhile, in Pakistan, rumors spread that India had retaliated with its own covert operations, sending commandos deep into Pakistan territory,but these rumors were later determined to be unfounded.

Neutral assessments

There have been several neutral assessments of the losses incurred by both India and Pakistan during the war. Most of these assessments agree that

India had the upper hand over Pakistan when ceasefire was declared. Some of the neutral assessments are mentioned below –

- According to the Library of Congress Country Studies conducted by the Federal Research Division of the United States – The war was militarily inconclusive; each side held prisoners and some territory belonging to the other. Losses were relatively heavy—on the Pakistani side, twenty aircraft, 200 tanks, and 3,800 troops. Pakistan's army had been able to withstand Indian pressure, but a continuation of the fighting would only have led to further losses and ultimate defeat for Pakistan. Most Pakistanis, schooled in the belief of their own martial prowess, refused to accept the possibility of their country's military defeat by "Hindu India" and were, instead, quick to blame their failure to attain their military aims on what they considered to be the ineptitude of Ayub Khan and his government.
- Former *New York Times* reporter Arif Jamal wrote in his book *Shadow War* – This time, India's victory was nearly total: India accepted cease-fire only after it had occupied 740 square miles, though Pakistan had made marginal gains of 210 square miles of territory. Despite the obvious strength of the Indian wins, both countries claim to have been victorious.
- Devin T. Hagerty wrote in his book *"South Asia in world politics"* – The invading Indian forces outfought their Pakistani counterparts and halted their attack on the outskirts of Lahore, Pakistan's second-largest city. By the time United Nations intervened on September 22, Pakistan had suffered a clear defeat.
- In his book *"National identity and geopolitical visions"*, Gertjan Dijkink writes – The superior Indian forces, however, won a decisive victory and the army could have even marched on into Pakistani territory had external pressure not forced both combatants to cease their war efforts.
- An excerpt from Stanley Wolpert's *India*, summarizing the Indo-Pakistani War of 1965, In three weeks the second Indo-Pak War ended in what appeared to be a draw when the embargo placed by Washington on U.S. ammunition and replacements for both armies forced cessation of conflict before either side won a clear victory. India, however, was in a position to inflict grave damage to, if not capture, Pakistan's capital of the Punjab when the cease-fire was called, and controlled Kashmir's strategic Uri-Poonch bulge, much to Ayub's chagrin.
- In his book titled *The greater game: India's race with destiny and China*, David Van Praagh wrote – India won the war. It gained 1,840 km^2 (710 sq mi) of Pakistani territory: 640 km^2 (250 sq mi) in Azad Kashmir,

Pakistan's portion of the state; 460 km^2 (180 sq mi) of the Sailkot sector; 380 km^2 (150 sq mi) far to the south of Sindh; and most critical, 360 km^2 (140 sq mi) on the Lahore front. Pakistan took 540 km^2 (210 sq mi) of Indian territory: 490 km^2 (190 sq mi) in the Chhamb sector and 50 km^2 (19 sq mi) around Khem Karan.

- Dennis Kux's *"India and the United States estranged democracies"* also provides a summary of the war, Although both sides lost heavily in men and material, and neither gained a decisive military advantage, India had the better of the war. New Delhi achieved its basic goal of thwarting Pakistan's attempt to seize Kashmir by force. Pakistan gained nothing from a conflict which it had instigated.
- *"A region in turmoil: South Asian conflicts since 1947"* by Robert Johnson mentions – India's strategic aims were modest – it aimed to deny Pakistani Army victory, although it ended up in possession of 720 square miles (1,900 km^2) of Pakistani territory for the loss of just 220 square miles (570 km^2) of its own.
- An excerpt from William M. Carpenter and David G. Wiencek's *"Asian security handbook: terrorism and the new security environment"* – A brief but furious 1965 war with India began with a covert Pakistani thrust across the Kashmiri cease-fire line and ended up with the city of Lahore threatened with encirclement by Indian Army. Another UN-sponsored cease-fire left borders unchanged, but Pakistan's vulnerability had again been exposed.
- English historian John Keay's *"India: A History"* provides a summary of the 1965 war – The 1965 Indo-Pak war lasted barely a month. Pakistan made gains in the Rajasthan desert but its main push against India's Jammu-Srinagar road link was repulsed and Indian tanks advanced to within a sight of Lahore. Both sides claimed victory but India had most to celebrate.
- Uk Heo and Shale Asher Horowitz write in their book *"Conflict in Asia: Korea, China-Taiwan, and India-Pakistan"* – Again India appeared, logistically at least, to be in a superior position but neither side was able to mobilize enough strength to gain a decisive victory.
- According to the Office of the Historian within the U.S Department of State: Conflict resumed again in early 1965, when Pakistani and Indian forces clashed over disputed territory along the border between the two nations. Hostilities intensified that August when the Pakistani army attempted to take Kashmir by force. The attempt to seize the state was unsuccessful, and the second India-Pakistan War reached a stalemate.

Ceasefire

The United States and the Soviet Union used significant diplomatic tools to prevent any further escalation in the conflict between the two South Asian nations. The Soviet Union, led by Premier Alexei Kosygin, hosted ceasefire negotiations in Tashkent (now in Uzbekistan), where Indian Prime Minister Lal Bahadur Shastri and Pakistani President Ayub Khan signed the Tashkent Agreement, agreeing to withdraw to pre-August lines no later than 25 February 1966.

With declining stockpiles of ammunition, Pakistani leaders feared the war tilting in India's favor. Therefore, they quickly accepted the ceasefire in Tashkent. Despite strong opposition from Indian military leaders, India bowed to growing international diplomatic pressure and accepted the ceasefire. On 22 September, the United Nations Security Council unanimously passed a resolution that called for an unconditional ceasefire from both nations. The war ended the following day.

India's Prime Minister, Shastri, suffered a fatal heart attack soon after the declaration of the ceasefire. As a consequence, the public outcry in India against the ceasefire declaration transformed into a wave of sympathy for the ruling Indian National Congress.The ceasefire was criticised by many Pakistanis who, relying on fabricated official reports and the controlled Pakistani press, believed that the leadership had surrendered military gains. The protests led to student riots. Pakistan State's reports had suggested that their military was performing admirably in the war – which they incorrectly blamed as being initiated by India – and thus the Tashkent Declaration was seen as having forfeited the gains. Some recent books written by Pakistani authors, including one by ex-ISI chief titled "The Myth of 1965 Victory", reportedly exposed Pakistani fabrications about the war, but all copies of the book were bought by Pakistan Army to prevent circulation because the topic was "too sensitive".

India and Pakistan accused each other of ceasefire violations; India charged Pakistan with 585 violations in 34 days, while Pakistan countered with accusations of 450 incidents by India. In addition to the expected exchange of small arms and artillery fire, India reported that Pakistan utilized the ceasefire to capture the Indian village of Chananwalla in the Fazilka sector. This village was recaptured by Indian troops on 25 December. On 10 October, a B-57 Canberra on loan to the PAF was damaged by 3 SA-2 missiles fired from the IAF base at Ambala. A Pakistani Army Auster AOP was shot down on 16 December, killing one Pakistani army captain; on 2 February 1967, an AOP was shot down by IAF Hunters.

The ceasefire remained in effect until the start of the Indo-Pakistani War of 1971.

INTELLIGENCE FAILURES

Strategic miscalculations by both India and Pakistan ensured that the war ended in a stalemate —

Indian miscalculations

Indian military intelligence gave no warning of the impending Pakistan invasion. The Indian Army failed to recognize the presence of heavy Pakistani artillery and armaments in Chumb and suffered significant losses as a result.

The "Official War History - 1965", drafted by the Ministry of Defence of India in 1992, was a long suppressed document that revealed other miscalculations. According to the document, on 22 September when the Security Council was pressing for a ceasefire, the Indian Prime Minister asked commanding Gen. Chaudhuri if India could possibly win the war, were he to delay accepting the ceasefire. The general replied that most of India's frontline ammunition had been used up and the Indian Army had suffered considerable tank losses. It was determined later that only 14% of India's frontline ammunition had been fired and India held twice the number of tanks as Pakistan. By this time, the Pakistani Army had used close to 80% of its ammunition.

Air Chief Marshal (retd) P.C. Lal, who was the Vice Chief of Air Staff during the conflict, points to the lack of coordination between the IAF and the Indian army. Neither side revealed its battle plans to the other. The battle plans drafted by the Ministry of Defence and General Chaudhari, did not specify a role for the Indian Air Force in the order of battle. This attitude of Gen. Chaudhari was referred to by ACM Lal as the "Supremo Syndrome", a patronizing attitude sometimes held by the Indian army towards the other branches of the Indian Military.

Pakistani miscalculations

The Pakistani Army's failures started with the supposition that a generally discontented Kashmiri people, given the opportunity provided by the Pakistani advance, would revolt against their Indian rulers, bringing about a swift and decisive surrender of Kashmir. The Kashmiri people, however, did not revolt. Instead, the Indian Army was provided with enough information to learn of Operation Gibraltar and the fact that the Army was battling not insurgents, as they had initially supposed, but Pakistani Army regulars.

The Pakistani Army also failed to recognize that the Indian policy makers would order an attack on the southern sector in order to open a second front. Pakistan was forced to dedicate troops to the southern sector to protect Sialkot and Lahore instead using them to support penetrating into Kashmir.

"Operation Grand Slam", which was launched by Pakistan to capture Akhnoor, a town north-east of Jammu and a key region for communications between Kashmir and the rest of India, was also a failure. Many Pakistani commentators criticised the Ayub Khan administration for being indecisive during Operation Grand Slam. These critics claim that the operation failed because Ayub Khan knew the importance of Akhnur to India (having called it India's "jugular vein") and did not want to capture it and drive the two nations into an all-out war. Despite progress being made in Akhnur, General Ayub Khan relieved the commanding Major General Akhtar Hussain Malik and replaced him with Gen. Yahya Khan. A 24-hour lull ensued the replacement, which allowed the Indian army to regroup in Akhnur and successfully oppose a lackluster attack headed by General Yahya Khan. "The enemy came to our rescue", asserted the Indian Chief of Staff of the Western Command. Later, Akhtar Hussain Malik criticised Ayub Khan for planning Operation Gibraltar, which was doomed to fail, and for relieving him of his command at a crucial moment in the war. Malik threatened to expose the truth about the war and the army's failure, but later dropped the idea for fear of being banned.

Some authors have noted that Pakistan might have been emboldened by a war game – conducted in March 1965, at the Institute of Defence Analysis, USA. The exercise concluded that, in the event of a war with India, Pakistan would win. Other authors like Stephen Philip Cohen, have consistently commented that the Pakistan Army had "acquired an exaggerated view of the weakness of both India and the Indian military ... the 1965 war was a shock".

Pakistani Air Marshal and Commander-in-Chief of PAF during the war, Nur Khan, later said that the Pakistan Army, and not India, should be blamed for starting the war. However propaganda in Pakistan about the war continued; the war was not rationally analysed in Pakistan, with most of the blame being heaped on the leadership and little importance given to intelligence failures that persisted until the debacle of the Indo-Pakistani War of 1971.

INVOLVEMENT OF OTHER NATIONS

The United States and the United Kingdom had been the principal suppliers of military materiél to India and Pakistan since 1947. Both India and Pakistan were Commonwealth republics. While India had pursued a policy of nominal non-alignment, Pakistan was a member of both CENTO and SEATO and a purported ally of the West in its struggle against Communism. Well before the conflict began, however, Britain and the United States had suspected Pakistan of joining both alliances out of opportunism to acquire advanced weapons for a war against India. They had therefore limited their military aid to Pakistan to maintain the existing balance of power in the subcontinent. In 1959, however, Pakistan and the United States had signed an Agreement of Cooperation in 1959 under which the United States agreed to take "appropriate action, including the use of armed forces" in order to assist the Government of Pakistan at its request. By 1965, American and British analysts had recognised the two international groupings, CENTO and SEATO, and Pakistan's continued alliance with the West as being largely meaningless.

Following the start of the 1965 war, both the United States and Britain took the view that the conflict was largely Pakistan's fault, and suspended all arms shipments to both India and Pakistan. While the United States maintained a neutral stance, the British Prime Minister, Harold Wilson, condemned India for aggression after its army advanced towards Lahore; his statement was met with a furious rebuttal from India.

Internationally, the level of support which Pakistan received was limited at best. Iran and Turkey issued a joint communiqué on 10 September which placed the blame on India, backed the United Nations' appeal for a cease-fire and offered to deploy troops for a UN peacekeeping mission in Kashmir. Pakistan received support from Indonesia, Iran, Turkey, and Saudi Arabia in the form of six naval vessels, jet fuel, guns and ammunition and financial support, respectively.

Since before the war, the People's Republic of China had been a major military associate of Pakistan and a military opponent of India, with whom it had fought a brief war in 1962. China had also become a foreign patron for Pakistan and had given Pakistan $60 million in development assistance in 1965. During the war, China openly supported the Pakistani position. It took advantage of the conflict to issue a strongly worded ultimatum to India condemning its "aggression" in Tibet and hinting at nuclear retaliation by China (China had exploded its first nuclear device the previous year). Despite strong fears of Chinese intervention on the side of Pakistan, the Chinese government ultimately exercised restraint. This was partly due to the logistical difficulties of a direct Chinese military intervention against India and India's improved military strength after its defeat by China in 1962. China had also received strong warnings by the American and Soviet governments against expanding the scope of the conflict by intervening. In the face of this pressure,

China backed down, extending the deadline for India to respond to its ultimatum and warning India against attacking East Pakistan. Ultimately, Pakistan rejected Chinese offers of military aid, recognising that accepting it would only result in further alienating Pakistan internationally. International opinion considered China's actions to be dangerously reckless and aggressive, and it was soundly rebuked in the world press for its unnecessarily provocative stance during the conflict.

India's participation in the Non-Aligned Movement yielded little support from its members. Support given by Indonesia to Pakistan was seen as a major Indian diplomatic failure, as Indonesia had been among the founding members of the Non-Aligned Movement along with India. Despite its close relations with India, the Soviet Union was more neutral than other nations during the war, inviting both nations to peace talks under its aegis in Tashkent.

AFTERMATH

India

Despite the declaration of a ceasefire, India was perceived as the victor due to its success in halting the Pakistan-backed insurgency in Kashmir. In its October 1965 issue, the TIME magazine quoted a Western official assessing the consequences of the war –

Now it's apparent to everybody that India is going to emerge as an Asian power in its own right.

In light of the failures of the Sino-Indian War, the outcome of the 1965 war was viewed as a "politico-strategic" victory in India. The Indian premier, Lal Bahadur Shastri, was hailed as a national hero in India.

While the overall performance of the Indian military was praised, military leaders were criticised for their failure to effectively deploy India's superior armed forces so as to achieve a decisive victory over Pakistan. In his book *"War in the modern world since 1815"*, noted war historian Jeremy Black said that though Pakistan "lost heavily" during the 1965 war, India's hasty decision to call for negotiations prevented further considerable damage to the Pakistan Armed Forces. He elaborates –

India's chief of army staff urged negotiations on the ground that they were running out ammunition and their number of tanks had become seriously depleted. In fact, the army had used less than 15% of its ammunition compared to Pakistan, which had consumed closer to 80 percent and India had double the number of serviceable tanks.

In 2015, Marshal of the Indian Air Force Arjan Singh, the last surviving armed force commander of the conflict, gave his assessment that the war ended in a stalemate, but only due to international pressure for a ceasefire, and that India would have achieved a decisive victory had hostilities continued for a few days more:

For political reasons, Pakistan claims victory in the 1965 war. In my opinion, the war ended in a kind of stalemate. We were in a position of strength. Had the war continued for a few more days, we would have gained a decisive victory. I advised then prime minister Lal Bahadur Shastri not to agree for ceasefire. But I think he was under pressure from the United Nations and some countries.

As a consequence, India focussed on enhancing communication and coordination within and among the tri-services of the Indian Armed Forces. Partly as a result of the inefficient information gathering preceding the war, India established the Research and Analysis Wing for external espionage and intelligence. Major improvements were also made in command and control to address various shortcomings and the positive impact of these changes was clearly visible during the Indo-Pakistani War of 1971 when India achieved a decisive victory over Pakistan within two weeks.

China's repeated threats to intervene in the conflict in support of Pakistan increased pressure on the government to take an immediate decision to develop nuclear weapons. Despite repeated assurances, the United States did little to prevent extensive use of American arms by Pakistani forces during the conflict, thus irking India. At the same time, the United States and United Kingdom refused to supply India with sophisticated weaponry which further strained the relations between the West and India. These developments led to a significant change in India's foreign policy – India, which had previously championed the cause of non-alignment, distanced itself further from Western powers and developed close relations with the Soviet Union. By the end of the 1960s, the Soviet Union emerged as the biggest supplier of military hardware to India. From 1967 to 1977, 81% of India's arms imports were from the Soviet Union. After the 1965 war, the arms race between India and Pakistan became even more asymmetric and India was outdistancing Pakistan by far.

Pakistan

At the conclusion of the war, many Pakistanis considered the performance of their military to be positive. 6 September is celebrated as Defence Day in Pakistan, in commemoration of the successful defence of Lahore against the Indian army. The performance of the Pakistani Air Force, in particular, was praised. However, the Pakistani government was accused by foreign analysts of spreading disinformation among its citizens regarding the actual consequences of the war. In his book *"Mainsprings of Indian and Pakistani foreign policies"*, S.M. Burke writes –

After the Indo-Pakistani war of 1965 the balance of military power had decisively shifted in favor of India. Pakistan had found it difficult to replace the heavy equipment lost during that conflict while her adversary, despite her economic and political problems, had been determinedly building up her strength.

Most observers agree that the myth of a mobile, hard hitting Pakistan Army was badly dented in the war, as critical breakthroughs were not made. Several Pakistani writers criticised the military's ill-founded belief that their "martial race" of soldiers could defeat "Hindu India" in the war. Rasul Bux Rais, a Pakistani political analyst wrote –

The 1965 war with India proved that Pakistan could neither break the formidable Indian defences in a blitzkrieg fashion nor could she sustain an all-out conflict for long.

The Pakistan airforce on the other hand gained a lot of credibility and reliability among Pakistan military and international war writers for successful defence of lahore and other important areas of Pakistan and heavy retaliation to India on the next day. The alertness of the airforce was also related to the fact that some pilots were scrambled 6 times in less than an hour on indication of Indian air raids. The Pakistan airforce along with the army is celebrated on Defence day and Airforce day in commemoration of this in Pakistan (6 and 7 September respectively).

Moreover, Pakistan had lost more ground than it had gained during the war and, more importantly, failed to achieve its goal of capturing Kashmir; this result has been viewed by many impartial observers as a defeat for Pakistan.

Many senior Pakistani officials and military experts later criticised the faulty planning of Operation Gibraltar, which ultimately led to the war. The Tashkent declaration was also criticised in Pakistan, though few citizens realised the gravity of the situation that existed at the end of the war. Political leaders were also criticised. Following the advice of Zulfikar Ali Bhutto, Pakistan's foreign minister, Ayub Khan had raised very high expectations among the people of Pakistan about the superiority – if not invincibility – of its armed forces, but Pakistan's inability to attain its military aims during the war created a political liability for Ayub. The defeat of its Kashmiri ambitions in the war led to the army's invincibility being challenged by an increasingly vocal opposition.

One of the farthest reaching consequences of the war was the wide-scale economic slowdown in Pakistan. The war ended the impressive economic growth Pakistan had experienced since the early 1960s. Between 1964 and 1966, Pakistan's defence spending rose from 4.82% to 9.86% of GDP, putting a tremendous strain on Pakistan's economy. By 1970–71, defence spending comprised a whopping 55.66% of government expenditure. According to veterans of the war, the war greatly cost Pakistan economically, politically, and militarily.

Nuclear theorist Feroze Khan maintained that the 1965 war was a last conventional attempt to snatch Kashmir by military force, and Pakistan's own position in the international community, especially with the United States, began to deteriorate from the point the war started, while on the other hand, the alliance with China saw improvements. Chairman joint chiefs General Tariq Majid claims in his memoirs that Chou En-Lai had longed advised the government in the classic style of Sun Tzu: "to go slow, not to push India hard; and avoid a fight over Kashmir, 'for at least, 20–30 years, until you have developed your economy and consolidated your national power'." General Majid maintained in *Eating Grass* that the "sane, philosophical and political critical thinking" was missing in Pakistan, and that the country had lost extensive human resources by fighting the war.

Pakistan was surprised by the lack of support from the United States, an ally with whom the country had signed an Agreement of Cooperation. The US turned neutral in the war when it cut off military supplies to Pakistan (and India); an action that the Pakistanis took as a sign of betrayal. After the war, Pakistan would increasingly look towards China as a major source of military hardware and political support.

Another negative consequence of the war was growing resentment against the Pakistani government in East Pakistan (present day Bangladesh), particularly for West Pakistan's obsession with Kashmir.Bengali leaders accused the central government of not providing adequate security for East Pakistan during the conflict, even though large sums of money were taken from the east to finance the war for Kashmir. In fact, despite some Pakistan Air Force attacks being launched from bases in East Pakistan during the war, India did not retaliate in that sector, although East Pakistan was defended only by an understrengthed infantry division (14th Division), sixteen planes and no tanks. Sheikh Mujibur Rahman was critical of the disparity in military resources deployed in East and West Pakistan, calling for greater autonomy for East

Pakistan, an action that ultimately led to the Bangladesh Liberation War and another war between India and Pakistan in 1971.

REFUGEES

According to Sumantra Bose, Muslims in the Rajouri and Poonch districts of Jammu and Kashmir suffered greatly due to the war. The Indian Army reportedly arrested 'truckloads' of Muslim men for suspect loyalties and took them away to Jammu for interrogation where many were brutalized and some were killed. 100,000 Hindus and Sikhs fled Chhamb-Jaurian area in south-western Jammu when the Pakistan army invaded it and 70,000 Muslims from Rajouri and Poonch crossed over into Azad Kashmir because of harassment by the Indian army and local Hindus and Sikhs, although people were 'largely' able to return to their homes after the war.

There was another cross-border migration in the Thar Desert. An estimated 3,500 Muslim families migrated from the Indian part of the Thar Desert to the Pakistani section of the Thar Desert, with reports of harassment of Muslims in Indian border villages by the Indian Army. Hindu upper castes and their retainers also fled from the Pakistani part of the Thar to the Indian side.

AS 2006 ARRIVES, TRAVEL BACK TO 1966

In early January 1966, Indian Prime Minister Lal Bahadur Shastri and Pakistan's President Mohammad Ayub Khan met at a summit in the Soviet city of Tashkent, today the capital of an independent Uzbekistan. Having seen their armies clash in a stalemate of a war in September of the previous year, the two leaders came together per courtesy of Soviet Premier Alexei Kosygin, the objective being the shaping of a deal that would take the two nations back to the territorial positions they occupied prior to the seventeen-day war in September 1965.

The talks began in something of drama, with Ayub and Shastri entering the summit hall through different doors at the same time, the purpose being to preclude either one of them feeling hurt by coming in after the other has already stepped inside. On hand to receive the two men was, of course, Kosygin. Over a period of seven days beginning on 4 January, Ayub and Shastri tried hammering out a deal and finally did so late on 10 January.

A few hours later, early on 11 January, the Indian leader died of a heart attack, thus casting a damper on what would have been a joyous occasion. An excited Aziz Ahmed, Pakistan's foreign secretary, roused his sleeping foreign minister Zulfikar Ali Bhutto to tell him, 'Sir, the bastard is dead'.

Bhutto, rather groggy-eyed, countered, 'Which one?' The initialling of the Tashkent Declaration had not been to Bhutto's liking, particularly when towards the end both Kosygin and his foreign minister Andrei Gromyko insisted that Bhutto be kept out of the talks because of the spoiler's role he appeared intent on playing. On that night in Tashkent, Bhutto's displeasure was as much directed at Ayub as it was at Shastri.

Shastri's demise quickly led to a situation where, in the latter part of January, Indira Gandhi was elected India's new prime minister. The Congress syndicate of old men led by party president K.Kamaraj reasoned that the untried daughter of Jawaharlal Nehru (and that despite her having been president of the Congress in the late 1950s and information and broadcasting minister in Shastri's cabinet) would prove easy to dominate, with power remaining in its hands.

Things did not quite happen that way, as later events were to show. As prime minister, Mrs. Gandhi travelled to Washington a few months after assuming office to see President Lyndon Johnson, who did not lose the opportunity of berating her over her country's poverty. On her way back home, the prime minister vowed to her delegation that never again would India allow itself to be bullied by foreigners. She embarked on wide-ranging projects, such as ensuring food autarky and developing a green belt across the arid wastes of Rajasthan.

India would never be the same again. Indira Gandhi made sure of that. In neighbouring Pakistan, Bhutto grumbled and whispered (and the whisper was a lie, of course) about how his president had sold out Pakistan's interests at Tashkent. At one point, President Ayub Khan was forced to deny that there was any rift between him and the foreign minister. But in mid-June, Bhutto went on long leave, making sure that he would take the train from Rawalpindi all the way, through such cities as Lahore, to his native Larkana. At Lahore railway station, a huge group of slogan-chanting students gave him a rousing welcome, clearly looking upon him as a future leader of the country. Tears came to Bhutto's eyes and as soon as he had wiped them on his handkerchief, an enthusiastic admirer snatched the handkerchief away from his hands. It had turned into a memento. By the end of July, however, Ayub had got exasperated with his young minister, enough to ask him to resign or face dismissal from the government. Bhutto showed every sign of wanting to stay and Ayub displayed all his readiness to see the back of the foreign minister. Bhutto eventually resigned and was replaced by the attorney general Syed Sharifuddin Pirzada.

For Pakistan's Bengalis, inhabiting the province that used to be known as East Bengal before it was rechristened East Pakistan, 1966 was a watershed in history. On 5 February, at a national conference called by Pakistan's opposition political parties in Lahore, Sheikh Mujibur Rahman, general secretary of the Awami League, presented what was clearly a radical demand for autonomy for East Pakistan. Known as the Six Points, the demand pitted traditionalists and modernisers in the country's politics against one another. Mujib was soon being vilified by men who thought he had attacked the very basis of Pakistan's foundations.

President Ayub Khan went to the extent of threatening the Bengali leader and his followers with what he called the language of weapons. In May, Sheikh Mujibur Rahman, not yet Bangabandhu to his people, was taken into custody under the Defence of Pakistan Rules. At around the same time, most senior leaders of the Awami League were carted off to prison by the regime and its loyalist governor Abdul Monem Khan. That left the young Mizanur Rahman Chowdhury and Amena Begum, Awami League figures yet outside the police dragnet, free to organise a province-wide general strike or hartal in support of the Six Points on 7 June. The strike was a resounding success and for the first time demonstrated the clear prospects of a rise of Bengali nationalism in East Pakistan.

In 1966, former US vice president Richard Nixon went travelling around the world, cultivating his ties with such grandees as France's Charles de Gaulle. At home, he went on a sustained campaign to promote the candidacies of his fellow Republicans at the mid-term elections. The results were a positive achievement for a party that had been out of power since Nixon's defeat at the hands of John F. Kennedy at the 1960 election. The credit for the gains of 1966 were placed at Nixon's door, who would thenceforth plan a second run for the White House. Meanwhile, President Johnson, having won the presidency in his own right against the 'warmonger' Barry Goldwater in 1964, now found himself doing in Vietnam precisely what he had accused his rival of planning to do. He was bombing North Vietnam and sending increasing numbers of American soldiers to Saigon to prop up the South Vietnamese regime. In 1966, President De Gaulle kept up his opposition to British entry into the Common Market, a position that would not change as long as he remained in office. The French leader also took his country out of the military structure of NATO, a clear demonstration of his faith in a restoration of French grandeur in world affairs independent of outside influence.

The Chinese, eight years after the Great Leap Forward of 1958, enthusiastically launched what they called a Cultural Revolution in 1966.

Clearly a move by Chairman Mao Zedong to reassert his authority over the communist party and the state, the revolution threw up young Mao supporters known as Red Guards. These young went around overturning values, revolting against their parents and informing on them to the party. The Cultural Revolution would in time see such respected men as President Liu Shaoqi removed, physically beaten up by mobs and hauled away to jail. Liu and his wife would die in a dark cell, unbeknownst to the world, three years later. Another communist figure, Deng Xiao-ping, would be purged because he was, in the eyes of the purists, a capitalist roader. Deng's fall came about because of his view that it did not matter if a cat was black or white as long as it caught mice.

In 1966, Nigeria went haywire with the bloody coup, the first of many, that left the urbane and accomplished Prime Minister Abubakr Tafawa Balewa dead. Politics would not be the same for the country again, for decades. In the same year, Ghana's President Kwame Nkrumah was ousted from power by his army even as his aircraft was coming in to land at Beijing, where he would be on a state visit. From China, Nkrumah made his way to Guinea, where his friend Sekou Toure, the president of the country, somewhat quixotically declared that the deposed Ghanaian leader would with him be co-president of Guinea. The position did not amount to much.

In Indonesia, President Ahmed Sukarno was in decline, with almost all his powers now exercised by General Suharto. The army, months after what had been touted as an attempted coup by the country's communists in September of the previous year, went on hunting down suspected leftists. By 1967, the body count in the massacre would go up to a million people. Former foreign minister Subandrio was tried and sentenced to death in 1966. In 1966, West Germany's Christian Democrats and Social Democrats, neither able to come by a clear majority at the elections, forged a grand coalition. The CDU's Kurt-Georg Kiesinger took over as chancellor, with the SPD's Willy Brandt assuming office as vice chancellor and foreign minister.

ON TO WEAPONS DEVELOPMENT: 1960-1967

With the two projects to necessary to provide the materials for nuclear weapons underway, the Cirus production reactor and the Trombay plutonium plant, Dr. Bhabha then turned his attention to acquiring information about nuclear weapons and initiating preliminary studies of weapon physics.

During the early sixties India's anxieties regarding China greatly increased. Tensions over the border disputes with China rose from 1959 onward, leading to large scale troop deployments by both sides in early 1962. By 1961 India had become aware of China's nuclear program which gave greater impetus to India's efforts. In January 1962 Bhabha set up a formal study group in high pressure physics at TIFR, headed by Prof. A.K. Asundi, to explore equations of state in the megabar range, a necessary step for designing implosion weapons. This group did its work in secret, submitting its papers to Bhabha for review.

A number of public indications show India's increasing interest in nuclear arms. On 9 January 1961 Nehru stated that

We are approaching a stage when it is possible to for us... to make atomic weapons. A few weeks later, on 2 February, Bhabha was asked how long this would take and he responded "about two years I suppose". In September 1962, at Bhabha's urging, Nehru passed the revised Atomic Energy Act giving the central government strict control over all decisions on atomic energy and futher tightening secrecy (this act can perhaps be likened to the U.S. Atomic Energy Act of 1954). This act explicitly linked atomic energy and its control to national security, scarcely mentioning civilian applications.

Following India's humiliating defeat by China in the Indo-Chinese border war of October-November 1962, the first formal demand for the development of nuclear weapons was made in Parliament, by the Jana Singh party, in December 1962. Bhabha, well aware that a Chinese nuclear test was not far off (his estimate was then 12 to 18 months), also began secretly agitating for a vigorous effort to match China's, going so far as to ask Nehru to authorize a nuclear test in Ladakh on the Chinese border.

Nehru died on 27 May 1964 and was succeeded by Lal Bahadur Shastri who took office on 2 June. That summer and fall expectations of a Chinese nuclear test steadily increased. PM Shastri, a Gandhian, was strongly opposed to pursuing the Indian nuclear option, and Bhabha began making public statements in favor intended to increase public support and political pressure. On 4 October Bhabha repeated his estimate publicly that India could build a bomb within 18 months of the decision to do so. Interestingly, a U.S. National Intelligence Estimate issued on 16 October thought India capable of developing a weapon in one to three years.

India's prime nuclear facilities were having growing pains though. Cirus operated erratically after going critical, and India had problems supplying fuel rods of the required purity. Cirus did not reach full power until 16 October 1963. Likewise the Phoenix plant at Trombay operated unreliably with only a fraction of its rated capacity when it began receiving spent fuel from Cirus in mid-1964 (for example experiencing an explosion during its first several months of operation). It was officially inaugurated 22 January 1965, but produced very little plutonium for years, taking India until *circa* 1969 to acquire sufficient plutonium for a single device.

The much anticipated Chinese test finally came on 16 October 1964. Shastri's initial reaction was to reiterate his opposition to India following the same path. But on 24 October 1964 Bhabha made a now famous speech on Indian radio. Bhabha argued that "atomic weapons give a State possessing them in adequate numbers a deterrent power against attack from a much stronger State". He further claimed that such weapons were remarkably cheap citing cost estimates provided by the U.S. AEC for projected Plowshare (peaceful nuclear explosive) devices-$350,000 for a 10 kt device, and $600,000 for a 2 Mt device. From this he estimated that "a stockpile of some 50 atomic bombs would cost under $21 million and a stockpile of 50 two-megaton hydrogen bombs something of the order of $31.5 million " [Perkovich 1999; pg. 67]

It seems Bhabha could not have been unaware of how inappropriate such cost estimates were to the circumstances of India. The U.S. Plowshare cost figures were based on the incremental cost of producing devices by a vast industrial complex costing tens of billions of dollars, which had already manufactured nuclear weapons numbering in the tens of thousands. And even so, it is very questionable that the U.S. Plowshare estimates-made by Plowhare advocates-constituted anything like full cost accounting for the usage of this vast infrastructure. And this also ignored the fact that the delivery systems for nuclear weapons typically cost several times as much as the weapons themselves. The real cost to India for any nuclear weapon program would be orders of magnitude greater than Bhabha's claims (China had spent over $4 billion in then-year dollars up to 1964 for its program).

Nonetheless his claims fuelled debate about the desirability of India initiating a weapons program, and undermined support for Shastri and his "no weapon" policy within his own Congress party. With Bhabha continuing to campaign both publicly and behind the scenes, Shastri eventually found himself in an untenable position. The enormous public stature of Bhabha, and the tight control over nuclear information, left no effective scientific voice to act as a counterweight.

A two day debate in the Lok Sabha (Parliament) on 23-24 November 1964 showed that the Congress party was split with a bare majority favoring pursuing a weapons program. On 27 November the most vocal advocate of pursuing nuclear weapons, the Jana Sangh party, introduced a motion in the Lok Sabha calling for the manufacture of nuclear weapons. It was voted down in a voice vote. But in his speech following the vote Shastri made a crucial change in his position. He mentioned that he had just come from a meeting with Bhabha, and stated that Bhabha actually desired that India pursue the development of peaceful nuclear devices for future engineering use. Then he indicated that he and Bhabha were now in full agreement that work should be conducted on such devices — that is, Shastri authorized the development of nuclear explosives.

There is a saying in the nuclear non-proliferation community: "The difference between a peaceful nuclear explosive and a bomb are the tail fins." Bhabha knew (and in fact had said so publicly in the past) that nuclear explosives for peaceful and weapon use were essentially the same, and he had suceeded in bringing Shastri around to supporting their development. The gain for Shastri was that now that he had Bhabha's support the lobby for an explicit weapon program was neutralized. At that time India was very vulnerable to the sanctions that an acknowledged weapon program would produce, and a "peaceful nuclear explosive" or PNE program was the only feasible way that weapons could be openly pursued. This fiction of a "PNE" would be maintained through India's first nuclear test in 1974 and up until 11 May 1998, after its second round of nuclear testing, when India finally acknowledged the objective of obtaining nuclear arms.

Despite the nationalistic rhetoric emphasizing Indian self-reliance that had characterized the nuclear debate, the first actions of both Shastri and Bhabha after their reconciliation was to seek outside assistance. In December Shastri publicly appealed vaguely to the existing nuclear powers for some sort of nuclear security umbrella for non-nuclear nation, a proposal that India never clearly defined or marshalled support for, and which slowly faded away over the next several months.

In February Bhabha visited Washington and implied to Undersecretary of State George Ball that he was interested in obtaining U.S. assistance in building nuclear explosives. Ball reported that "Dr. Bhabha explained that if India went all out, it could produce a device in 18 months; *with a U.S. blueprint it could do the job in six months.*"

U.S. reports written in March indicate a request was received for an actual Plowshare device. In April Glenn Seaborg, chairman of the U.S. AEC, indicated that Bhabha had inquired "whether we would be prepared to make a moderate amount of plutonium available for research and development."

Curiously a number of U.S. officials and agencies also became interested after the Chinese test in providimg Plowshare devices, technology, and even (under some conditions) nuclear weapons to India. The U.S. AEC discussed undertaking a cooperative Plowshare program with India in November 1964.

And Assistant Secretary of Defense for International Security Affairs John McNaughton prepared a proposal to initiate a program to train and equip Indian forces to use nuclear weapons, and create a stockpile to disperse to India in times of crisis.

This caught the U.S. at a turning point in the evolution of U.S. policy. Up until the mid 1960s, although non-proliferation had been a U.S. interest, it had been distinctly secondary to efforts to promote the peaceful use of nuclear power (e.g. "Atoms for Peace" and Plowshare) and to strengthen the defenses of non-communist nations (e.g. the Multi-Lateral Force proposal to share nuclear weapons with other NATO nations). But a landmark event occurred on 21 January 1965 with the Gilpatric Committee on Nuclear Proliferation delivered its report to Pres. Johnson. This report took an uncompromising stand on non-proliferation, establishing the trend for non-proliferation concerns to dominate all others which continues to the present day.

In April Shastri gave Bhabha formal approval to move ahead with nuclear explosive development. On 5 April 1965 Bhabha initiated the effort by setting up the nuclear esplosive design group Study of Nuclear Explosions for Peaceful Purposes (SNEPP). Bhabha selected Raja Ramanna-Director of Physics at AEET-to lead the effort.

That spring Bhabha met with T.S. Murthy, bright student then undergoing training at the French nuclear laboratory at Saclay, in Paris. Bhabha confided that Shastri had approved of conducting a nuclear test, and that he was prospecting for a test site. Then Bhabha suggested he scout out the French for useful information, especially regarding polonium technology used for first generation neutron initiators for weapons. By mid year test were conducted with large amounts of high explosives to calibrate seismographs used for nuclear test monitoring.

Evidence suggests that India's new interest in the nuclear option was of great concern to Pakistan. Reports from the fall of 1964 into mid 1965 indicate considerable concern by President Ayub Khan, and his Foreign Minister Zulfikar Ali Bhutto (later President). In March both men met with Chou En-lai in Beijing, a meeting both felt had very positive results and developed Chinese support for Pakistan. It was in mid-1965 that Bhutto made his famous remark that is India acquired nuclear weapons: "then we should have to eat grass and get one, or buy one, of our own." Under Bhutto's later presidency the foundations of Pakistan's nuclear program would be laid. Thus in 1965, the seeds of the Indo-Pakistani nuclear confrontation of three decades later had been sown.

George Perkovich suggests that it was fear of the changes in the balance of power that India's nuclear weapon program would bring that motivated Pakistan to initiate the Second Indo-Pakistani War that summer.

This war, the second major war in three years involving India, was fought in three phases. First Pakistani forces moved in to the Indian marshland of the Rann of Kutch in April. India attempted to repulse the incursion, but the rainy season threatened isolation of Indian troops, and they withdrew. Thus emboldened by this first probe Pakistan attacked an Indian outpost in Kargil, Kashmir. India counterattacked and seized territory that had been held by Pakistan. Shastri agreed to a ceasefire and withdrew from Pakistani territory, and adopted a conciliatory stance regarding the Rann of Kutch-a stance widely regarded in India as weak. It was apparently similarly regarded in Pakistan, because on 1 September Pakistan launched a massive armoured assault on Kashmir. This attack pushed into Indian held Kashmir and threatened Srinagar but then ground to a halt. Then on 6 September India counterattacked south of Kashmir driving 15 miles into Pakistan, threatening Lahore.

Despite superior U.S. supplied arms in Pakistani hands (especially armour), India maintained a strong position on the battlefield. Then on 17 September China, which had supported Pakistan throughout the conflict-even alleging Indian aggression in the face of a Pakistani assault, attempted to involve itself directly by threatening Indian positions on the Tibetan border. India firmly resisted Chinese pressure, supported by both the U.S. and the USSR.

The outcome of the war did a great deal to strengthen India's long-term resolve to acquire nuclear weapons. The alliance between U.S. armed Pakistan and nuclear-armed China presented India with a security threat that they could not ignore. Although India did find some support from the Superpowers with respect to Chinese pressure, India found that when faced with unprovoked attack-foreign "even handedness" cut off supplies and aid to both, indicating that India could not expect outside aid if threatened in the future.

It seems clear that at this point Bhabha felt he had authority to go ahead with developing and perhaps even testing an actual nuclear device, since in the wake of the war he seemed satisfied with the program then authorized. Homi Sethna, then head of the IAEC, has stated that Shastri told Bhabha during the war to go ahead with development but to hold off testing unless he had clearance from the cabinet.

This initial effort to develop a "peaceful nuclear explosive" (PNE) existed almost entirely as an unwritten personal understanding between Dr. Bhabha and PM Shastri.

On 11 January 1966, just hours after he had signed the Tashkent Declaration formalizing the end of hostilities in the war with Pakistan, PM Shastri died of a heart attack. Just two weeks later on January 24, and the very day Shastri's successor Indira Gandhi was sworn in as Prime Minister, Dr. Homi Bhabha was killed while on a trip to Europe when the plane in which he was flying collided with Mount Blanc. India's impressively large nuclear establishment was suddenly left without any official plan or policy, to give it direction.

But Bhabha had by now shaped India's nuclear establishment and policy making environment to such an extent that the patterns he established would persist for decades after this death. Under Bhabha, the drive toward building the infrastructure for nuclear explosives, and the advocacy for developing such explosives had come from the nuclear scientists themselves-not the civilian government, and certainly not from the Indian military which virtually no role in the planning or decision making.

The advance of the nuclear explosives program would also be conducted without any serious public debate over the decisions taken, and without consultation of parliament. The desire of weapons developers to continual advance the program would be offset though by the fact that the support for the program was not based on a broad consensus among key decision makers. Thus the program's fortunes were hostage to the personal preferences of the Chairman of the IAEC, and the mood and attention of the Prime Minister.

Some of the numerous positions held by Bhabha were distributed among his top scientists working on SNEPP, like Ramanna and Sethna, but the principal successor to Bhabha was Vikram Sarabhai personally chosen by Indira Gandhi to be Chairman of the IAEC, and Secretary of the Department of Atomic Energy. Sarabhai was a follower of Mohandas Gandhi and a pacifist who opposed nuclear arms. His selection was probably politically motivated as Sarabhai hailed from a rich and politically powerful family.

At the beginning of June 1966 Sarabhai ordered a halt to SNEPP, and the confiscation of the papers that had been generated on the project. It appears that this was Sarabhai's personal decision, rather than a reflection of PM Gandhi's policies at this time, and he may not have even consulted with her on it. That this was possible illustrates the vulnerability of a program not based on a broad consensus among key decision makers. It did not altogether mean the end of Indian progress toward acquiring nuclear weapons however. The development of the necessary infrastructure proceeded apace, and the cadre of scientists that Bhabha personally recruited did not forget their objective (as they would demonstrate less than 18 months later). And the logic of India's strategic situation continued to push India toward exercising this option.

In 1966 India's diplomatic policy towards nuclear weapons made a fateful shift. While international interest in non-proliferation, focusing on restricting the spread of nuclear weapons to *any* additional states, India's Nehruvian policy of broadly opposing nuclear arms developed a pointed new emphasis. Indian negotiator V.C. Trivedi adopted the stance advocating non-proliferation and nuclear disarmament as long as it was universal-that no club of permanent nuclear powers should be permitted. As long as existing nuclear powers resisted disarmament, they left other nations no choice but to pursue the same option as they saw necessary. The quid pro quo was clear-India would not eschew nuclear arms unless the existing nuclear states did also. This fundamental logic led to India refusing to sign the Nuclear Non-Proliferation Treaty and voting against it on 12 June 1968, and has informed Indian nuclear diplomacy ever since.

INDO-PAKISTANI WAR OF 1947

After rumours that the Maharaja supported the annexation of Kashmir by India, militant Muslim revolutionaries from western Kashmir and Pakistani tribesmen made rapid advances into the Baramulla sector. Maharaja Hari Singh of Kashmir asked the government of India to intervene. However, India and Pakistan had signed an agreement of non-intervention. Although tribal fighters from Pakistan had entered Jammu and Kashmir, there was no iron-clad legal evidence to unequivocally prove that Pakistan was officially involved. It would have been illegal for India to unilaterally intervene in an open, official capacity unless Jammu and Kashmir officially joined the Union of India, at which point it would be possible to send in its forces and occupy the remaining parts.

The Maharaja desperately needed military assistance when the Pakistani tribals reached the outskirts of Srinagar. Before their arrival into Srinagar, India argued that the Maharaja must complete negotiations for ceding Jammu and Kashmir to India in exchange for receiving military aid. The agreement which ceded Jammu and Kashmir to India was signed by the Maharaja and Lord Mountbatten of Burma. In Jammu and Kashmir, National Conference volunteers worked with the Indian Army to drive out the Pakistanis.

The resulting war over Kashmir, the First Kashmir War, lasted until 1948, when India moved the issue to the UN Security Council. Sheikh Abdullah was not in favour of India seeking UN intervention because he was sure the Indian Army could free the entire State of invaders. The UN had previously passed resolutions for setting up monitoring of the conflict in Kashmir. Following the set-up of the United Nations Military Observer Group in India and Pakistan

(UNCIP), the UN Security Council passed Resolution 47 on 21 April 1948. The resolution imposed an immediate cease-fire and called on the Government of Pakistan 'to secure the withdrawal from the state of Jammu and Kashmir of tribesmen and Pakistani nationals not normally resident therein who have entered the state for the purpose of fighting.' It also asked Government of India to reduce its forces to the minimum strength, after which the circumstances for holding a plebiscite should be put into effect 'on the question of Accession of the state to India or Pakistan.' However, both India and Pakistan failed to arrive at a Truce agreement due to differences in interpretation of the procedure for and extent of demilitarisation one of them being whether the Azad Kashmiri army is to be disbanded during the truce stage or the Plebiscite stage.

In November 1948, The Indian and Pakistani governments agreed to hold the plebiscite, but Pakistan did not withdraw its troops from Kashmir, thus violating the conditions for holding the plebiscite. In addition, the Indian Government distanced itself from its commitment to hold a plebiscite. India proposed that Pakistan withdraw all its troops first, calling it a precondition for a plebiscite. Pakistan rejected on the grounds that the Kashmiris may not vote freely given the presence of Indian army and Sheikh Abdullah's friendship with the Indian Prime Minister, Jawaharlal Nehru. However, Pakistan proposed simultaneous withdrawal of all troops followed by a plebiscite under international auspices, which India rejected. Hence Pakistan didn't withdraw its forces unilaterally In addition, the Indian Government distanced itself from its commitment to hold a plebiscite. Over the next several years, the UN Security Council passed four new resolutions, revising the terms of Resolution 47 to include a synchronous withdrawal of both Indian and Pakistani troops from the region, per the recommendations of General Andrew McNaughton. To this end, UN arbitrators put forward 11 different proposals for the demilitarization of the region. All of these were accepted by Pakistan, but rejected by the Indian government. The resolutions were passed by United Nations Security Council under Chapter VI of the United Nations Charter. Resolutions passed under Chapter VI of the UN charter are considered non-binding and have no mandatory enforceability, as opposed to the resolutions passed under Chapter VII.

Sino-Indian War

In 1962, troops from the People's Republic of China and India clashed in territory claimed by both. China won a swift victory in the war, resulting in the Chinese annexation of the region called Aksai Chin, which has continued since then. Another smaller area, the Trans-Karakoram, was demarcated as the Line of Control (LOC) between China and Pakistan, although some of the territory on the Chinese side is claimed by India to be part of Kashmir. The line that separates India from China in this region is known as the "Line of Actual Control".

1965 and 1971 Wars

In 1965 and 1971, heavy fighting broke out again between India and Pakistan. The Indo-Pakistani War of 1971 resulted in the defeat of Pakistan and the Pakistani military's surrender in East Pakistan, leading to the creation of Bangladesh. The Simla Agreement was signed in 1972 between India and Pakistan. By this treaty, both countries agreed to settle all issues by peaceful means using mutual discussion in the framework of the UN Charter.

Bibliography

Agarwal, S. P., and Aggarwal, J. C.: *Educational and Social Uplift of Backward Classes: At What Cost and How? Mandal Commission and After,* Concept Publishing Co., New Delhi, 1979.

Ahir, D.C.: *Dr. Ambedkar, Buddhism and Social Change,* BR Publishing, Delhi, 1993.

Ambedkar, B. R.: *Annihilation of Caste: An Undelivered Speech,* Arnold Publishers, New Delhi, 1990.

Anthony, J. Parel : *Hind Swaraj or Indian Home Rule,* Cambridge University Press, 1925.

Asghar Ali.: *Mandal Commission Controversy,* Ajanta Publications, Delhi, 1991.

Ashton, S.R.: *British Policy Towards the Indian States, 1905-1939,* London: Curzon, 1982.

Barill, C.: *Social and Political Ideas of B.R. Ambedkar,* Aalekh Publishers, Jaipur, 1977.

Benjamin, Joseph: *Scheduled Castes in Indian Politics and Society,* Ess Ess Publications, New Delhi, 1989.

Bhattacharya, Sabyasachi : *Vande Mataram : The Biography of a Song,* New Delhi, Penguin, 2003.

Bose, Sipra: *Social Mobility Among Untouchables,* Cohesion and Conflict in Modern India, New Delhi, 1978.

Bourai, Himanshu : *Gandhi and Modern Indian Liberals,* Delhi, Abhijeet Pub., 2004.

Chakrabarti, Santosh : *Studies in Tagore : Critical Essays,* New Delhi, Atlantic, 2004.

Chatterjee, Partha: *Caste and Subaltern Consciousness,* Oxford University Press, Delhi, 1994.

Chaudhary, M.: *Partition and the Curse of Rehabilitation,* Calcutta, Bengal Rehabilitation Organization, 1964.

Dan Nabudere: *The Political Economy of Imperialism,* London, 1977.

Engineer, Asghar Ali.: *Mandal Commission Controversy,* Ajanta Publications, Delhi, 1991.

Galanter, Marc.: *Competing Inequalities: Law and the Backward Classes in India,* University of California Press, CA, 1984.

Gaur, Mahendra : *Indian Political Parties Annual,* Delhi, Kalpaz Pub., 2006.

Ghosh, Ila : *Rgvedic Rsikas : Life and Philosophy,* Eastern Book Linkers, Delhi, 2007.

Gopal, S. : *Selected Works of Jawaharlal Nehru,* New Delhi, 1994.

Hasan, Mushirul: *India's Partition: Process, Strategy and Mobilization,* New Delhi, Oxford UP, 1993.

Ishwaran, K.: *Shivpur: A South Indian Village,* Routledge, London, 1968.

Jaffrelot, Christophe: *Dr. Ambedkar and Untouchability: Fighting the Indian Caste System,* New York, Columbia University Press, 2005.

Jha, Prem Shankar: *India: A Political Economy of Stagnation*, Bombay, Oxford University Press, 1980.

Joan V.: *Conquest of Violence; The Gandhian Philosophy of Conflict*, University of California Press, Berkeley, 1965.

John Noyce. *Lal Bahadur Shastri: an English-language bibliography*. Lulu.com, 2002.

Juergensmeyer, Mark: *Religion as Social Vision: The Movement Against Untouchability in 20th Century Punjab*, University of California Press, Berkeley, 1979.

Kamble, J. R.: *Rise and Awakening of Depressed Classes in India*, National Publishers, New Delhi, 1979.

Khairmode, C.B.: *Dr. Bhimrao Ramji Ambedkar*, Pratap, Bombay, 1978.

Lobo, C.H.J.J.: *Dr B.R. Ambedkar: The Champion of Social Democracy in India*, Hilerina Publishers, Bangalore, 1984.

Mahar, Michael J.: *The Untouchables in Contemporary India*, University of Arizona Press, Arizona, 1972.

Maheshwari, Shriram: *Rural Development in India: A Public Policy Approach*, New Delhi, Sage, 1995.

Mallik, Suneila: *Social Integration of the Scheduled Castes*. Abhinav, New Delhi, 1979.

Maw, Martin: *Visions of India*, Vertag Perer Lang, London, 1990.

Michel, A. A.: *The Indus Rivers: A Study of the Effects of Partition*, New Haven, Yale UP, 1967.

Mishra, Anil Dutta : *Challenges of 21 Century : Gandhian Alternatives*, New Delhi, Mittal Pub., 2003.

Murthi, R.K. : *Discovery of Nehru*, Indian Pub., Delhi, 1993.

Narula, Sanjay : *Indian Politics*, New Delhi, Murari Lal and Sons, 2007.

Pavan Choudary and Anil Shastri. *Lal Bahadur Shastri: Lessons in Leadership*. Wisdom Village Publications, 2014

Punekar, S.M.: *Harijan Contribution to Medieval Thought*, Prasaranga, Bangalore University, Bangalore, 1991.

Rajasekharaiah, A.M.: *B.R. Ambedkar: the Politics of Emancipation*, Sindhu Publications, Bombay, 1971.

Ram, Jagivan: *Caste Challenge in India*, Vision Books, New Delhi, 1980.

Sarkar, J.: *Caste, Occupation and Change*, B. R. Publishing Co., Delhi, 1984.

Sharma, G. S.: *Legislation and Cases of Untouchability and Scheduled Castes in India*, Allied Publishers, Bombay, 1975.

Shashi B.R.: *Ambedkar and Human Rights*, KK Publishers, New Delhi, 1981.

Silverberg, James: *Social Mobility in the Caste System in India*, Mouton Publishers, The Hague, 1968.

Singh, L.P. : *Portrait of Lal Bahadur Shastri*, Delhi: Ravi Dayal Publishers, 1996.

Yogesh, A.: *The Changing Frontiers of Caste*, National Publishing House, Delhi, 1968.

Zelliot, Eleanor: *From Untouchable to Dalit: Essays on the Ambedkar Movement*, Manohar, New Delhi, 1992.

Index

❑❑❑